Obesity in the News

Obesity is a pressing social issue and a persistently newsworthy topic for the media. This book examines the linguistic representation of obesity in the British press. It combines techniques from corpus linguistics with critical discourse studies to analyse a large corpus of newspaper articles (36 million words) representing ten years of obesity coverage. These articles are studied from a range of methodological perspectives, and analytical themes include variation between newspapers, change over time, diet and exercise, gender and social class. The volume also investigates the language that readers use when responding to obesity representations in the context of online comments. The authors reveal the power of linguistic choices to shame and stigmatise people with obesity, presenting them as irresponsible and morally deviant. Yet the analysis also demonstrates the potential for alternative representations which place greater focus on the role that social and political forces play in this topical health issue.

GAVIN BROOKES is Senior Research Associate in the ESRC Centre for Corpus Approaches to Social Science at Lancaster University. His research interests include corpus linguistics, discourse studies, health communication and multimodality. He is Associate Editor of the *International Journal of Corpus Linguistics*.

PAUL BAKER is Professor of English Language at Lancaster University. He has written twenty books on various aspects of language, discourse and corpus linguistics. He is the commissioning editor of the journal *Corpora*, an associate editor of the Cambridge Elements in Corpus Linguistics series and a fellow of the Royal Society of Arts.

Obesity in the News

Language and Representation in the Press

Gavin Brookes

Lancaster University

Paul Baker

Lancaster University

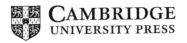

CAMBRIDGE
UNIVERSITY PRESS

CAMBRIDGE
UNIVERSITY PRESS

University Printing House, Cambridge CB2 8BS, United Kingdom

One Liberty Plaza, 20th Floor, New York, NY 10006, USA

477 Williamstown Road, Port Melbourne, VIC 3207, Australia

314–321, 3rd Floor, Plot 3, Splendor Forum, Jasola District Centre,
New Delhi – 110025, India

103 Penang Road, #05–06/07, Visioncrest Commercial, Singapore 238467

Cambridge University Press is part of the University of Cambridge.

It furthers the University's mission by disseminating knowledge in the pursuit of
education, learning, and research at the highest international levels of excellence.

www.cambridge.org
Information on this title: www.cambridge.org/9781108836395
DOI: 10.1017/9781108864732

© Gavin Brookes and Paul Baker 2021

First published 2021

Printed in the United Kingdom by TJ Books Limited, Padstow Cornwall

A catalogue record for this publication is available from the British Library.

Library of Congress Cataloging-in-Publication Data
Names: Brookes, Gavin (Linguist), author. | Baker, Paul, 1972– author.
Title: Obesity in the news : language and representation in the press / Gavin Brookes,
    Paul Baker.
Description: Cambridge, United Kingdom ; New York, NY : Cambridge University
    Press, 2021. | Includes bibliographical references and index.
Identifiers: LCCN 2021025801 (print) | LCCN 2021025802 (ebook) |
    ISBN 9781108836395 (hardback) | ISBN 9781108818971 (paperback) |
    ISBN 9781108864732 (epub)
Subjects: LCSH: Obesity–Press coverage–Great Britain. | Overweight persons–Press
    coverage–Great Britain. | Obesity–Public opinion. | Overweight persons–Public
    opinion. | Public opinion–Great Britain. | Overweight persons–Great Britain–Social
    conditions–21st century. | Discrimination against overweight persons–Great Britain. |
    BISAC: LANGUAGE ARTS & DISCIPLINES / Linguistics / General |
    LANGUAGE ARTS & DISCIPLINES / Linguistics / General
Classification: LCC PN5124.O217 B76 2021 (print) | LCC PN5124.O217 (ebook) |
    DDC 072.4/49616398–dc23
LC record available at https://lccn.loc.gov/2021025801
LC ebook record available at https://lccn.loc.gov/2021025802

ISBN 978-1-108-83639-5 Hardback
ISBN 978-1-108-81897-1 Paperback

Contents

Figures

Tables

Acknowledgements

The research reported in this book is based on the project 'Representations of Obesity in the News', undertaken within the ESRC Centre for Corpus Approaches to Social Science (CASS) at Lancaster University (Grant reference ES/R008906/1).

We would like to thank the anonymous reviewers for their constructive comments which have helped us to improve this monograph. We would also like to thank Andrew Hardie for his technical assistance throughout the project and Isobelle Clarke for her support in collecting data for Chapter 9. We also wish to thank Andrew Winnard, Isabel Collins and Rebecca Taylor at Cambridge University Press for their support.

1 Introduction

Obesity, the News and This Study

Introduction

FAT TESTS FOR TOTS Kids as young as two should be weighed annually to fight obesity epidemic, experts claim

(Sun, 26 March 2019)

Supermarket special offers contribute to obesity, says report

(Guardian, 26 March 2019)

These headlines were taken from two articles about obesity printed by different newspapers in the United Kingdom. The first comes from the *Sun*, a right-leaning tabloid, while the second is from the left-leaning broadsheet, the *Guardian*. Both articles were published on the same day in response to statistics published by Public Health England showing that the country's rates of childhood obesity had increased in the previous 12 months.[1] They each support their claims by referring to outside, expert sources. Despite being about the same issue and having been written at the same time and within the same social and political context, these headlines offer decidedly different takes on obesity. For the *Sun*, the increased incidence of obesity constitutes an 'epidemic' which needs to be 'fought' through regular weighing of children. On the other hand, there is no metaphorical language in the *Guardian* headline, which instead foregrounds the role of supermarket special offers in contributing to the purportedly rising levels of childhood obesity. These differences entail distinct perspectives on the issue of obesity. For the *Sun*, obesity is a medical problem – an *epidemic* – that resides within individuals and can therefore be addressed through closer measurement and monitoring of the body. Further into the article from which this headline was taken, it is also suggested that such annual weighing is carried out by medical practitioners, thereby situating obesity and those with it firmly under medical jurisdiction. For the *Guardian*, on the other hand, obesity appears to be a problem

---

[1] www.gov.uk/government/statistics/ncmp-and-child-obesity-profile-academic-year-2017-to-2018-update#history.

associated with wider social structures, transcending individuals and their bodies. In this case, it is supermarkets which are framed as being responsible for rising levels of childhood obesity, with the implication that this trend could be arrested through tighter regulation.

These differences could be explained by the differing formats in which either newspaper is published; as a tabloid, the *Sun* could be more inclined to use metaphorical language and to present issues in more sensationalistic terms. Furthermore, the individualisation of obesity in the *Sun*, and the neo-liberal perspective inherent within that, could also be interpreted as reflecting the free market values associated with the (centre-)right of the British political spectrum, a position advocated by right-leaning newspapers such as this. Left-leaning newspapers such as the *Guardian*, on the other hand, might be more likely to bring into focus the failings of the right-leaning Conservative government in regulating industries which it views as being culpable for increasing rates of obesity, as well as being critical of big business. Readers of either of these headlines (and their attendant articles) will therefore access different perspectives on the topic of obesity and, through sustained exposure to either perspective, will likely form differing views on it, on people living with it, and on whether and how it should be addressed.

Whatever the reasons for these differences, and whatever the impact on their respective readerships might be, an important point to note is that they exist as evidence for the potential for variability in the ways that obesity can be *represented* – and that is the focus of this book. Hall (1997: 61) defines *representation* as 'the process by which members of a culture use language [. . .] to produce meaning. Already this definition carries the important premise that things – objects, people, events in the world – do not have in themselves any fixed, final or true meaning. It is us – in society, within human cultures – who make things mean, who signify'. Hall's definition captures several important features of representation with which we are sympathetic and want to highlight here.

The first is that representations are accomplished through 'language', which Hall defines broadly as 'any system which deploys signs, any signifying system' (*ibid.*). Incidentally, Hall's definition applies to forms of communication – or 'signifying systems' – that include but also go beyond language, including images. As (corpus) linguists, we are particularly interested in the capacity of language to represent, in this case its capacity to represent obesity, and though we do not focus on imagery (discussed later in relation to limitations), we are nevertheless cognisant of the power of modes other than language to represent health and illness (see, for example, Harvey and Brookes 2019).

In this book, we interpret the language used to represent obesity in terms of *discourses*. The study of 'discourse' is now a significant activity across numerous humanities and social science disciplines which involve the analysis of language and text, such as linguistics, psychology, philosophy and cultural studies (Fairclough 2003). A consequence of this multidisciplinary interest is that a multitude of definitions for discourse have been put forward (see Baker 2006). In this book, we adopt a broadly social constructionist view of discourse and obesity, wherein the former is taken to have the power to constitute societal understandings and indeed experiences of the latter; Foucault (1972: 52) uses the term 'discourse' to refer to 'practices that systematically form the objects of which they speak'. While being sympathetic with this position, for the purposes of this book we also adopt a dual focus on 'discourse', using the term to refer both to linguistic practice (i.e. 'contextually sensitive written and spoken language produced as part of the interaction between speakers and hearers and writers and readers' (Candlin et al. 1999: 321)) and, in the social constructionist sense, to social practice ('as ways of structuring areas of knowledge and social/institutional practices' (*ibid.*: 323)). From this view, the concept of discourse can be applied both to forms of text and to the concepts that are referred to in the text. For example, press discourse involves the social practices and language use that occur around newspapers as a genre or register. Social practices would include aspects relating to the creation and consumption of newspapers ranging from the use of printing presses, the hiring of journalists, the use of investigative practices to gather information relating to stories and procedures set up to handle complaints about articles. We could also consider discourse in relation to the texts that press journalists create – how articles are laid out in relation to one another to form an edition of a newspaper, the ways that individual articles are structured (use of headline, leader, paragraphs, etc.) and also the language content and style of the articles, e.g. how news values (Galtung and Ruge 1965; discussed later in this section) may privilege certain topics or stances along with the use of linguistic conventions such as terms like 'exclusive'. On the other hand, we could conceive of discourses around a concept such as obesity. Again, this would involve both social practices and language use. Social practices here might relate to the contexts within which it is seen as appropriate or not to refer to obesity, while language use might refer to the narratives, metaphors and arguments that people use in order to represent obesity in particular ways.

This view of discourse as constituting not only stretches of language use but also ways of structuring knowledge and practices is, as noted, particularly close to the view of discourse advanced by Foucault and brings us to the next feature of representation highlighted by Hall; that is, that 'objects, people, events in the world [...] do not have in themselves any fixed, final or true meaning. It is us – in society, within human cultures – who make things mean' (1997: 61). Put another way, there is no reality that is wholly independent of discourse, for our understandings and experiences of all things in the world are, to a greater and lesser extent, enabled but also constrained by the very discourses that we use to represent them. In this book, we also conceive of discourse as not merely reflecting 'entities and relations in social life' (Candlin et al. 1999: 323), including obesity, but as actively contributing towards their constitution (Fairclough 1992). This is because our understandings and experiences of health- and illness-related phenomena, such as obesity, are based not just in the "biological realities" of our bodies but also in the language that we use to talk about them (Brookes et al. 2021). This point is articulated by Fox (1993: 6), who argues that 'illness cannot be just illness, for the simple reason that human culture is constituted in language [. . .] and that health and illness, being things which fundamentally concern humans, and hence need to be "explained", enter into language and are constituted in language, regardless of whether or not they have some independent reality in nature' (see also Gwyn 2002). Indeed, as the headlines reproduced at the beginning of this chapter demonstrate, obesity is not a unanimously agreed-upon phenomenon but, rather, is subject to a wide range of competing discourses and representations, all of which entail different conceptualisations of what obesity actually is and if and how it should be responded to.

Third and finally, Hall (1997: 61) attributes agency in the creation of representations to those 'members of a culture' who produce the language – the *discourses* – that are used to communicate about things in the world. The referent of 'members of a culture' is suitably broad, as the discourses used to represent things in the world are often contributed by a wide range of social actors and institutions. Indeed, Brookes et al. (2021) argue that the centrality of discourse to health is reflected in the range of texts in which communication about health and illness is present. The topic of this book, obesity, is no exception to this. We regularly encounter discourses around obesity across a wide range of contemporary texts and sites, including public health information, television, advertising and literature. In this study, we focus, in the British press, on just one type of text produced in just one (geographical) context. We should bear in mind, then, that obesity discourses are produced and consumed within a wider range of contexts than this, and that these discourses are likely to be culturally contingent. Our decision to focus on the press only captures part of the picture but is driven by practical and theoretical considerations. On a practical level, newspaper texts, unlike, for example, broadcast media and television, can be downloaded in very large quantities in rapid fashion. Moreover, the utility of online newspaper databases (described below) makes it possible for researchers to search for and retrieve all news articles mentioning a particular topic (i.e. obesity), ensuring both size and comprehensiveness in data that would be unlikely to be obtainable for other types of texts. Theoretically, though the print press is in decline in the United Kingdom in economic terms, the news media still constitutes a powerful shaper of knowledge and social attitudes, with empirical research demonstrating the capacity of the news to shape individuals' attitudes to social issues and groups (Lynott et al. 2019). Moreover, and of particular relevance to this book, the news media still represents a primary source of health information for populations across the world.

Yet, the representations offered by the media do not constitute a transparent 'window' on society. That is to say, none of the representations of obesity provided by the newspapers we examine in this book provide an 'objective' account of the issue but are instead partial accounts that are shaped by 'a number of competing forces of differing strengths and directions' (Iggers 1999: 100). This includes contextual factors at the sociocultural and institutional levels (e.g. editorial practices), as well as the affordances and constraints of the mode and linguistic grammar in which the discourses are rendered (Fowler 1991).

A key consideration in the creation of news – and one of the 'competing forces' described by Iggers (1999: 100) – is the audience. Reporters' and editors' understandings of who constitutes their audience informs the selection of what is presented as 'the news' and the tone and style of presentation, including how a story is constructed as being newsworthy for a particular audience (Richardson 2007: 90–91). Relevant to this process is the concept of news values, which can be defined as follows,

> News values are the criteria employed by journalists to measure and therefore to judge the "newsworthiness" of events. [. . .] News values are meant to be the distillation of what an identified audience is interested in reading or watching, the "ground rules" for deciding what is merely an "event" and what is "news". Journalists use these ground rules to select, order and prioritise the collection and production of news.
>
> (Richardson 2007: 91)

While the 'ground rules' of news values 'may not be written down or codified by news organisations [. . .] they exist in daily practice and in knowledge gained on the job' (Harcup and O'Neill 2001: 261; see also Cotter 2010). The most influential list of 'news values' was provided by Galtung and Ruge (1965) who identified twelve criteria which, they suggest, are employed by journalists to gauge the newsworthiness of events. These are usefully summarised by Richardson (2007: 91–92) as

1. frequency (daily news needs daily stories);
2. threshold (the scale or intensity of the event);
3. unambiguity (whether the event can be easily described);
4. meaningfulness (the cultural proximity to the story);
5. consonance (events people expect or want to happen);

6. unexpectedness (the scarcity or rarity of the event);
7. continuity (follow-up stories);
8. composition (a balance of stories across the paper);
9. reference to elite peoples;
10. reference to elite nations;
11. personification (about or directly affecting people); and
12. negativity (if it bleeds it leads!)

This set of news values has been highly influential in discourse studies of the media and, for our purposes, provides a useful set of principles for understanding and interpreting how obesity-related events may be represented in ways that render them more newsworthy to particular audiences. However, there are a few caveats to bear in mind when drawing on the news values in this list. The first is that Galtung and Ruge's (1965) original study was based on reportage surrounding three international crises (Congo 1960, Cuba 1960 and Cyprus 1964). It has thus been argued that their taxonomy does not adequately capture the news values that are applied to the coverage of more mundane, particularly domestic, news events (Harcup and O'Neill 2001, 2017). Second, Galtung and Ruge's original study was published in 1965 (55 years ago, at the time of writing), and it is important to acknowledge that news values can change over time (Richardson 2007: 93). Finally, more recent research on news values has highlighted their constructed nature (Bednarek and Caple 2017); that is, the notion that news values do not necessarily guide the selection of events for news reporting but can also be applied to an event during the process of news creation. In this sense, discursive choices made in the creation of a news text can serve to present an event in a way that the text producers think will make it appear more newsworthy – and thus more interesting – to their target audience. All of these points are worth bearing in mind as we consider the influence of news values at various points throughout our analysis.

Our interpretation of obesity discourses in the British press is thus related to contextual factors at the sociocultural, institutional and textual levels. In this sense, our analytical approach, which is described in more detail later, can be located within the discipline of Critical Discourse Studies (CDS). CDS can be conceptualised as a perspective on discourse analysis which broadly seeks to examine and critique the ways in which power relations are established, negotiated, challenged and exploited through discourse in context (Fairclough 1995, 2015). CDS is a methodologically eclectic and often interdisciplinary research paradigm characterised by a range of complementary approaches to discourse. The approach we take in this book can be characterised as one that combines principles from CDS with techniques from corpus linguistics. Corpus linguistics is broadly a set of methods, but also a field of research, which analyses linguistic patterns based on large collections of naturally occurring language (McEnery and Wilson 2001). Such a collection of texts is called a corpus (the Latin word for 'body', plural *corpora*).

We describe and evaluate our methodological approach later in this chapter. For now, we note that in taking a broadly social constructionist approach to the topic of obesity, we do not aim to document or describe any empirical reality of obesity, its causes, epidemiological patterns or health effects. Neither do we seek to recommend any cures or 'solutions' for obesity. Rather, we are interested in examining the discourses that are used to represent obesity in the press, mindful that such representations can contribute to our experiences and very understandings of what obesity is within society, and that these representations can be empowering or disempowering towards certain social groups or types of people. A broad question that critical discourse researchers try to keep in mind is, 'who benefits from a particular discourse?'. CDS has an emancipatory agenda; as well as viewing discourse and texts as being contingent upon their contexts of production and consumption, it seeks to highlight structures within societies that can result in abuses of power and to consider the perspectives and voices of those who are often not regarded. To this end, our book is especially concerned with identifying practices around newspaper reporting of obesity that may not be beneficial to less powerful people in society.

To gauge a more accurate and representative picture of press coverage of obesity, we base our analysis on a large corpus of British newspaper articles about the topic (43,878 articles, 36,053,221 words) published over a ten-year period (2008–2017). By studying a dataset of this size and span, our analysis is able to account for a wider range of discursive patterns in obesity representation and is better able to explore change and stability over time, thereby illuminating the ways in which emerging discourses might respond to or even instigate social change, as well as how the presence of more sustained representations could have an incremental effect in shaping people's perceptions and views of obesity over longer periods of time. Claims relating to the potential for the news to not only reflect but also shape individuals' views and experiences of obesity are not simply inferred from the content of the articles themselves but are also triangulated with analysis of readers' responses in below-the-line comments accompanying online articles (Chapter 9), to consider how readers might support but also challenge the discourses and attendant representations in the articles. We describe our data and methodological approach in more detail later. Before that, we provide a more comprehensive introduction to the topic of obesity, including outlining prominent definitions of it; describing its prevalence, associated health risks, perceived causes and current responses; and reviewing existing research into its media representations.

Obesity: Background

As a socially constructed phenomenon that is subject to a range of discourses and constructions from a multitude of perspectives (e.g. medicine, public health, academia, activism), the phenomenon of obesity defies straightforward definition. We will use this space mostly to outline the biomedical view of obesity, since this presently dominates in the societal context on which this study is based and within which this work was carried out (i.e. the UK). However, in keeping with the social constructionist perspective set out in the previous section, we acknowledge that this is just one perspective on and way of 'constructing' obesity, albeit a dominant and influential one. At this point, it is worth noting that despite the claims to certainty and truth that are backed up by seemingly 'neutral' science and statistics made by experts who view and study obesity through the lens of biomedicine, almost all aspects of obesity are poorly understood. Yet, as Lupton (2018: 28) points out, '[l]ike other powerful institutions, medicine and public health draw upon, reproduce and sometimes emphasize these beliefs and assumptions in ways of which the practitioners and researchers engaged in these institutions are often unaware'. In view of this, throughout this section we also aim to denaturalise the biomedical perspective on obesity, chiefly by discussing criticisms of it and by comparing it to alternative perspectives, such as fat activism.

The biomedical perspective is currently the dominant conception of obesity and other matters pertaining to the body and its ailments within Western societies. This paradigm locates illness and disease within the individual and considers effective treatments to be principally surgical or pharmacological. Biomedicine aims to explain disease 'mostly by mechanical causality and with reference to explanatory models as close to the molecular level as possible' (Filc 2004: 1275). Biomedicine is characterised by a realist ontology and a positivist epistemology which regard scientific data about the body and its ailments as being objective and independent from social processes (*ibid.*). In Western societies, the biomedical perspective on health and illness has long enjoyed dominant status regarding how these issues are talked about, conceptualised and indeed acted upon (Lupton 2013). The dominance of the biomedical perspective on obesity in particular has been observed by a plethora of researchers (Ritenbaugh 1982). From this perspective, obesity is viewed as a disease, as reflected in the World Health Organization's (WHO) widely cited (and accepted) definition of obesity as 'abnormal or excessive fat accumulation that presents a risk to health' (WHO 2019: online).

The classification of obesity as a disease by organisations such as the WHO is the result of a process by which larger bodies have become increasingly 'medicalised' over time. Medicalisation refers to the sociocultural process by which an ever-wider range of human experiences come to be defined, experienced and treated as medical conditions (Zola 1972; Conrad 2007). To demonstrate how bodies with large amounts of fat have become medicalised as 'obese', it is useful to consider alternative perspectives on such bodies which have emerged at different points in time. For example, Jutel (2009) describes recommendations to doctors working in the 1920s to interpret moderate fat accumulation as a sign of longevity. Jutel regards this as symptomatic of a wider 'historic fear' of thinness which originated from its association with wasting diseases, which were regarded as preventable and indeed curable through acquiring more body fat.

Vigarello (2013) traces the origins of the medicalisation of obesity to the beginning of the nineteenth century, at which point fat bodies began to be regarded as hazardous to health. Vigarello notes that although larger bodies had always attracted the interest of scientists and philosophers, it was at this point that these bodies generally came to be viewed differently; namely, in terms of numbers and quantification. Voigt et al. (2014: 25–26) describe the vagueness of early definitions of obesity, with some authors equating being overweight with physical bulk and even operating with social standards and perceptions as thresholds for determining whether a person was overweight. However, around the beginning of the nineteenth century, conceptions of overweight and obesity as simply constituting excessive body fat were supplanted by consideration of individuals' body mass or relative weight. Thus, researchers began to test measures of waist circumference, waist-to-hip ratio and body mass index as ways of defining and diagnosing obesity, as well as of assessing its associated health risks. Vigarello (2013) accordingly characterises knowledge about the body during this period as a 'flurry of numbers' (111), as the main way of learning about bodies and body parts was increasingly to measure them. This trend accelerated during the 1830s, as statisticians became increasingly interested in the human body. It was at this time that Belgian statistician Adolphe Quetelet developed scales comparing weight with height in an attempt to determine statistical body weight norms for persons of different heights. In the 1970s, this scale was revived and rebranded as the Body Mass Index (Levay 2014).

The Body Mass Index (BMI) is a scale used to quantify the amount of tissue mass (muscle, fat and bone) in an individual. The BMI measures weight relative to height. This measurement gives a BMI 'score', according to which a person's weight can be categorised as 'very severely underweight' (BMI <15), 'severely underweight' (BMI 15–16), 'underweight' (16–18.5), 'normal weight' (BMI 18.5–25), 'overweight' (BMI 25–30) and 'obese' (BMI 30+). Obesity diagnoses can be subdivided into six classes: (i) 'moderately obese' (BMI 30–35), (ii) 'severely obese' (BMI 35–40), (iii) 'very severely obese' (BMI 40–45), (iv) 'morbidly obese' (BMI 45–50), (v) 'super obese' (BMI 50–60) and (vi) 'hyper obese' (BMI 60+). By 1977, the BMI was recognised by the WHO as the authorised standard measure of ideal body weight for populations across the globe (Raisborough 2016: 35). Today, the BMI scale is circulated widely by health authorities such as the UK National Health Service (NHS) and is used by practitioners to 'diagnose' their patients as overweight or obese. This means that if an individual's BMI score exceeds 30 – thereby meeting the criteria for an obesity diagnosis – they are automatically viewed as having obesity (and being ill), irrespective of their actual state of health (*ibid.*).

Yet, from the social constructionist perspective introduced at the beginning of this chapter, 'obesity', along with concepts such as 'fat', 'overweight' and indeed 'normal', can be viewed as social categories that are, to an extent, arbitrary, as they vary across different historical, social and cultural contexts (Lupton 2018: 28–29). In terms of the BMI, the assignment of certain scores to different levels of obesity is born out of the statistical association between different body types and certain forms of ill-health. An assumption underpinning the BMI is that certain health risks materialise with excessive body fat and correlate positively with the amount of that body fat. The association between obesity and risk to health has been established by a large body of research, mostly carried out from a broadly biomedical perspective, which has demonstrated a link between obesity and a raft of diseases and forms of ill-health, such as cardiovascular disease, hypertension, diabetes and cancer (Kim and Popkin 2006). For example, in a study of obesity-attributable deaths in the United States, Allison et al. (1999) found that the risk of health hazards generally increased as BMI scores exceeded 25–27, with people with BMI scores of between 30 and 35 having a 50 per cent higher mortality rate than people with BMIs between 23 and 25.

Yet, associations between obesity and health risks have also been challenged, for example by fat activists, with such critics arguing that claims pertaining to the adverse health consequences of obesity are based on statistical associations that might falsely assume a direct causal relationship between obesity and co-occurring forms of ill-health. They argue that, although obesity might correlate with higher incidence of diseases such as diabetes and heart disease, correlation does not necessarily entail causation and that we should adopt a wider view and also consider the role of other factors (e.g. social, economic and political). Put another way, '"overweight" and "obesity" may sometimes be confounding factors that should therefore be displaced from the centre of our concern' (Voigt et al. 2014: 24–25). Such claims are often supported by studies evidencing the so-called healthy obese – that is, people whose BMI exceeds 30 (thereby making them diagnosable as having obesity) but whose metabolic health is comparable to that of individuals of so-called 'normal weight' (Blüher 2012). Similarly, some critics of the BMI point to research suggesting that physical health is more contingent on fitness than 'fatness' and that it is possible for people to have obesity and be healthy, so long as they are also *fit* (see Ortega et al. (2018) for a discussion). At the same time, some have pointed to individuals who are classifiable as 'normal weight' but exhibit evidence of poor metabolic health (Carnethon et al. 2012). All of this has prompted suggestions that obesity-related health risks should be measured not using indices of body fat but cardiorespiratory fitness (Atanasova et al. 2013: 2). A frequent criticism of the BMI in particular is that it does not account well for certain body types, for example people who are not particularly tall but are very muscular and so might weigh a lot for their height and as a result could meet the threshold for an obesity diagnosis.

Much of the critical counter-perspective on the health implications of obesity would therefore seem to be united behind Monaghan's claim that the 'actual extent of risks and deaths assumed to be due to fatness is scientifically indeterminable and, like any currency, subject to potentially massive inflation' (2005: 304). This 'inflation' has been attributed to such factors as studies conflating 'overweight' and 'obesity' and the problems and inaccuracies of the BMI (Gard and Wright 2005), while for others it signals a more insidious agenda 'designed to expand the territory dominated by obesity "experts", the diet industry and manufacturers of pharmaceutical treatments for weight problems' (Bonfiglioli et al. 2007: 54).

Whatever the case may be, like its very definition, the possible health implications of obesity would appear to be a contested issue. It is also clear that neither defining nor diagnosing obesity are straightforward, reflecting its contested nature and the variability of the discourses surrounding it. For all the criticisms made of it, being cognisant of the BMI is important for our purposes, as it underlies how obesity is diagnosed and defined in the context under study. With these definitional and diagnostic criteria in mind, we now move on to explore obesity's epidemiological characteristics.

Epidemiological studies have widely reported high and increasing rates of obesity across many parts of the world. As Brewis summarises

> In all but the poorest nations in sub-Saharan Africa, technically overweight and obese bodies are becoming the new biological norm [...]. From Fiji to Jamaica, and the United Arab Emirates to the United States, the average adult's body mass index ... is now well into the overweight range. In eight countries – four in the central Pacific and four in the Persian Gulf and North Africa – more than 75 percent of the adult population is overweight or obese.
>
> (Brewis 2017: 1)

Indeed, in 2018 the WHO published an online report indicating that in 2016 approximately two billion adults were overweight or obese (WHO 2018). Of adults aged 18 years or over, 39 per cent were overweight while 13 per cent were obese. A recent report by NHS Digital (2020) indicated that obesity was present in 26 per cent of adult men and 29 per cent of adult women in England, with these figures rising to 60 per cent and 67 per cent, respectively, when cases of overweight were considered too. When Brewis describes obese bodies as 'becoming the *new* biological norm' (our emphasis), she draws particular attention to obesity's rising prevalence. We will discuss the changing prevalence rates of obesity in the United Kingdom, focussing in particular on the ten years under study, at the beginning of Chapter 4, in which we examine changing obesity discourses over time.

It is important to note here that all groups are not affected by obesity to the same extent. Focussing again on the UK context, in terms of sex, approximately five in ten women and six in ten men are diagnosable as being overweight or as having obesity (National Obesity Observatory 2012). We will return to the influence of sex on obesity at the beginning of Chapter 7, in which we analyse gendered discourses. In terms of ethnicity, using the BMI as a measure, Sproston and Mindell (2006) found that, compared to the general population, obesity prevalence was higher among Black African, Black Caribbean and Pakistani women and lower among Chinese women. For men, obesity prevalence was found to be lower among men from Black African, Indian, Pakistani and Bangladeshi and Chinese backgrounds.

The statistics cited to this point relate to obesity in adults. However, obesity can also be diagnosed in children. Using National Child Measurement Programme data relating to primary school children, Public Health England (2020) report that more than one in five children can be diagnosed as overweight or as having obesity when they begin primary school, though this figure rises to one in three children by the time they leave. Social class is also identified as a decisive factor in the prevalence of obesity in children, with rates being highest in the most deprived 10 per cent of the population, approximately double what it is for the least deprived 10 per cent. Yet, social class is not just important for obesity in children but is also decisive for adults. While historically only the wealthiest and most powerful portions of the population had access to sufficient excess of food and leisure to develop obesity, more recently and in more developed countries this trend has reversed, such that people at the lower end of the socioeconomic cline are now affected most acutely by obesity (Brewis 2014). We return to the issue of social class, including its theorisation and the ways in which it has been observed to contribute to obesity, in Chapter 8 in advance of our analysis of discourses around obesity and social class.

Since the 1990s, governments and public health authorities have responded to the apparently rising prevalence of obesity and its associated ailments by declaring an 'obesity epidemic'. Lupton (2018: 3–4) observes how, although fat bodies have long been associated with ill-health, the period since the 1990s has 'witnessed an unprecedented intensification of focus by [. . .] experts and researchers on the negative health and economic effects of obesity', with the mid-2000s appearing to be 'a pivotal point at which concern about the "obesity epidemic" intensified and peaked'. Nowadays, the phrase 'obesity epidemic' is commonplace not only in medical and health policy descriptions of obesity prevalence but can also be found in other sites, such as entertainment and news media who capitalise on, but also construct and contribute towards, obesity's seemingly persistent newsworthiness (Boero 2007, 2012; Saguy et al. 2010). For Boero (2012: 7), the so-called 'obesity epidemic' constitutes a 'postmodern epidemic', which she defines as the process whereby 'partially and unevenly medicalised phenomena lacking a clear pathological basis get cast in the language and anxiety of more traditional epidemics'. This 'partial medicalisation', as Boero puts it, is in turn powered by the moral panic that is generated by experts and perpetuated by the media.

Despite the pervasiveness of the phrase 'obesity epidemic', not everyone agrees that obesity constitutes an epidemic, with critics arguing that claims pertaining to its range and scale are often exaggerated. As Gard and Wright (2005) point out, agreeing that there is a trend in weight increase is one thing but agreeing on the severity and extent of that trend is quite another. Many critics claim that what we are witnessing right now is actually a relatively small rise in the average weight of the population. They point to more recent data which indicates that obesity rates have actually ceased increasing (Campos et al. 2006). Others, such as Boero (2012), attribute rising rates of obesity not to any rise in the size of bodies in real terms but rather to the changing parameters – that is, to the 'diagnostic fluidity' (2012: 5) – of the BMI, which she argues has drastically increased the numbers of people who are diagnosable as overweight and obese. Arguably the most comprehensive critique of the 'obesity epidemic' is provided by Gard and Wright (2005) in their book, *The Obesity Epidemic*. They review the scientific and epidemiological literature surrounding obesity and identify what they interpret to be inaccurate and contradictory findings which have led to misleading assumptions and generalisations about obesity levels. These, they argue, have contributed to the notion of an 'obesity epidemic', leading to the conclusion that individuals' health will be adversely affected on the basis that their BMI score is above some arbitrarily defined norm. In a later book, titled *The End of the Obesity Epidemic*, Gard (2011) pays particular attention to the role of alarmist rhetoric in scientific research articles in establishing the 'obesity epidemic'. He argues that descriptions of obesity as 'burgeoning', 'exploding' and 'rampant' are all examples of hyperbolic language used to transform speculative ideas about obesity into scientific facts which have apocalyptic ends. Such critiques, offered by Gard and others, essentially argue that the reporting and interpretation of medical and epidemiological data relating to body mass have been shaped by different political agendas and certain pre-existing assumptions about the body and health. Regardless of the legitimacy of the 'obesity epidemic', such critiques highlight the way in which the 'obesity epidemic' has been constructed as a medical problem through the practices and knowledge claims of medical and public health researchers (Lupton 2018: 29–30).

Setting its legitimacy to one side, the 'obesity epidemic' has instigated a huge body of research trained on identifying obesity's 'risk factors', as well as how its epidemiological trends might be arrested or reversed. Beginning with its risk factors, the first thing to note is that, just as defining obesity is not straightforward, neither is explaining and accounting for its causes. The cause of obesity is often presented as resulting simply from energy or calorie intake exceeding energy expenditure over a period of time. Atanasova et al. (2013: 2) describe this as the 'energy equation'. So pervasive is this explanation and appealing in its simplicity that it seems to enjoy logical, even common-sense, status. Indeed, the WHO states that '[t]he fundamental cause of being obese or overweight is an energy imbalance between calories consumed and calories expended' (WHO 2018: online). We can also find evidence of the energy equation logic shaping public health messages relating to obesity. For example, the website of the NHS advises the public that '[o]besity is generally caused by eating too much and moving too little. If you consume high amounts of energy, particularly fat and sugars, but don't burn off the energy through exercise and physical activity, much of the surplus energy will be stored by the body as fat' (NHS 2019: online).

Despite its common-sense status in public health campaigns (discussed in more detail later in this section), the energy equation has received criticism from numerous quarters. Atanasova et al. (2013: 2) problematise the two sides of the energy equation of food intake and physical (in)activity when they draw attention to the fact that, although food consumption has received considerably more focus than (in)activity in medical research, patterns of consumption have not changed significantly over the recent past and so cannot alone account for any rise in obesity rates. This, they argue, points to physical (in)activity as the major public health challenge associated with obesity. Yet, even with an approach that is more balanced in its focus on consumption *and* (in)activity, the energy equation can still be criticised for over-simplifying the causal complexity of obesity, which is multifaceted and likely to include energy consumption relative to energy expenditure but also numerous other factors.

Although retaining a focus on the individual and individuals' backgrounds and behaviours, researchers have in recent years begun to place more emphasis on the role of social and physical environments in contributing to the purported 'obesity epidemic'. Arguably the most developed of these accounts is that of the 'obesogenic environment', where 'obesogen' refers to 'pollutants and chemicals that encourage obesity' (Voigt et al. 2014: 24). The 'obesogenic environment' perspective focusses on some of the socioeconomic factors which contribute to the development of obesity in populations, including the abundance of cheap, nutritionally poor and high kilojoule food; the spread of fast food outlets and advertising; the decline of healthy home-cooked meals (attributed in part to the increasing entry of women into the workforce); the amount of time that people – particularly children – spend engaged in sedentary pursuits such as watching television and playing video games; and a general decrease in physical mobility due to contemporary working and transport conditions (*ibid.*). The concept of the obesogenic environment is useful because it helps us to think about obesity as not merely a biological issue but also, crucially, a social one. Even if we subscribe to the view that obesity's primary cause is excessive calorie consumption and lack of energy expenditure, the obesogenic environment explanation asserts that we might expect to find significant levels of obesity in societies in which opportunities for physical activity are limited and low-calorie and nutritious food is less accessible and affordable than calorie-laden, sugary and nutrition-poor foods. This is not just a case of looking at differences across societies but also at differences (and disparities) *within* them, for the social, economic and political causes of obesity do not, as we have seen, impact all members of society equally. As Raisborough (2016: 3–4) argues, 'we may be alarmed to realize that the people most likely to encounter the risks [of obesity] are also those most unfavourably situated at the intersections of socially stratifying power relations . . . We may feel very uneasy when we acknowledge the sociological point that poverty, deprivation, and social inequalities drawn along the lines of social class, gender, and ethnicity, amongst others, are major drivers of ill health.'

The logical extension of the obesogenic environment argument is that any effective response to obesity needs to recognise and address the social, economic and political conditions under which obesity occurs. Indeed, campaign groups have lobbied for policymakers to tackle obesity by addressing the 'obesogenic environment', for example through tougher regulation on junk food manufacturing and marketing and by designing urban spaces which better facilitate exercise (e.g. including more cycle paths and parks). Yet, as Lupton observes, these structural factors can be very difficult to challenge or change, since they 'form part of a complex network of agribusiness, the processing, marketing and distribution of food as well as major social changes relating to working and everyday life' (2018: 15). Instead, rather than addressing the role of powerful institutions in contributing to the purported 'obesity epidemic', medical and public health authorities in the United Kingdom (and other countries) have responded by focussing on the transformation and regulation of individuals and their bodies. Specifically, these powerful institutions have designated obesity as the outcome of individual behaviours which tie in with the energy equation model introduced earlier; that is, obesity has been constructed as 'the outcome of individual risk behaviours such as sedentary living and consuming energy-dense, nutrient-poor foods' (Atanasova et al. 2012: 651–652; see also Glasgow 2012).

A contemporary example of a UK public health initiative employing this logic is the recent and ongoing *Change4Life* campaign. Launched in 2009, *Change4Life* is the UK Government's longest-running anti-obesity initiative. In collaboration with private sector partners, the campaign uses social marketing techniques to target children and parents of young children in a bid to influence lifestyle behaviours (Mulderrig 2018). Entering the *Change4Life* website (www.nhs.uk/change4life), users are greeted by the following short paragraph, situated on the homepage, which not only sums up the campaign's objectives but demonstrates aptly its personal and conversational tone.

> These days, 'modern life' can mean that we're a lot less active. With so many opportunities to watch TV or play computer games, and with so much convenience and fast food available, we don't move about as much, or eat as well as we used to.

This campaign is notable not only because it is the flagship anti-obesity public health campaign in the United Kingdom but also because it exemplifies the penchant for contemporary public health campaigns to attempt to encourage individuals to take up certain practices of self-regulation. Lupton (1995) contends that public health campaigns such as this are inherently pedagogical in the sense that they position themselves as sources of expert knowledge and scientific truth in order to inform their audiences and direct them towards behaviours that are more 'rational' from a public health point of view. Mulderrig (2018) argues that *Change4Life* and other such campaigns can be understood from the perspective of governmentality in the sense that they seek to manage populations by 'governing "at a distance", favouring self-disciplinary control over more coercive forms of state power' (40). Originally developed by Foucault (1976), governmentality is 'a theory of how expertise-led control over individual behaviour emerged as a technique of political rule. It encompasses the array of institutions, relations and practices through which the social and economic wellbeing of a territory and its population are managed' (Mulderrig 2018: 41). The enactment of governmentality varies historically and since the mid-twentieth century has taken the form of neoliberalism.

Neoliberalism is a contemporary political movement which advocates economic liberalisation, free trade and open markets (Harvey 2005). As a theory of political and economic practice, it proposes that 'human wellbeing can best be advanced by liberating individual entrepreneurial freedoms and skills within an institutional framework characterized by strong private property rights, free markets, and free trade' (Kwan and Graves (2013: 5–6). Neoliberalism has played an increasingly central role in the ways that Western societies are governed, which has led to social services (including health care), state-owned enterprises and indeed some aspects of government itself, working with, and in some cases being supplanted by, private industries operating in a context of economic deregulation and tax cuts. The neoliberal political project is both supportive of and supported by the reconfiguration of expert knowledge and power, whereby these are taken away from the 'bureau-professionals of the welfare state' and reassigned to managers, auditors, consumers and the market (Mulderrig 2018: 41). As a consequence, social relations are reshaped, with individuals repositioned as responsible and risk-prepared citizen-consumers, while the state acts as an enabling force that promotes a neoliberal political rationality which implores individuals to 'take responsibility' for their lives and their communities. Neoliberalism is thus underpinned by personal responsibility, for Foucault argued that neoliberal governments maintain social order and prosperity by relying on their citizens managing their bodies and their health voluntarily rather than having to be coerced or threatened with punitive measures (Foucault 1979). The *Change4Life* campaign serves as a particularly good example of what such a model of self-governance looks like in practice.

When applied to health, neoliberal governmentality positions individuals as active health consumers who are responsible for maintaining and enhancing their health and economic productivity by avoiding risky products and prac-tices. This can be particularly challenging in neoliberal societies in which the free market is given precedence and products and practices hazardous to health are available in abundance. Lupton considers how this applies to the manage-ment of weight risk and obesity specifically when she writes, '[t]here are highly established and profitable markets seeking to sell consumers products, such as fast foods and soft drinks, that are linked to being overweight, as well as products directed at losing weight. Within the free market, neoliberal society, both are encouraged: it is considered up to consumer/citizens to make wise choices about which products they should buy and use as part of the project of self-actualization and fulfilment' (2018: 34).

In terms of medical responses, the construction of obesity as a disease – and a life-shortening one at that – has resulted in the development of a range of medical treatments intended to 'cure' it, including the creation of specialist medical roles such as bariatricians who can offer counselling and advice, prescribe pharmaceutical remedies and perform surgical procedures designed to reduce body fat, such as gastrointestinal bypasses, bariatric surgery and gastroplasty (Markula et al. 2008: 4–5). In a context where individuals are held responsible for managing their obesity risk, procedures such as these are likely to offer useful – in some cases, essential – means for reducing body weight, thereby enabling individuals to fulfil their roles as responsible citizens. Yet, the impetus for individuals to manage their bodies and maintain a 'healthy weight' is not just evident in public health policies and the development of medical solutions but has been capitalised on by the food, fashion, fitness, pharmaceutical and cosmetic industries, as well as sections of the (news) media (Burns and Gavey 2008). Indeed, the pathologisation of large bodies has also provided fertile ground for the birth and subsequent growth of a weight-loss industry which continues to develop and market a multitude of weight-reducing products, ranging from exercise equipment and diet plans to wearable activity trackers and weight-loss pills (Wann 2009; Lupton 2017).

However, this industry has largely been regarded critically within the social science literature, where the declaration of an 'obesity epidemic' has been widely interpreted in terms of its more cynical, commercial motivations. One such critic is Lupton, who writes, '[i]t is certainly the case that there is a massive weight-loss industry which is devoted to appealing to the vulnerabilities, anxieties and fears of people who have been medically classified as overweight or obese, or who have defined themselves as "too fat"' (2018: 29; see also Gard and Wright 2005; Campos et al. 2006; Bonfiglioli et al. 2007). Raisborough, another critic, takes a broader perspective, shedding light on a wider range of industries that have profited from the so-called 'obesity epidemic'. She writes

> We may also start to feel uneasy about 'epidemic claims' once we consider too the vested interests that the global pharmaceutical, insurance, and diet industries have in the obesity epidemic [...]. We could feel a little troubled when we remember that fat makes for big business and not just for the enterprising few exploiting the market gap in oversized clothes, toilet seats, and caskets; food companies have quickly realized increased profitability in products that can boast their health-enhancement qualities alongside their low or no fat content.
>
> (Raisborough 2016: 4)

As well as its problematic relationship with commercial interests, another frequent criticism of the neoliberal approach to public health is its potential to invoke what Lupton (1995: 3) describes as a 'victim-blaming discourse' which, in placing all responsibility for ill-health on individuals, concomitantly shifts attention *away from* the structural, political and economic determinants of health, including obesity risk (as discussed earlier), over which individuals often have very little control (particularly at the lower end of the socioeconomic spectrum) (Baum and Fisher 2014). Campaigns such as *Change4Life* have been criticised for exhibiting a lack of sensitivity towards the complexities surrounding individuals' health-related behaviours, including not least the embeddedness of these within historical, economic, cultural and social contexts (Lupton 2018). Or, as Atanasova et al. (2012: 652) surmise, 'policies emphasising personal behaviour fail to grasp the following: when individuals behave in ways that may be damaging to their health, this may not necessarily be due to their lack of awareness about adverse health effects; rather, the constraints of their life experiences and environments may mean that they are simply unable to change their behaviours'. And this is likely to be one of the reasons why public health policies underpinned by neoliberal governmentality have generally failed to instigate significant health improvements in their populations (Glass 2000).

Although there is evidence of some proponents of the biomedical perspective paying greater attention to the social and structural dimensions of health, such as in the case of the 'obesogenic environment' perspective introduced earlier, even these emphasise the role of personal responsibility. As Lupton (2018: 34–35) points out, '[t]he obesogenic perspective makes the simplistic assertion that because food is more readily available in contemporary societies people therefore consume more of it, and become fat. It assumes that the "natural" state of the human body is to be thin (given the right environmental conditions) and that in this context of ready supply of poor quality food that all individuals may potentially become obese as they will be unable to resist the temptations or persuasions of over-eating or lack of exercise.' The risk of such a perspective is that it automatically implies greater susceptibility towards obesity of certain socially and economically disadvantaged groups, who are more likely to live in environments that are deemed to be more 'obesogenic'. Such prima facie assumptions could risk such groups being regarded as more 'at-risk', less knowledgeable and less responsible (Gard and Wright 2005).

In addition to its practical limitations, the victim-blaming inherent in the neoliberal approach can also result in the stigmatisation of individuals who become ill, as they may be perceived to have failed the imperative to remain healthy and fully economically productive. This is particularly the case for so-called lifestyle diseases, such as obesity, but also type 2 diabetes and others, which individuals are perceived to 'bring upon themselves' through poor lifestyle choices. Moreover, given the widely noted negative connotations attached to obesity, people with visibly larger, adipose bodies are also liable to experience stigma on the grounds that they are likely to contravene society's 'thin ideal' (Rich and Evans 2005). This type of stigma is widely referred to as 'weight stigma'.

As we have alluded at various points throughout this discussion, not all perspectives on obesity frame it as a problem. The strongest counter position to the biomedical perspective in this regard is the 'fat pride' or 'fat acceptance' position – a social justice movement which began in the United States in the form of the National Association to Advance Fat Acceptance, established in 1969, and was bolstered in the 1970s by the Fat Underground movement. The aim of these and similar other grassroots organisations is to establish resources for 'self-esteem, fitness, fashion, socialising, medical advocacy, and defense from discrimination' (Wann 2009: x), as well as to create 'theatre, dance, music, poetry, fiction, magazines, film, and art' which celebrate the 'fat' body and promote more positive attitudes towards it (*ibid.*).

In this section, we hope to have demonstrated how obesity, as a socially constructed phenomenon, is subject to a wide range of definitions and discourses. We have not been able to address all of these perspectives, so have instead focussed mostly on the biomedical viewpoint, underpinned by the intertwined institutions of medicine and public health, which presently dominates in the United Kingdom. In this sense, the foregoing discussion serves to illustrate the social and political context within which the newspaper articles analysed in this book were both produced and consumed. It is the very fact that obesity is not ubiquitous but open to discursive contest and negotiation which makes it worthy of study and interesting from the discourse analyst's viewpoint. So in this book, we are interested in studying how obesity is negotiated, through discourse, in the context of the British national press. Throughout the forthcoming chapters, we hope to show how, even in this relatively singular context, obesity is represented using a wide range of discourses which are themselves intertwined with an even wider range of discourses pertaining to the body, health, medicine and identity more broadly. Ours is not the first study to explore media representations of obesity and we will review some of this research, and situate our own work in relation to it, in the next section.

Obesity in the (News) Media

The first studies broadly concerned with the relationship between the media and obesity set out to address the role of the media in circulating and emphasising notions of slim embodiment. Most of this work was carried out by (critical) feminist scholars who focussed mainly on western media such as advertisements, fashion magazines, films and television, critiquing their tendencies to hold up slim and difficult-to-achieve body types as beautiful, sexually desirable and something to which all women should aspire (Orbach 1978; Bordo 1993). Work in this important vein continues to this day, with the critical scope expanded to interrogate an ever-widening range of media, more recently incorporating representations of (women's) bodies in new (social) media texts (Lupton 2017). Unrealistic depictions of the 'ideal' feminine body type have subsequently been linked to increased bodily dissatisfaction, with high levels of media exposure widely considered to be a factor in the development of eating disorders, continuous dieting and more general feelings of shame, anxiety and inadequacy in women whose bodies do not conform to such ideals (Lupton 2018).

Following this pioneering work and in response to increasing levels of press coverage of obesity (discussed in the previous section), the last two decades have witnessed a proliferation in the amount of social scientific research examining media representations of obesity (Boero 2007, 2013). Writing from a critical standpoint, social scientists have sought to problematise the media's coverage of obesity by elucidating its broadly negative and stigmatising portrayals of obesity and people with it, as well as by questioning the extent to which the purported 'obesity epidemic' is indeed a genuine public health crisis or rather a 'moral panic',[2] created in part by the media's alarmist reporting of the issue (Monaghan 2005; Campos et al. 2006; Kwan and Graves 2013; Raisborough 2016).

A significant portion of studies of obesity in the media have drawn on the sociological concept of framing (Goffman 1974), with the aim of explicating the various 'frames' through which obesity emerges as a social problem. Combining a number of conceptualisations, Atanasova and Koteyko (2017: 651) usefully define a frame as 'an organising principle [...], a central organising idea [...] or an interpretative package that enables individuals to make sense of issues by turning "meaningless" aspects "into something mean- ingful" (Goffman 1974: 21–22)'. In this context, media framing of obesity is understood as 'implicitly (or explicitly) promot[ing] a dominant viewpoint and tend[ing] towards [...] reinforcing existing cultural and political relations of power' (Boero 2013: 372).

Studies of media framing of obesity have generally identified three primary frames. The first is a medical frame which construes obesity as a disease, biological problem or genetic trait that is most effectively remedied through medical or surgical solutions (Saguy and Almeling 2008; Atanasova and Koteyko 2017). The second is a frame of societal responsibility, which fore- grounds the role of governments and certain industries in creating the condi- tions for obesity to thrive. This includes such factors as ineffective regulation of 'junk' food manufacturing and advertising, the costliness of nutritious food compared to more affordable but less nutritious alternatives, and the design of urban spaces in ways that make them less conducive to walking and cycling compared to driving or using public transport (Atanasova and Koteyko 2017). The final primary frame is one of personal responsibility, which constructs obesity as something that is caused by individuals' lifestyle choices and thus positions individuals as responsible for preventing and 'curing' obesity by

---

[2] Rohloff and Wright (2010: 404) define a moral panic as 'a sociological concept that seeks to explain a particular type of overreaction to a perceived social problem [whose] principal aim was to expose the processes involved in creating concern about a social problem; concern that bore little relationship to the reality of the problem, but nevertheless provided the basis for a shift in social or legal codes'.

making changes to their levels of physical activity and the types of food they consume (Boero 2007; Bonfiglioli et al. 2007; Shugart 2013; Atanasova and Koteyko 2017). Despite the increased presence of the social responsibility frame, this final frame of personal responsibility is widely observed to be most dominant in Western societies such as the United Kingdom. Boero (2013: 373) notes how this individualistic frame is 'often the frame of final recourse in reporting which initially seems to advance less individualistic frames'. Although we have presented the frames separately in this discussion, it is of course possible for them to be combined in the ways that obesity is conceptualised and talked about. A good example of this can be found in the websites of obesity charities and weight loss support groups which frame obesity as something that is problematic and so set out to encourage and support people in losing weight, akin to a neoliberal framework. At the same time, such organisations aim to be respectful towards people with obesity and so try to provide more positive representations of them (compared to, say, some sections of the mainstream media), even though they would not identify with the 'fat acceptance/pride' movement described earlier.

Several studies have highlighted the contradictory nature of the personal responsibility frame. For example, Boero's (2007) study of 751 articles about obesity published in US newspaper *The New York Times* between 1990 and 2001 found that obesity tended to be framed as something that was out of control, as a problem of culture and environment and couched in language associated with biomedical epidemics, yet was also construed as a problem that could be cured by relying on common-sense solutions. This theme, of obesity being represented in contradictory terms as, on the one hand, a medical, genetic, moral and/or environmental problem beyond individual control yet, at the same time, a problem that is caused by a lack of self-control and accordingly cured by individual willpower, has also been noted in more recent studies such as Saguy and Almeling's (2008) study comparing social problem frames of obesity in medical science and US news reporting and Shugart's (2013) examination of narratives of obesity in contemporary mainstream US media. Some studies have set out to denaturalise the personal responsibility frame. For example, Saguy and Gruys (2010) compared news reporting of eating disorders against that of obesity in the United States between 1995 and 2005 and found that while obesity was predominantly attributed to individuals' lifestyle choices, the cause of eating disorders tended to be located *outside* the individual, with wider social factors brought into sharper focus. The authors linked this difference to broader social structures within which high status is afforded to thinness while fatness is linked to low status and associated with sloth and gluttony.

As well as comparing the media coverage of obesity to that of other health issues, another way in which previous research has sought to denaturalise the dominant frames or discourses surrounding obesity has been to study changes in representation over time. An example of such a study was carried out by Caulfield et al. (2009), whose diachronic analysis of US newspaper articles published between 1990 and 2007 revealed a shift in focus *away from* the view of obesity as a disease and *towards* the view of obesity as a matter of personal responsibility. Shugart (2013) similarly noted a shift in emphasis towards personal responsibility but also observed a more recent, fatalistic framing of obesity as both unavoidable and inevitable – something which she argues not only upholds stigma surrounding obesity but also forecloses any complex discussion surrounding its social determinants. Although the personal responsibility frame has widely been observed as dominant in media coverage, diachronic studies such as these do at least serve to demonstrate that this was not always the case (or at least to the extent that it is now) and, as such, may not necessarily be the case in the future.

Another way of considering the situatedness of media 'frames' or discourses around obesity is to consider different cultural contexts. Most studies on media representations of obesity have focussed on the United States. However, a smaller number of studies have based their analyses on other cultural contexts, with some carrying out systematic comparisons of coverage between different countries. For example, Ries et al. (2011) compared press reporting of obesity policy in the United States, Canada and the United Kingdom, finding that while the media in all three countries tended to adopt a personal responsibility frame, they also expressed significantly different attitudes towards obesity policy, which the authors explain with recourse to the countries' respective economic structures and healthcare systems. Other studies have reported more pronounced differences between the media framing of obesity in the United States and other countries. For example, Saguy et al. (2010) found that the French media is more likely than the US media to foreground the social-structural forces underpinning rising rates of obesity, which were also often attributed to the so-called Americanization of French culture. In terms of the UK context, Atanasova and Koteyko (2017) compared obesity frames in British and German online newspapers, revealing a 'dominant cross-national framing of obesity in terms of "self-control", which places a more pronounced emphasis on individual responsibility' (2017: 650). These comparative studies are valuable because they demonstrate how media frames of obesity are not universal but rather are shaped by national economic and social structures which can, in turn, influence the development and implementation of social policies relating to obesity and health(care) more widely.

More recently, a small number of studies have explored how particular groups are represented in media texts about obesity, paying particular attention to the portrayal of racial and ethnic minorities and economically disadvantaged groups (Gollust et al. 2009). The framings identified in such studies have tended to mirror those reported in relation to more general populations, specifically a focus on the role of individuals and the assignment of negative moral evaluations. However, most studies examining the representation of particular groups affected by obesity have focussed on children and the phenomenon of childhood obesity (Boero 2007; Saguy and Almeling 2008). These studies have highlighted an important difference between the representation of obesity in children and adults, whereby in media discussions of childhood obesity, blame is assigned not to the children affected by obesity (as it is in representations of adults) but to their parents, schools and, in some cases, the media itself.

As noted, the media plays an important role in communicating health information and scientific research to the public. With regard to obesity-related research, the media has been found to selectively report on studies that provide the most dramatic content, and which thus lend themselves more easily to sensationalist headlines. For example, in a study comparing the obesity frames in scientific studies against their corresponding press releases and news articles, Saguy and Almeling (2008) reported that although there was overlap between the two samples, the media texts were more inclined to present the studies' findings and implications in more dramatic terms than the original scientific papers did and were also more likely to foreground individual blame for obesity. The authors trace this in part to the tendency of the news media to report on studies producing the most alarmist and 'individual-blaming' findings. Another theme identified in this body of work pertains to the media's lack of scepticism regarding the validity of the findings they reproduce, as well as contradictions in media coverage of scientific research (Boero 2007, 2012).

A relatively recent area of focus in studies of obesity in the media relates to the representation of obesity policy. Ries et al. (2011) found that even if countries framed the issue of obesity itself in similar ways, they could still differ in the ways they framed policy issues. All of this was found to depend on each country's national political context, with advocates of certain policies using the media as a vehicle to promote their initiatives and circulate them among a wider audience (Boero 2012).

The studies discussed so far in this section have all adopted a mono-modal perspective on their data, focussing just on the use of language. However, in recent years, a small but growing body of studies have also considered how news articles' linguistic framings combine with accompanying imagery in the ways they represent obesity and people with it. In separate studies of photographs and videos featured on US news websites, Heuer et al. (2011) and Puhl et al. (2013) reported that people with obesity were depicted in stigmatising ways, as lazy and lacking self-discipline, often with their heads cut out of images and/or being pictured wearing ill-fitting clothes. Examining visual representations of obesity in 583 photographs taken from British and German newspapers published between 2009 and 2011, Atanasova et al. (2013) reported that over half of the images in their data portrayed obesity and people with it in stigmatising ways, for example showing tools for weighing or measuring bodies, exercise equipment, food and drinks and evidence of TV viewing or gaming, all of which, they argued, had the potential to cue readers'/viewers' moral judgements. They noted no significant differences between the British and German data, suggesting that audiences in both contexts were exposed to similar visual discourses of obesity. More recently, Lupton (2018: 52) described how the bodies of people with obesity are frequently portrayed in news media as 'bulging and distended, often using close-up camera effects to distort their bodies beyond the reality of their fleshiness'. Lupton also notes the frequent use of 'strategies of exposure and shaming', with people with obesity 'often shown as gorging themselves with food, invariably food designated as "unhealthy", such as hamburgers or chips' (2018: 52).

To summarise, then, research into media representations of obesity has revealed a range of frames or discourses, with representations emphasising personal responsibility emerging as dominant in most studies and across most media contexts (although we should also note the dominance of studies focussing on the global west and on the United States in particular). Atanasova et al. (2012) argue that the predominance of the personal responsibility frame can be interpreted as reflecting wider developments in public health, which in many western societies is now driven by a neoliberal logic which, as we have described, responsibilises individuals into managing their own health and risks of ill-health through their lifestyle choices (see also Crawford 1980; Brown and Baker 2012). Meanwhile, Kwan and Graves (2013: 5) suggest that the dominance of the personal responsibility frame reflects a longer tradition in which victim blaming and individualistic discourses exist in relation to many social issues, including obesity and health.

Existing research on media representations of obesity provides an unquestionably rich set of insights on the topic which, as the forthcoming chapters will show, are useful for explaining and comparing our findings. However, we also aim to build on this work by adopting new types of data and analytical perspectives, as well as by pursuing fresh areas of analytical focus. In terms of data, most existing studies are, as noted, based on US media. Although British newspapers have been studied more than those of many other countries, our focus on press data originating in the United Kingdom adds to the still relatively slim body of existing work based on this context. As will be described in the next section, our data also represents the most comprehensive and recent dataset of its type, with a date range that begins at the start of 2008 and runs to the end of 2017. This is an important consideration, since most studies of media representations of obesity are based on older datasets, with most studies carried out during the early 2000s. However, given that press coverage of obesity in the United Kingdom and elsewhere has, as we will see, risen in recent years, there is a pressing need for research that keeps up to date with this coverage and any attendant changes to the discourse. As Boero (2013) asserts, '[t]here is no doubt that the amount of media attention to obesity will continue to grow as researchers secure more funding to come up with solutions, as more obesity policy is debated and enacted, and as governments continue to need to individualize responsibility for public health. The task of social scientists will [be] not only to keep up with this reporting but also to sharpen their critical focus' (377–378). As well as the size and recency of our data, our study can also be distinguished from the majority of research on obesity representation by its linguistic focus; where most studies on obesity representation have described the content of the texts in their data (i.e. *what* is said), our study is based on systematic linguistic analysis of recurring word choices (i.e. *how* it is said) and the discourses and resultant representations these evoke.

Aside from analysing the articles themselves, another way in which this book advances on previous research is by examining representations of obesity in readers' comments accompanying a sample of online articles in our data. Reader responses to media representations of obesity have received relatively scant attention to-date. This observation is made by Atanasova et al. (2012), who identify this as an area for future study in media representations of obesity, noting that such data-sites provide hitherto 'untapped opportunities to analyse how readers respond to obesity news stories' (2012: 557).

Furthermore, Lupton (2017) discusses the potential for social media spaces such as reader comments sections to allow dominant perspectives on obesity put forward by the articles to be challenged by readers, providing space for less dominant perspectives such as fat activism and body positivity to be advanced instead. Although such comments are unlikely to offer a transparent window into individuals' understandings, beliefs or opinions, adopting this novel perspective nevertheless helps us to engage with such issues in an unprecedented way, allowing us to examine previously unexplored perspectives on media representations of obesity and thus to test and potentially expand on findings from the types of audience response studies discussed earlier. Having begun to consider some of the ways in which our data and approach advance on existing studies of obesity representation, we now provide a more detailed account of our corpus and introduce the main corpus linguistic techniques that we use to analyse it.

Data and Approach

The study reported in this book is based on a methodology which combines corpus linguistics with CDS. As noted, CDS can be understood broadly as a perspective on discourse analysis which seeks to examine and critique the ways in which power relations are established, negotiated, challenged and exploited through discourse in context. The term *corpus linguistics*, meanwhile, largely refers to a collection of methods which use specialist computer programs to analyse linguistic patterns in large, digitised collections of naturally occurring language data. These programs offer methods that can help human analysts to identify frequent or salient features of the language in the texts contained in the corpus, which must then be subjected to a detailed analysis carried out by the human researcher. In this section, we describe the design and compilation of our corpus of news articles about obesity, before outlining the main analytical techniques we use to study representations of obesity within it. We will then conclude this section by setting out some of the main strengths and limitations, as we see them, of our data and approach.

The majority of the analysis in this book is based on a purpose-built corpus comprising all UK national press articles containing at least one mention of *obese* or *obesity*, published between 2008 and 2017 (inclusive). This constitutes the decade leading up to our point of data collection. Articles were collected using the online news repository *LexisNexis*, which archives both online and print versions of newspapers. To avoid skewing frequencies, duplicate articles from the same newspaper were removed. Table 1.1 shows the newspapers represented in the corpus, along with the number of articles and words contributed by each. Note that in this table, online and print

Table 1.1. *Breakdown of the corpus by newspaper*

Newspaper	Articles	Words	Mean article length (in words)
Express	5,193	3,265,741	629
Guardian	5,008	5,238,062	1,046
Independent	4,336	3,303,269	762
Mail	12,805	11,890,340	929
Mirror	3,398	2,202,323	648
Morning Star	152	63,641	419
Star	1,072	370,818	346
Sun	2,286	1,082,808	474
Telegraph	5,680	4,804,351	846
Times	3,948	3,831,868	971
Total	**43,878**	**36,053,221**	**822**

versions of newspapers have been combined under one heading, as have sister/ Sunday editions (e.g. *Guardian* and *Observer* are under the heading *Guardian*; *Mirror* and *People* are under the heading *Mirror*; and *Independent* and *i* are under the heading *Independent*). However, when citing examples from the corpus we will refer to the specific newspapers from which they originate, rather than using the general headings in this table.

As Table 1.1 shows, the corpus is not equally balanced in terms of the number of articles and words contributed by each newspaper. One newspaper, the *Mail*, comprises around 30 per cent of the words in the corpus, while the contribution of the *Morning Star* is marginal. Average article length also varies considerably, with the *Guardian*'s average being more than double that of tabloids such as the *Star* and *Sun*. This imbalance represents the real-life press landscape and specifically the corresponding imbalance in terms of how much obesity coverage is provided by each newspaper. To capture as much obesity coverage in our analysis as possible, we decided against removing or reducing texts simply for the purpose of achieving a more balanced corpus. While this imbalance does not pose too much of an issue for most of our analysis, as we compare different newspapers and sections of the press using relative rather than raw frequencies, we nevertheless need to note that any analysis of the corpus as a whole is based on an imbalanced sample, with language use in some newspapers, foremost the *Mail*, over-represented relative to other newspapers.

The corpus we analyse in this book constitutes, to our knowledge, both the largest and most recent collection of newspaper articles about obesity assembled for research. Existing studies of news media representations of obesity have based their insights on datasets that are considerably smaller than that assembled for this book, amounting, at most, to hundreds (rather than thousands) of articles. However, when we consider how many articles are published about obesity every year, and thus the sheer mass of newspaper data that is available for study, then these previous datasets are not very widely representative. As well as being larger and more representative than data used in previous studies, our corpus is also structured in a way that facilitates insights into aspects of obesity representation that have rarely (if ever) been explored in prior studies (Atanasova et al. 2012: 556). This includes carrying out systematic comparisons of articles according to their format (i.e. broadsheets vs. tabloids), political leaning (i.e. left-leaning vs. right-leaning) and date of publication (i.e. similarity and change over time). Finally, the corpus analysed in this book not only represents *print* versions of obesity articles, but also online articles published on the respective newspapers' websites. This marks another area of expansion on existing research, which has focussed, in the main (and in the context of the United Kingdom, exclusively), on printed newspapers only. This is a significant gap to address, prompting Atanasova et al. (2012) to propose that studies of obesity press representations analyse online versions of news articles, since '[t]he current focus on print diverges from the general attentiveness in media studies to the topic of the online presence, convergence and the successful adoption of social media features by many print editions' (2012: 557).

A crucial feature of modern corpus linguistics research is that corpora are stored in a machine-readable format so that they can be analysed using a computer. Specialist computer programs are available for this purpose, such as *AntConc*, *WordSmith Tools* and the tool we use in this study, *CQPweb* (Hardie 2012). Such programs allow human researchers to carry out tasks that would otherwise be impractical to perform manually on such vast datasets, for example searching for every occurrence of a word or combination of words, generating frequency information about linguistic phenomena of interest (e.g. words, chains of words, grammatical types) and performing statistical tests on those frequencies (i.e. to measure the significance or strength of relationships). Moreover, these programs offer the practical advantage that they can perform frequency counts and complex statistical calculations with greater speed and reliability than would be possible using a purely manual approach to (critical) discourse analysis.

There is no standard set of procedures in corpus linguistics, and there is some variability in terms of the procedures and statistical measures afforded by different programs or tools. This notwithstanding, our analysis makes use of four techniques that have become established in corpus research; namely, frequency, keywords, collocation analysis and concordance analysis, all of which we accessed using *CQPweb* (Hardie 2012). We will provide brief introductions to each of these in this section. However, since we use these techniques in different ways across the forthcoming chapters, we will provide more precise details regarding their parameters and cut-offs as and when these are relevant throughout our analysis.

Frequency provides a list of all the words that are present in the corpus or a user-determined section of the corpus, along with their frequency of occurrence. Frequency information can provide a useful starting point for corpus analysis, as it affords a rapid overview of the linguistic landscape of the texts in the corpus, as well as allowing users to search for the frequency of particular words or sequences of words of interest. For example, we use frequency in Chapter 5, as part of our analysis of the shaming and reclaiming of obesity in the press, specifically as a means of identifying nouns that are frequently used to denote people with obesity and verbs that tend to be attributed to them. We also use frequency to adopt a similarly targeted approach in Chapter 6, in which we examine the discourse surrounding the terms *diet*, *body*, *healthy* and *exercise*. In Chapter 7, we use frequency information to compare mentions and uses of gender-marked nouns and pronouns, and then in Chapter 8 when examining the representation of different social class groups. Throughout the book, then, we utilise frequency as an inductive measure to pinpoint the occurrence of particular words or phrases that are relevant to our analysis and as a means of carrying out more focussed analysis by sampling texts from our corpus on the basis that they mention a particular topic, theme or social group.

Another, more statistically robust way of accessing words that are characteristic of the texts in our corpus is keywords. Put simply, keywords are words that occur with a significantly higher frequency in one corpus when compared against another. The corpus against which we compare the corpus under analysis is termed the 'reference corpus' and this typically represents a 'norm' for the type of language being analysed. In the keywords procedure, the frequency of each word in the corpus we are analysing is compared against its equivalent in the reference corpus. If these frequencies are judged to be significantly different (according to the statistical measure(s) chosen by the user), then that word will be flagged as a keyword by the computer. Words which have a significantly higher relative frequency in our corpus compared to the reference corpus are 'positive keywords', while words with a significantly lower relative frequency (including potentially being absent altogether) are 'negative keywords'. Positive keywords are thus words that are overused in our corpus relative to the norm represented by the reference corpus, and so can be interpreted as being characteristic of the texts we are analysing, while negative keywords, conversely, represent words that are underused relative to what we might expect based on the reference corpus. In this book, we focus on positive keywords – that is, words that are especially frequent in our corpus (or a section or sample of it) compared against a reference corpus.

The choice of reference corpus, statistic and cut-off point are all crucial in determining the number and type of words that will be flagged as key by the computer. In this book, we use log-likelihood (Dunning 1993). This is a measure which assigns to keywords scores that indicate the level of confidence the user can have that a word is indeed key and has not arisen as such due to a sampling error. This is important to bear in mind, as it means that the keywords we examine in this book are ranked by *confidence*, rather than degree or *strength* of keyness, for which we would require an effect size measure such as log ratio. Different cut-offs can be applied, but a log-likelihood score of 3.84 indicates a confidence level of 95 per cent (standard in social sciences (McEnery 2006)); a score of 6.63 indicates a confidence level of 99 per cent; and a score of 15.13 or more indicates a confidence level of 99.99 per cent. While our use of log-likelihood is consistent across the analysis, our choice of reference corpus and cut-off varies across chapters depending on each chapter's focus and, on a more practical level, the amount of space we have to analyse the keywords. We use the keywords approach in Chapters 2 and 3, respectively, to explore similarities and differences across different sections of the corpus when we divide it up according to newspapers' political leaning and publication type (i.e. left-leaning broadsheets, left-leaning tabloids, right-leaning broadsheets, right-leaning tabloids). We also use keywords in our analysis of change over time in Chapter 4, specifically obtaining keywords by comparing each year of the corpus against the rest and then by comparing articles published in a particular month (e.g. in January across all years) against all other months grouped together. Keywords also feature in the second half of Chapter 7 when, following our analysis of the discourse around gender-marked nouns, we examine the keywords that emerge when comparing a sample of press weight loss narratives about women against a reference corpus containing a sample of weight loss narratives about men, and vice versa. Finally, in Chapter 9 we use keywords to compare both a sample of articles and their corresponding reader comments against the same reference corpus as a way of exploring similarities and differences between those articles and their accompanying comments.

Collocation is a linguistic device whereby words, by associating strongly with one another, become bearers of meaning. Collocation analysis, then, is a word association measure that tells us how often two or more words occur alongside each other across the texts in the corpus, and whether this association is notable as a sizeable effect. Corpus linguists have long sought to learn about words' meanings and patterns of use by examining their patterns of co-occurrence, or 'collocations', across corpora. Analysing those words with which a word of interest frequently collocates can help to shed further light on the discourses that surround and constitute it and the concept it denotes (Brookes and McEnery 2020). As with keywords, the volume and type of collocates identified by the analytical software will depend on user-determined parameters, including span (words to the left and right of the search word within which candidate collocates will be considered), minimum frequency threshold, and choice of statistic and cut-off. Collocation is used in Chapters 2, 3, 4 and 8, mainly to provide an impression of a word's discourse prosody, at which points we focus mainly on those words' most frequent (lexical) collocates. Collocation analysis is utilised more systematically in Chapter 5, where we use it to identify adjectival collocates of words referring to people with obesity, in Chapter 6 to explore the discourse around the words *healthy*, *body*, *diet* and *exercise*, and then in Chapter 7 to analyse the discourse around gender-marked nouns and pronouns. In Chapter 5, collocates are ranked by frequency, with adjectival collocates then extracted for closer analysis. However, in Chapters 6 and 7 we rank collocates using the cubed version of the Mutual Information statistic (MI^3). Mutual Information (MI) measures collocation strength by comparing the observed frequency of each collocational pairing against what would be 'expected' based on the relative frequency of each word and the overall size of the corpus. The difference between the observed and expected frequencies of co-occurrence is then converted into a score, with higher scores assigned to stronger collocations (Gablasova et al. 2017). While traditional MI assigns higher scores to exclusive and unusual word combinations involving low-frequency items (Evert 2008), MI^3 assigns higher scores to collocates which have a higher frequency of co-occurrence and so tend to be 'more established in the discourse' (Brezina et al. 2015: 160), arguably making it better suited to corpus-aided discourse studies such as ours.

While collocation can help us to better apprehend words' patterns of use in the news articles in our corpus, to interpret the discourses that such words and collocational patterns signal, and to understand how these discourses contribute to representations of obesity in these contexts, we have to analyse them within their wider textual surroundings using the final technique we introduce here – concordance analysis. Concordancing is essentially a way of viewing corpus data that allows the analyst to study every occurrence of a user-determined word or phrase in the corpus within its wider contexts of use. As an illustrative example, Figure 1.1 shows a concordance output for some of the occurrences of the word *obesity* in our corpus, obtained using *CQPweb*.

With the search-word running down the centre of the screen and a few words of context displayed to the left and right, the concordance output provides a way for the analyst to examine patterns of use that might be less obvious during linear, left-to-right readings of the texts in the corpus. The rows of text – or 'concordance lines' – can also be sorted randomly or, to help the analyst to spot patterns, alphabetically according to the words to the left or right of the search-word. Yet even the concordance output offers a relatively

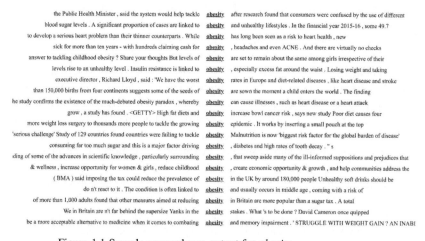

Figure 1.1 Sample concordance output for *obesity*

narrow view of the contexts in which words or phrases occur. To fully apprehend the discourses that are signalled by a particular word or phrase, it was therefore necessary to analyse expanded samples of articles and sometimes articles in their entirety. The concordance technique therefore affords a way of adopting a more qualitative perspective on the texts in a corpus, and was used in the interpretation of words and larger linguistic patterns across all the forthcoming analytical chapters. Given the size of our data, many of the words and patterns we analyse occur many thousands of times. For example, the word *obesity* occurred 64,673 times. In such cases, it was not practical for us to examine every single occurrence across our corpus. Therefore, we resolved to closely analyse a random sample. For this purpose, we experimented with different sample sizes and found that 100 cases proved sufficient for uncovering a range of different uses, including in most cases clearly indicating majority and minority patterns, while on a practical level being small enough to keep our analysis manageable.

Although, as noted, these techniques are used in various ways depending on the research questions and foci addressed in each chapter, all were utilised in a cyclical approach that first involved engaging with the corpus or a subset of it using frequency or keywords to identify themes or texts containing words or phrases of interest, before using collocation analysis to develop an understanding of frequent patterns of use, and then finally examining concordance lines and entire texts in order to interpret the attested patterns in terms of the obesity discourses they constitute. It is at this final stage that our analysis is most critical, as we interpret the identified discourses in terms of their power to represent obesity and people with it and we also explain their use and possible effects in relation to the contexts in which they have been produced and consumed. Crucial to this approach, then, is the combination of computational and statistical measures with human-led, context- and theory-sensitive readings of the data. The latter not only allowed us to adopt a critical perspective on the texts in our corpus but was also enriched by our knowledge and contact, as researchers, with the journalistic practices and social and healthcare contexts of which these media texts and the discourses they contain are constitutive and by which they are themselves constituted.

The benefits, but also challenges, of integrating corpus linguistics with (critical) discourse studies are by now well documented (Baker 2006; Baker et al. 2008). Therefore, we will not rehearse all of these arguments here but instead outline some of the main strengths and limitations of this methodological synergy, focussing on those that are most relevant to our study. One of the main appeals of combining corpus linguistics with CDS is that the greater size and representativeness of corpora, relative to the often small datasets analysed in CDS, can make critical analyses more comprehensive, allowing analysts to base their insights on larger and more representative patterns of language use. Relatedly, by allowing analysts to hone their focus on the most frequent or statistically salient linguistic features in the texts under study, corpus techniques can help critical analysts to guard against the charge that the texts or features they address in their analysis are 'cherry-picked' by the human researcher because they support a preconceived argument or position (Widdowson 2004). This increased objectivity is also supported by corpus linguistics' commitment to methodological transparency, which is under-pinned by two guiding principles: (i) no systematic bias in the selection of texts included in the corpus (i.e. do not exclude a text because it does not fit a pre-existing argument or theory) and (ii) total accountability (all data gathered must be accounted for) (McEnery and Hardie 2012). Indeed, frequency and statistical salience offer more objective analytical routes into corpus data. However, the corpus approach is not completely objective, as the human analyst must select which techniques to use, decide on their parameters (discussed in this section) and then interpret the output, typically with recourse to more subjective, human-led analysis of samples of the data. Introducing the corpus linguistic perspective into CDS can also bear analytical benefit, as the option to analyse a large collection of texts, especially which span a long period of time, can help the analyst to better interpret the relative statuses of discourses (i.e. as dominant or marginalised). It can also account for dis-courses' incremental effects; that is, some discourses can appear to be used marginally or sparingly in one or two texts but appear more established or dominant when used across a large number of texts and/or over a long period of time.

Of course, many of these analytical benefits apply not only to the use of corpus linguistic methods in CDS but are also relevant to other areas of linguistics and discourse analysis. Indeed, the volume of linguistic research which draws on corpus linguistic methods is now vast and continues to grow apace. One area of application that is relevant to this book is the rapidly expanding field of corpus-based health communication research (Crawford et al. 2014; Brookes et al. 2021). In addition to the benefits described previ-ously in this section, it has been argued that corpus linguistic methods can be particularly appealing to researchers working within the domain of health (care), as they can help analyses to come closer to the 'gold standard' of evidence-based approaches that are underpinned by statistical patterns rather than purely qualitative observations based on small-scale data alone (Crawford et al. 2014). Indeed, as part of the project on which this book is based, we have worked with a range of external stakeholders, including obesity charities, who have been particularly impressed by the capacity of corpora to represent media language data on a vast scale, as well as by the range of insights that such a dataset (and the methods used to analyse it) can provide. Yet corpus linguistic methods can also be particularly useful for studying the discourses around *contested* health issues (Hunt and Brookes 2020), such as obesity. This is because the option of building and analysing a corpus containing a large number of texts from a large number of authors (in our case, all of the obesity-related articles published by all of the United Kingdom's national newspapers over a ten-year period) can better represent the wide range of varied and even conflicting discourses that typically attend to such contested health phenomena (*ibid.*). With the aid of a corpus, these discourses can not only be accounted for more comprehensively by the analyst but can also be studied in terms of how they relate to and compete with each other to become the dominant way of explaining and communicating about the health issue in question (Brookes 2018). In our case, then, the option of examining a corpus of newspaper articles about obesity will help us to produce an analysis that covers a wider range of competing discourses around obesity and that is arguably more sensitive to how these discourses might be positioned in relation to one another, for example as dominant or minority, in this context.

Having focussed on some of the ways in which corpus linguistics methods can enhance (critical) studies of discourse, it also worth acknowledging some of the limitations of the corpus approach. One long-standing criticism of corpora pertains to their limited capacity to represent context. As Widdowson (2000: 7) argues, '[t]he texts which are collected in a corpus have only a reflected reality', for '[r]eality [. . .] does not travel with the text'. In the case of the articles in our corpus, the texts are, of course, divorced from the contexts in which they were originally produced and consumed, so any arguments or conclusions relating to why a particular discourse was drawn on in a text and how it was received by readers are necessarily hypothetical (though in Chapter 9 we come closer to the latter as we analyse readers' online comments). To an extent, this is true of most studies of discourse. Yet, of particular relevance to corpus studies is the at-present limited capacity of corpora to represent the non-linguistic (i.e. visual) aspects of written texts. The corpus introduced in this section represents only the linguistic parts of the obesity articles sampled. As such, our analysis does not account for the possible use of imagery nor the amount of page space a particular story took up, or whether it appeared on the front page or was buried half-way into the newspaper, where it would be likely to get much less attention. In recent years, researchers have begun to experiment with ways in which such visual elements could be feasibly represented in a corpus and then incorporated into a corpus linguistic analysis. However, no approach seems as yet to be suited to representing the images in a corpus the size of ours. For now, we accept that our analysis is confined to the linguistic but note that the analysis of corpora of media texts stands to benefit from the further development of multimodal corpora and techniques of analysis in the future.

Following this introductory chapter, our analysis begins with large-scale examinations of keywords that were obtained by dividing the corpus into four sections representing a cross-section of newspapers' formats and political leanings (i.e. broadsheet left, broadsheet right, tabloid left, tabloid right). Chapter 2 considers keywords that are shared across all four sections, thus focussing on aspects of language that are found reasonably consistently across the whole corpus, whereas Chapter 3 takes each of the four sections separately, considering the keywords that arise when they are compared against each other, thus focussing on words and discourses that are particularly characteristic of each. These two chapters therefore function as companions to one another, taking into account both similarity and difference. Then, Chapter 4 examines change over time, in terms of tracing how different keywords change year by year, as well as looking at differences between months. Chapters 5 to 8 each focus on salient aspects of the corpus which were identified in the earlier chapters, as well as in previous research on obesity representation on other datasets. Chapter 5 considers shaming representations and Chapter 6 looks at the discourse around four frequent words: *healthy*, *body*, *diet* and *exercise*. These chapters both approach the discourse of personal responsibility from different angles, then, while Chapters 7 and 8 are also related to one another, with each one focussing on how a particular aspect of social identity is represented within press discourse on obesity. Chapter 7 takes gender into account, focussing on representations of obesity in relation to men and women, whereas Chapter 8 looks at social class, enabling us to indirectly examine the extent of discourse which relates to political and social framings around obesity. As mentioned earlier, Chapter 9 analyses readers' comments to a set of online articles from the *Mail*, while in Chapter 10 we reflect on our findings across the book and consider where and how obesity coverage could be improved in the future. But let us now turn to the next chapter, which considers the language which is consistently common across the entire corpus, thus giving us a broad overview of what is most typical in UK press reporting on obesity.

2   The Way In
Shared Keywords in the Press

Introduction

In this first analytical chapter, we begin our examination of our corpus of obesity news articles by using the keywords technique to obtain an overview of the most characteristic language across the data, linking this to salient discourses and themes in the overall representation of obesity. As a reminder, keywords, as defined in corpus linguistics research, are those words that are especially frequent in one corpus compared against another corpus (known as the reference corpus). In this chapter, rather than generate keywords for the entire corpus, we focus on words that emerge as key across all sections of the press, spanning format and political leaning, thereby ensuring that our analysis accounts for words and patterns that are truly characteristic across all types of newspaper coverage. We refer to these as *shared keywords*. The shared keywords obtained from our corpus provide a 'way in' to our data and are unpacked in terms of their associated obesity discourses to an extent in this chapter but also in future chapters. Before presenting our analysis, we begin by providing a more detailed account of how we structured our data to help widen the representativeness of our keywords. This methodological discussion and the resultant decisions taken are relevant not only to this chapter but also the following chapter, in which we retain this data structure for the purposes of exploring differences in the obesity discourses drawn on by newspapers of differing formats and political persuasions.

The shared keywords approach

One way we could have approached the objectives of this chapter (described in the previous section) would have been to generate keywords by comparing our corpus in its entirety against a suitable general reference corpus. However, because our corpus is not evenly balanced in terms of the different newspapers and sections of the press that it contains (for example, one of the newspapers in our corpus, the *Mail*, comprises a third of it), keywords obtained from the corpus as a whole would risk over-representing what is characteristic of those sections of the press that constitute a greater proportion of the corpus. Therefore, such an approach would likely reveal less about what is characteristic of obesity coverage in sections of the press that make up a comparatively smaller section of the data. For this reason, we instead decided to adopt a more refined approach, dividing our corpus into a series of subsets (or 'sub-corpora') representing different sections of the press, before focussing on those words that were key across all of these sections (when compared against the same reference corpus), and so were characteristic of all types of newspapers.

There are a great number of examples of corpus studies of print media which have divided their data according to newspapers' political leaning or publication type. Such studies have tended to utilise keywords for contrastive purposes – to search for differences, rather than similarities, between the different sections of their corpora. For example, in an analysis of press representations of Islam, Baker (2010a) obtained keywords by comparing articles from tabloids against broadsheets, and vice versa. While studies such as this have quite logically tended to organise their corpora by publication format *or* political leaning, if we divide up our corpus of obesity newspaper articles in either of these ways, we again run into potential problems surrounding the representativeness of our keywords, with certain types of publication being over-represented and others being under-represented. For example, a sub-corpus containing all articles from the tabloids would consist almost entirely of words from right-leaning publications (88 per cent), with the keywords from such a sub-corpus thus likely to offer a strong representation of characteristic language in right-leaning tabloids at the expense of left-leaning tabloids. The same issue emerges if we group our data according to political leaning, too. For example, a sub-corpus containing all articles from right-leaning newspapers would be made up mainly of words from tabloids (66 per cent).

To overcome these issues and produce an analysis that was sensitive both to newspapers' publication formats *and* political leanings, we decided to group newspapers according to both these variables. This resulted in four sub-corpora: left-leaning broadsheets (Broadsheet Left), right-leaning broadsheets (Broadsheet Right), left-leaning tabloids (Tabloid Left) and right-leaning tabloids (Tabloid Right). The newspapers assigned to each of these sub-corpora, along with their number of texts and words, are shown in Table 2.1.

Having organised our data in this way, we then wanted to identify similarities between the characteristic language of each of these sub-corpora, as these similarities could point to general themes and discourses in the representation of obesity across the press as a whole. Although corpus linguistics approaches to (critical) discourse studies have traditionally been considered inherently contrastive in nature (Partington 2009), in recent years increasing attention has been paid to the ways in which corpus techniques can also be used to study similarity (C. Taylor 2013). For this analysis, we identified similarities

Table 2.1. *Breakdown of sub-corpora by format and political leaning*

Broadsheet Left				Broadsheet Right		
Newspaper	Texts	Words		Newspaper	Texts	Words
Guardian	5,008	5,238,062		*Telegraph*	5,680	4,804,351
Independent	4,336	3,303,269		*Times*	3,948	3,831,868
Total	**9,344**	**8,541,331**		**Total**	**9,628**	**8,636,219**

Tabloid Left				Tabloid Right		
Newspaper	Texts	Words		Newspaper	Texts	Words
Mirror	3,398	2,202,323		*Express*	5,193	3,265,741
Morning Star	152	63,641		*Mail*	12,805	11,890,340
Total	**3,550**	**2,265,964**		*Star*	1,072	370,818
				Sun	2,286	1,082,808
				Total	**21,356**	**16,609,707**

between these sub-corpora in terms of what we are referring to as *shared keywords*. This involved subjecting each sub-corpus to an independent keyword analysis; comparing each one against the written component of the British National Corpus (BNC); and then focussing on those words that were key across all four datasets and so could be considered characteristic of all sections of the press. The BNC is a 100 million-word corpus of contemporary general British English usage during the 1990s. The corpus can be divided into two parts. The written component, which is 90 million words in size, consists of language from newspapers, research journals, periodicals and books. The spoken component, which makes up the remaining 10 million words, consists of transcriptions of spontaneous conversation and context-governed speech, for example in lectures. For this analysis, we obtained keywords by comparing each of our four sub-corpora displayed in Table 2.1 against the *written* section of the BNC.[1] This choice of reference corpus helped to ensure that our keywords would represent words that were characteristic of the obesity newspaper articles compared against more general written British English and thus help to control for the differences between written and spoken language overly

[1] Researchers at Lancaster University are developing an updated version of the BNC. However, at the time of writing, the written section of this updated corpus was not available. Therefore, we decided to use the older version of the BNC, accepting that while it represents modern written English, at around thirty years old, the texts in our reference corpus do not fully represent contemporary written British English.

influencing the keywords produced (Biber and Conrad 2009). In the section that follows, we present the results of this procedure and begin our analysis of the shared keywords it produced.

Analysis: Shared keywords

Having generated keywords for each sub-corpus, we ranked each list by log-likelihood score and extracted the top fifty keywords from each.[2] This was an arbitrary cut-off, chosen because it gave us a manageable number of keywords for qualitative analysis. We then compared the four lists of fifty keywords side-by-side, removing all keywords that did not occur across all four lists. This left us with a total of twenty-seven shared keywords, which are displayed, along with their normalised frequencies in each sub-corpus, in Table 2.2.

Having obtained these shared keywords, we then qualitatively analysed how each contributed to the representation of obesity across random samples of 100 articles taken from each sub-corpus (i.e. 400 articles per keyword). During this phase, we identified a wide range of representations. As such, many of these keywords and their attendant discourses are explicated more fully in forthcoming chapters. For now, we focus just on the most frequent patterns surrounding them, as well as minority counter-examples where we have found these, with the aim of giving an impression of how each keyword tended to contribute to representations of obesity in the corpus. We should also note that although these keywords were statistically salient across all four sub-corpora, this does not necessarily equate to similarity in the ways that they were used in these different sections. As such, while our focus in this chapter is mainly on similarity, we also note major differences in the discourses surrounding these terms where these occur.

Medical keywords

The first point we want to note about Table 2.2 is that several of the shared keywords provide evidence of the press's tendency to employ medical terminology and, by extension, medical concepts and frameworks, in its coverage of obesity. This includes keywords that constitute medical labels for and relating to obesity, such as *obese*, *obesity* and *overweight*, but also terms such as *BMI*, *disease* and the names of specific diseases (i.e. *cancer*, *diabetes* and *heart* [*disease*]). The emergence of *obese* and *obesity* as shared keywords is not particularly surprising, given that both correspond to the search-words used to

---

[2] *CQPWeb* counts punctuation marks as tokens, meaning that they can also be flagged as keywords by the computer. However, because they were not particularly useful for this part of our analysis, we excluded these items from the keyword lists examined in this chapter.

Table 2.2. *Shared keywords with normalised frequencies in each sub-corpus*

	Normalised frequencies (per million words)			
Keyword	**Broadsheet Left**	**Broadsheet Right**	**Tabloid Left**	**Tabloid Right**
BMI	128.08	170.21	247.58	268.88
calories	285.08	347.03	552.08	643.60
cancer	636.08	592.27	1,030.47	1,084.85
children	1,602.68	1,703.75	1,631.54	1,628.32
diabetes	646.50	633.49	1,035.32	1,249.57
diet	598.62	772.10	1,349.98	1,373.71
disease	646.50	595.17	798.34	1,067.99
drinks	551.32	377.60	605.48	517.95
eat	492.66	665.22	986.78	894.72
eating	549.45	665.80	1,115.64	1,036.56
exercise	587.96	525.23	641.67	740.77
fat	379.80	1,078.94	1,599.32	1,543.68
food	797.77	1,463.60	1,880.88	1,746.09
foods	1,979.20	345.17	500.89	552.39
health	358.84	1,853.36	2,071.52	2,145.19
healthy	2,495.04	585.21	1,049.44	946.07
heart	556.24	623.42	951.91	1,104.53
lifestyle	502.26	206.69	313.77	327.46
NHS	181.94	656.77	860.12	704.89
obese	845.42	871.21	1,499.14	1,291.96
obesity	749.30	1,601.40	1,906.47	1,900.58
overweight	1,750.90	554.29	852.18	862.87
people	486.34	2,459.87	2,646.56	2,751.04
risk	2,922.61	741.88	1,194.64	1,500.69
says	1,320.17	1,338.55	1,416.62	1,283.65
sugar	971.75	911.28	1,272.75	1,156.55
weight	884.17	1,158.26	3,106.40	2,694.75

sample articles for the corpus. However, the same cannot be said for *over-weight*. Though the emergence of *overweight* as key is not too surprising, its statistical salience across all sections of the press nevertheless provides evidence of the newspapers adopting medical terminology and concepts in their descriptions of people with larger bodies. At the semantic level, the term *overweight* derives its meaning from the shared understanding that there is a weight norm or standard that can be exceeded (i.e. that people can be 'over' and, conversely, 'under'). This standard is determined by the *BMI*, another shared keyword. As a reminder, in Chapter 1 we introduced the BMI as a medical framework used by practitioners, epidemiologists, public health officials and others to ascertain whether or not a person is of a 'normal' or 'healthy' weight for their height. The influence of this medical scale is evidenced not only in the adoption of terminology such as *overweight* but is most explicit in cases where the adjective shared keyword *obese* is directly preceded, and thus pre-modified, by the adverbs *morbidly* (2,448 occurrences) and *clinically* (874). Similarly, the adjective *morbid* directly precedes the keyword *obesity* 288 times. While *clinically* might imply that the person or people being represented have received a clinical diagnosis of obesity, *morbidly* is unquestionably lifted straight from the terminology developed as part of the BMI metric. In the samples we analysed for each of these words, we found that they were used in a wide variety of ways but mostly when reporting on obesity's prevalence, causes and possible health implications.

The press's reliance on medical categories, and BMI categories specifically, also manifested in more explicit ways, namely through uses of the shared keyword *BMI* itself. Like the medical labels mentioned previously, *BMI* could be used in the citation of obesity-related statistics, including about prevalence but also in relation to increased susceptibility to certain diseases and health complications associated with obesity. In such instances, providing *BMI* scores allowed the press to reproduce quantified conceptions of the body, as well as of the risks associated with certain body types. This extract from the *Mail*, for example, contains four separate mentions of *BMI*, as well as mentions of two other shared keywords, *risk* and *heart*, which we explore in more depth later.

> Compared with men who had a **BMI** of between 18.5 and 20 as 18-year-olds, those with a **BMI** of 20 to 22.5 had a 22 per cent increased risk of heart failure. For those with a **BMI** between 22.5 and 25 the risk doubled, while it more than tripled for men with a **BMI** of 25 to 27.5.
>
> (*Mail*, 17 June 2016)

The keyword *BMI* was also used to define *obesity* and explain the differences between categories such as *obese* and *overweight*, as well as underweight (although this was not a keyword) and to establish what could be considered a normal or 'healthy' body size,

> **BMI** is the measure of a person's weight in kilograms divided by the square of height in metres. A healthy adult **BMI** range is estimated to be 18.5 to 24.9. Above this is considered overweight, and above 30 obese.
>
> (*Telegraph*, 2 October 2015)

> Your **BMI** reading is split into a range of categories: **BMI** under 18.5 – Underweight **BMI** 18.5 to 25 – Healthy range **BMI** 25 to 30 – Overweight **BMI** 30 or over – Obese There are plenty of arguments against **BMI** as a good measure (it doesn't work so well if you're very tall, or carry a lot of muscle) but it can be a reasonable starting point for setting a target weight.
>
> (*Times*, 6 January 2015)

The second example, from *the Times*, notably acknowledges one of the criticisms of the BMI we considered in the first chapter when it points out, in brackets, that '(it doesn't work so well if you're very tall, or carry a lot of muscle)'. Although this counter-perspective is undercut somewhat by the conclusion that the BMI nevertheless provides a 'reasonable starting point for setting a target weight', this extract does at least give space to a more critical take on this metric. We found evidence of these kinds of critical perspectives on the BMI in other articles spanning all four sub-corpora. However, this was a minority discourse, and tended to occur more in the broadsheets than the tabloids. To give an impression of the scale of this trend, across four samples of 100 articles mentioning *BMI* (one from each sub-corpus), its utility was explicitly challenged in 14 per cent of left-leaning broadsheet articles and 17 per cent of the articles from the right-leaning broadsheets, and just 3 per cent of the sample of left-leaning tabloids and 4 per cent of the articles from the right-leaning tabloids. In the tabloid samples, we found that this counter-discourse could also manifest in articles which gave examples of slim and muscular celebrities who would be categorised as *overweight* or *obese* on the basis of their *BMI*, as if to highlight what the newspapers appeared to perceive as the incredulity of the metric. These articles consistently featured images of the celebrity in question, depicted, for example, in swimwear to display their bulging muscles and slim waistlines, providing a visual contrast between such images and the verbal descriptions of them as *obese* in the articles.

> 'If you look at my **BMI**, I'm OBESE!' Bachelor star Tim Robards opens up about his physique . . . and reveals how his 7:2:1 diet rule could be the key to your best body yet. Ex-Bachelor star, Tim Robards, speaks to FEMAIL about his fitness Tim says you need to focus less on the numbers and more on how you feel.
>
> (*Mail*, 26 October 2016)

So, this counter-discourse is present across the data, but it is a minority discourse and is more likely to be found in the broadsheets than the tabloids. In the main, *BMI* is used in a relatively uncritical way.

Taken together, we might be tempted to interpret the medical terminology keywords as indicating medicalising discourses around obesity. In Chapter 1, we introduced medicalisation as the sociocultural process by which some human experiences come to be regarded as 'normal' and others as 'abnormal', 'deviant' and requiring medical intervention (Zola 1972; Conrad and Schneider 1980; Conrad 2007). In that chapter, we also considered how Western medical institutions, along with global health authorities such as the World Health Organisation, have contributed to the increasing medicalisation of high body weight (as obesity). According to Conrad (2007: 211), medicalisation is realised through a range of activities which include 'defining a problem in medical terms, using medical language to describe a problem, adopting a medical framework to understand a problem, or using a medical intervention to "treat" it'. The keywords we've looked at so far certainly provide evidence of the adoption of medical language (e.g. *obese, obesity, overweight*), while in the majority of cases the BMI framework, lexicalised through the shared keyword *BMI*, affords the press with the discursive means with which to not only explain obesity and what it is, but also to categorise and quantify (readers') bodies and the health risks that are associated with certain (larger) body types. When drawn on in this uncritical sense, the use of *BMI* not only rests on medical conceptions of the body and weight but, crucially, it helps to legitimate this perspective. Legitimation is defined by van Leeuwen (2008: 20) as the 'reasons that either the whole of a social practice or some part of it must take place, or must take place in the way that it does', he elaborates, '[t]exts not only represent social practices, they also explain and legitimate (or delegitimate, critique) them' (see also: van Leeuwen and Wodak 1999; van Leeuwen 2007). Grounded, as it is, in numbers and statistics, the BMI metric provides exactly the type of 'scientific instrument', as Lupton (2018: 28) puts it, required to legitimate the medicalising perspective which seeks to patholo-gise obesity and to present it as a medical problem.

Another way in which the press construed obesity as a medical problem was by discursively linking it to other, more established and less contested dis-eases, such as *cancer, diabetes, heart disease, liver disease* and *kidney disease*, among others. The relationship between obesity and these diseases could be one of causation – with obesity described as heightening susceptibility to them (this was the case mostly for *diabetes* and *heart disease*).

> The Health Select Committee member also suggested the Government's failure to tackle the child obesity crisis could lead to more kids getting **cancer** and **heart disease** later in life. She said: "Adults who are obese are at increased risk of **diabetes**, **heart disease** and **cancer**."
>
> (*Mirror*, 3 October 2016)

> Without action, almost nine in 10 adults and two-thirds of children will be overweight or obese by 2050 and at risk of **diabetes**, **cancer**, **heart disease** and other health problems
>
> (*Guardian*, 24 January 2008)

The second most frequent pattern in articles mentioning diseases was the discursive grouping of obesity with other diseases, not as a cause but as an equivalent. Such passages often took the form of lists, with obesity cited alongside the aforementioned diseases in particular in the context of articles reporting on the social and economic implications of certain forms of ill-health.

The organisation urges local authorities to crack down on vehicle use, by such means as charging and traffic calming. The guidance was commissioned by the Department of Health, motivated by the **obesity**, **cancers** and **heart disease** that can accompany the sedentary lifestyle.

(*Guardian*, 23 January 2008)

It is vital that coordinated policies are implemented to tackle the shared risk factors and complications of chronic diseases such as **obesity** and **diabetes**.

(*Mail*, 29 November 2017)

In their study of management documents produced by Swedish universities, Ledin and Machin (2015) explore the power of lists to recontexualise otherwise disparate elements so that they appear to be connected or equivalents of one another. As they put it, '[i]n a list, the elements are represented as being of the same order where items or components on the list are "equal" and belong to a common paradigm' (469).

Earlier in this section, we noted that we might be 'tempted' to interpret the prevalence of medical terminology among our shared keywords as signalling the presence of medicalising discourses. However, and as our use of 'tempted' implies, the picture is a little more complex than that. As well as referring to diseases *other than* obesity, we were interested in the capacity for the keyword *disease* to refer to obesity itself. Analysis of this keyword was not productive to this end, as it tended to yield references to other diseases – namely those aforementioned. When we consider the fifty most frequent L1 collocates of *disease* – that is, words occurring directly before it – we find a plethora of words which denote diseases *other than* obesity. The top collocate is *heart* (12,034), but others included *cardiovascular* (1,953), *liver* (1,855), *kidney* (413), *chronic* (318), *coeliac* (262), *artery* (177), *lung* (144), *bowel* (129), *respiratory* (95), *vascular* (88), *pulmonary* (76), *autoimmune* (57), *coronary* (55), *lyme* (49), *neurone* (39), *arteria* (37) and *cardiac* (33). The frequency with which these terms alone collocate with *disease* totals 17,814 (58.45 per cent of the uses of *disease*), with the bigram *heart disease* constituting the vast majority of these occurrences. This means that the majority (at least 58.45 per cent) of uses of *disease* in our corpus refer to health problems *other than* obesity. Indeed, the word *disease* was very rarely used in reference to obesity itself. Analysis of 100 random uses of *disease* in each section of the corpus shows that it denotes obesity in just 2 per cent of cases in the left-leaning broadsheets, 3 per cent of the right-leaning broadsheets, 1 per cent of the left-leaning tabloids, and 2 per cent of the right-leaning tabloids. Therefore, all sections of the press are unlikely to label obesity explicitly as a *disease*.

In an attempt to isolate that minority of cases in which *disease* was used to refer to obesity specifically, we narrowed our focus further and searched for cases where the noun *disease* was directly preceded by the definite and indefinite articles, respectively *the* and *a*, as this filtered out the types of bigrams noted previously. The bigram *the disease* occurs 4,182 times, while *a disease* occurs just 583 times. Taken together, these bigrams account for just 16.2 per cent of uses of *disease* (much lower than the combined 58.45 per cent of cases referring to other illnesses noted previously). Yet, in reality, the difference is even starker, as analysis of the more frequent of these two bigrams, *the disease*, showed that this barely ever referred to obesity. We examined 100 random cases of *the disease* in each sub-corpus and found that it referred to obesity just once in the left-leaning tabloids and not at all in the other sections of the press. Therefore, the less frequent pairing, *a disease*, was more productive for analysing cases where obesity was referred to as a disease.

The bigram *a disease* occurred 142 times in the left-leaning broadsheets (16.63 times per million words (PMW)), 119 times in the right-leaning broadsheets (13.78 PMW), 35 times in the left-leaning tabloids (15.45 PMW) and, finally, 287 times in the right-leaning tabloids (17.28 PMW). So, in relative terms, *a disease* occurs with comparable frequency across the different subcorpora. When preceded by the indefinite article, *a*, the noun *disease* was more semantically flexible and could be used in statements that obesity is or is not 'a disease' in the way that 'the disease' couldn't. This bigram also has the option of featuring in hypothetical and conditional statements, such as 'if obesity is a disease', rendering it more amenable to debate. Indeed, the bigram 'a disease' was used to discuss obesity but also featured in debates around the medical status of other contested health conditions, including addiction, ADHD and eating disorders, as well as ageing. In the left-leaning broadsheets, 22 out of 100 uses of *a disease* referred to obesity, of which the majority (sixteen cases) occurred in passages arguing that obesity is a disease. As this example shows, these consistently featured in quotes attributed to scientists and celebrities.

> "Obesity is **a disease**, not a choice made by parents or their children," said Dr Nikhil Dhurandhar, president of the Maryland-based Obesity Society. "Many known and unknown biological factors, in addition to personal nutrition and physical activity decisions, may interfere with weight loss, reinforcing the fact that we can't treat obesity solely by placing the blame on parents or individuals."
>
> (*Guardian*, 8 March 2015)

The remaining cases feature in passages which explicitly address the status of obesity as 'a disease'. In other words, most of the uses of *a disease* in this section argue that obesity is a disease, while a minority are concerned with the debate about obesity's disease status, but none explicitly argue that obesity is *not* a disease.

The picture is more complex in the left-leaning tabloids, though. All mentions of *a disease* in this section occur in the *Mirror*, of which ten refer to obesity. Of these, four uses argue that obesity is a disease. However, three of these are found in one article, again quoting a scientist

> Dr Harry Rutter, from London School of Hygiene and Tropical Medicine, added at a briefing: "Obesity starts in a country as **a disease** of the rich. Then it becomes **a disease** across all of society It then becomes **a disease** of the poor."
>
> *(Mirror*, 10 October 2017)

More commonly, the bigram *a disease* featured in the *Mirror* in passages arguing that obesity is *not* a disease. This accounted for the remaining six uses in this part of the corpus. Again, and as this example shows, scientists and scientific research could also be used to legitimate the argument that obesity is *not* a disease, as were celebrities (there was another example, for instance, in which actor and comedian Ricky Gervais is quoted as stating that obesity is not a disease).

> Finally, a sensible study that says if you tell fat people obesity is **a disease** they'll believe they have no control over it – and just keep eating. But the truth is most fat people already know obesity isn't **a disease**. However, they choose to believe it is because then they don't have to take responsibility for a self-induced and totally avoidable condition that comes from stuffing your face with too many chips and doughnuts.
>
> *(Mirror*, 1 February 2014)

As this extract shows, consistent across such articles is the construction of obesity as something that is a matter of personal responsibility. Such arguments rely on – and in some cases reproduce – an opposition between obesity being a disease on the one hand and something that is preventable (and, by extension, over which people have control) on the other. Yet we should acknowledge at this point that something being a disease and being preventable are not mutually exclusive qualities; for example, some forms of cancer are widely regarded as preventable but are not considered not to be diseases because of this. Moving onto the right-leaning press, and the broadsheets first, and 13 out of 100 uses of *a disease* in this section of the corpus refer to obesity. The proportions of those uses construing obesity as being or not being a disease are fairly evenly split, with seven uses construing it as not a disease and the remaining six uses construing it as a disease, as in these examples.

> If you haven't yet read Max Pemberton's Spectator cover story Obesity Is Not **A Disease** I urge you to do so. It describes a social problem of

> quite grotesque, wobble-jowled saggy-bottomed enormousness: the vast sums of money – 5 billion a year – being funnelled from our pockets in order to pay for the extra healthcare costs of the clinically obese.
>
> *(Telegraph,* 20 October 2013)

> Prof Pinki Sahota, deputy chairman of the Association for the Study of Obesity, said the study "confirms much greater effort is needed to educate people about the fact obesity is **a disease**".
>
> *(Telegraph,* 14 May 2015)

Moving onto the tabloids, and a similarly split picture emerges; 24 per cent of uses of *a disease* in this section refer to obesity. Like the left-leaning tabloids, this section of the press was split, with 58 per cent construing obesity as not a disease (see extract) and the remaining 42 per cent construing it as something that is.

> The more you tell fat people that their bulging guts are the consequence of an "illness", the less likely they are to do anything about it. Tell the fatties that obesity is **a disease** and they suddenly become less interested in trying out that novel idea – "a diet".
>
> *(Sun,* 30 January 2014)

So, the use of *a disease* across the different sections of the press shows a complex and contradictory set of discourses that reflect the nature of societal debates about obesity's disease status. While in the left-leaning broadsheets it tends to signal a discourse which presents obesity as something that *is* a disease, the picture is more complex across all other sections of the press, with both arguments being presented but those that hold obesity as *not* a disease being slightly more frequent. We will return to this feature of the data in the concluding section of this chapter.

Risk and responsibilisation

The next shared keyword we want to consider is *risk*. As well as being a computational keyword, *risk* can be considered a cultural keyword, in the sense originally described by Raymond Williams (1976). In 1992, sociologist Ulrich Beck argued that we were now living in a 'risk society' (Beck 1992). This view is shared by Mythen and Walklate (2006: 1), who describe the pervasiveness of risk in contemporary society when they write, 'in contemporary culture, risk is a ubiquitous issue that stretches over a range of social activities, practices and experiences. In Britain, current debates about welfare, crime, national security, food safety, employment and sexuality are all underscored by risk.' Giddens and Pierson (1998: 209) argue that as societies become more advanced, they become better at assessing our capacity for risk (for example, through measurements such as the BMI), while modernisation itself results in human societies creating new risks (such as junk food) and regulations around them (e.g. a 'sugar tax'). The notion of risk is important to our understandings of health and illness, with researchers noting how 'news and lifestyle media reports of risk, as well as citizen activist literature and social marketing campaigns, represent it as something to be avoided in the interests of preserving good health and well-being' (Lupton 2013: 15). Although risk is widely researched within the social sciences, it remains a rather ill-defined concept. Indeed, Mythen and Walklate (2006: 1) rightly describe risk as 'opaque and disputed'. Linguistic studies of the meaning of *risk* have noted the propensity for this term to be used in different ways depending on the topic and context of communication (Hamilton et al. 2007). However, Petruck (1997) characterises the semantic frame of RISK in terms of two sub-frames: CHANCE (which tends to have positive valence) and HARM (which tends to have negative valence). Across all four of our sub-corpora, *risk* was used overwhelmingly in the latter sense identified by Petruck (1997); that is, to connote harm.

Across each of the sections of our corpus, *risk* was used in two related ways which map onto a 'chain' of risk, wherein the articles could refer to risk either in terms of (i) the risk of developing obesity or (ii) obesity heightening risk of other health problems. Although both of these senses could be found across all four sections of the corpus, we noted a preference for one or the other depending on the newspapers' formats and political leanings, with a particularly notable distinction between tabloids and broadsheets. Specifically, in broadsheets *risk* tended to be presented in terms of the risk factors associated with the development of obesity (73 per cent of cases in the left-leaning data and 67 per cent of cases in the right-leaning data).

> The children's commissioner, Al Aynsley-Green, called for "a firm commitment ... to introduce a 9pm watershed on junk food TV adverts to further limit young people's exposure to unhealthy foods". There will be attempts to identify families whose children are at **risk** of obesity. The government plans a 75m campaign aimed primarily at helping parents of babies and young children to improve their diet and exercise.
>
> (*Guardian*, 24 January 2008)

On the other hand, the tabloids tended to refer to *risk* in the sense of presenting obesity as a risk factor for the development of other health problems such as diabetes, heart disease, dementia and some types of cancer (56 per cent of cases in the left-leaning data and 59 per cent of cases in the right-leaning data).

Past studies have revealed a link between being obese or overweight and an increased **risk** of developing Alzheimer's.

(*Mail*, 1 September 2015)

While the broadsheets were therefore much more likely to focus on risk in terms of the risk factors that could be attributed to individuals' developing obesity, the tabloids were more likely to present obesity itself as a factor in individuals' developing other health problems. We also note that there is tentative evidence for differences according to newspapers' political leanings, with the left-leaning newspapers exhibiting a slightly higher preference for focus on risk factors in obesity development and the right-leaning newspapers being slightly more likely to focus on risks of other health problems associated with obesity. These differences are much smaller than those between broadsheets and tabloids, though. The differences in how the tabloids and broadsheets tend to conceptualise risk in relation to obesity could be explained by differences in style, whereby the former tend to present stories on health issues in ways that sensationalise their threat – in this case by constructing obesity as a cause of a range of (potentially fatal) diseases. For the broadsheets, their marginal tendency to refer to risks in terms of causes of obesity could be viewed as an outcome of their propensity to report on the wider social and political determinants of ill-health, as in the previous example from the *Guardian*, as well as what individuals themselves can do to reduce their risks (explored more in the next chapter). We have carried out a more comprehensive analysis of the discourses around *risk* in news coverage of obesity in Brookes and Baker (2021), where we have found that the use of *risk* has increased, in relative terms, over time.

Whatever the case, the rhetoric of risk can be linked to discourses of personal responsibility (Lupton 1995), for we can find evidence across all newspapers of individuals being more and less subtly implored to monitor and reduce their risk of obesity and then, in turn, the health problems that are purported to follow from it. Typically, these risk-reducing actions and behaviours orient to consumption practices and what people eat and drink, as indicated by shared keywords denoting food and drink (*calories, drinks, food, foods, sugar*) and verbs denoting consumption (*diet, eat, eating*). As well as focussing on *what* individuals consume (with a particular focus on high calorie and sugary food and drink), the use of these keywords in context also reveals a focus on *how* people eat and *when*. By way of demonstrating this, it is useful to take a closer look at another shared keyword, *diet*.

Inspecting the collocates of *diet* within a window of five words to the left and right (otherwise expressed as: −/+ 5), we find that it has a tendency to co-occur with words which perform an ostensibly evaluative or stance-marking function, contributing broadly to either a positive or negative evaluative or discourse prosody (Stubbs 2001). *Diet* tends to be evaluated negatively when it collocates with words such as 'poor' (1,084), 'high-fat' (598) and 'unhealthy' (375). In these cases, a poor or unhealthy *diet* – typically characterised by consumption of high calorie and sugary food and drink – is represented as causing obesity. Collocates indicating a more positive evaluation of *diet*, such as 'healthy' (2,375), 'balanced' (1,195) and 'strict' (488) – a collocate which taps into ideas of discipline and self-restraint – are framed as ways of overcoming obesity or of reducing one's risk of becoming obese.

> **Poor diet** leading cause of obesity, heart disease and various cancers
> *(Mail,* 22 June 2016)

> Eating plenty of fruit and vegetables as part of a **healthy diet** also helps you avoid obesity, which has knock-on protection against heart attacks, strokes, diabetes and cancer.
> *(Guardian,* 1 January 2008)

Taken together, the keywords denoting dieting and consumption, along with some uses of *risk*, can be interpreted as signalling responsibilising discourses (Burchell 1993), according to which obesity is construed as something that is caused by individuals' lifestyle choices and can therefore also be averted or solved by individuals modifying those choices. Similar patterns could be observed around the shared keywords *lifestyle* and *exercise*, with unhealthy lifestyles and a lack of exercise framed as causes of obesity and, conversely, adopting a healthy lifestyle and taking up exercise being presented as means for individuals to lower their risk of obesity. Taken together, implorations to readers to *diet, exercise* and adopt a *healthy lifestyle* tend to feature in articles propagating a position which situates the responsibility, for not just developing obesity but also for addressing it and reducing one's risk, firmly at the feet of individuals. Consistent with their shared keyness here, discourses around food, drink and consumption pervade the corpus and enter our analysis at various points, with discourses around diet and healthy lifestyles in particular forming the focus of the analysis in Chapter 6.

For now, we note that evidence of responsibilising discourses can be found through the use of these shared keywords across all sections of the press and that their use broadly conveys a sense in which individuals can and should assume responsibility for their obesity *risk* through the lifestyle choices they make. Personal responsibility and choice are foundational principles in neo-liberal societies (Harvey 2005), which rest on the assumption that individuals can and should reduce their health risks in order to remain economically productive and reduce the burden that they place on healthcare systems. This brings us, then, to our next shared keyword – *NHS*.

Seemingly ever topical, it is not too surprising to encounter the keyword *NHS* in our corpus of obesity articles. This is not just because obesity is a health issue with relevance to the NHS but because, presumably on account of its status in UK society and the general strength of feeling about it among members of the British public (R. Taylor 2013), the NHS seems to be eminently and self-evidently newsworthy in the UK media. This keyword featured in a range of contexts to which we cannot do justice here. However, one pattern that was shared by all sections of the press and which has direct relevance to the foregoing analysis was the focus on the strain – economic and otherwise – that obesity is purported to place on the *NHS*. Obesity itself could be presented as the direct cause of this economic strain, as in the following example.

> Health Minister Ivan Lewis said: "It is essential we take healthy eating options to these stores and reach those families who are at the greatest risk of poor health due to a poor diet." He explained that poor diet puts people at serious risk of heart disease and diabetes and that dealing with the effects of obesity costs the **NHS** 4.2 billion annually.
>
> (*Morning Star*, 14 August 2008)

However, and as the next three examples show, this burden could also be characterised in terms of the extra strain that obesity places on healthcare as well as other emergency services (e.g. the fire service). Obesity's associated causes and consequences (e.g. physical inactivity and diabetes) could also be presented as placing strain on the NHS.

> Steven Ward, chief executive of ukactive, said: "We know physical activity is key to weight management by burning calories, but it's a win-win that reaching for your gym shoes means you're less likely to reach for the snack cupboard." With obesity and physical inactivity placing unprecedented strain on the **NHS**, it's essential our next government tackles the root of the problem by getting more people, more active, more often.
>
> (*Telegraph*, 18 May 2017)

> Mr Burnham said that unless firm action is taken to halt the rise in obesity and diabetes, the cost of diabetes to the **NHS** will rise from 10 billion to 17 billion a year by 2035.
>
> (*Mail*, 15 January 2015)

> Fire service 'called out to obese'; News in brief HEALTH Fire engines have been called out once a day on average for the past five years to rescue people too fat to move. Most of the calls have come from the **NHS** struggling to cope with obese patients.
>
> (*Independent*, 13 March 2009)

We would argue that if obesity is, as the press represents it, a health problem, then there is surely something illogical about the argument that it in some way constitutes a waste or misuse of the NHS and its funds. So perhaps it is the case that the press regards obesity differently to some other health problems. The construal of obesity as constituting a burden on healthcare, and in our case on the NHS, rhymes with the representations identified in critical discourse studies of UK press representations of immigrants, who are frequently framed by sections of the media as a drain on the country's economic, welfare and healthcare resources (Baker et al. 2013; Brookes and Wright 2020). Such depictions rest on the construal of such groups as outsiders or deviants; that is, as the 'Other'. The patterns observed in the foregoing analysis could indicate that similar strategies are being applied in the representation of people with obesity. We will return to this consideration briefly at the end of this chapter and in more detail in our analysis of shaming discourses in Chapter 5.

Fat

The final shared keyword we want to consider in this section is *fat*. This is a somewhat nebulous term which has an array of meanings and cultural associations. As Lupton (2018: 3) observes

> In and of itself, fat has no meaning. It is the specific historical, social and cultural contexts in which fatness is lived, experienced, portrayed and regulated which give it meaning, just as other bodily attributes or features such as skin or hair colour, youth and height take on certain meanings depending on their contexts. These meanings are dynamic and shifting, subject to change as the context changes. In explaining these phenomena around fatness, wider interests and issues concerning human bodies and selfhood are brought into play.

Setting to one side the various attitudes and values that surround this word in society, at the semantic level the term *fat* can function as a noun to refer to either bodily tissue or a nutrient that we find in food and drink. Meanwhile, the adjective form can be used to describe people with larger bodies. In everyday language, these different senses of *fat* are often conflated, with a consequence for health literacy being the assumption that a person cannot become *fat* if they do not consume *fat* in terms of what they eat and drink (Smith-Stvan 2013: 81). With these multiple meanings in mind, we analysed a sample of 100 uses of *fat* in each sub-corpus, noting the different senses in which this word was used, as well as its potential to contribute to the broader types of obesity representations considered so far in this chapter. We grouped our findings into four categories: (i) Adjective; (ii) Noun – body tissue; (iii) Noun – nutrient; (iv) Other. The number of cases of each, identified across the four samples, are shown in

Table 2.3. *Uses of* fat *across samples from the four sub-corpora*

	Broadsheet Left%	Broadsheet Right%	Tabloid Left%	Tabloid Right%
Adjective	13	10	38	36
Noun – body tissue	37	39	27	32
Noun – nutrient	34	31	22	20
Other	16	20	13	12

Table 2.3. Since these are samples of 100 uses, these numbers could also be interpreted as percentages.

As the table shows, each section of the press used *fat* in all senses. If we combine results from all the samples together, we find that overall *fat* was used most often to denote body tissue, accounting for 33.75 per cent of the total sample. Second-most common was *fat* as a nutrient found in food and drink (total: 26.75 per cent), followed by *fat* as an adjective used to describe and label people (24.25 per cent). Finally, 'other', which accounts for the uses of *fat* that did not fall into any of the aforementioned categories, made up just 15.25 per cent of the total cases analysed. Although these mean percentages help us to look at the most typical uses of *fat*, they also tell only part of the story. If we look more closely at the numbers in each column, we see that the semantic preferences of *fat* can be fairly reliably split between broadsheets and tabloids. In both of the broadsheet sub-corpora, *fat* was used most frequently to mean body tissue (average: 38 per cent), followed by nutrient (average: 32.5 per cent). Then, curiously, bucking the trend in the total sample, the category 'other' accounted for an average of 18 per cent of the broadsheet samples, with uses of *fat* as an adjective being least common: just 11.5 per cent on average. On the other hand, in a reverse of the broadsheets, in both of the tabloid sub-corpora, *fat* is used most frequently as an adjective to label people (average: 37 per cent), then as a noun denoting body tissue (average: 29.5 per cent), then as a noun denoting the nutrient (average: 21 per cent), with the 'other' category the least common (average: 12.5 per cent). While there are not huge variances between most of these figures, the most striking difference is that the tabloids were on average more than three times as likely than the broadsheets to use *fat* as an adjective to describe a person.

As well as differences in frequency, our analysis also revealed some differences in how the tabloids and broadsheets used these various senses of *fat* in the articles. For example, when using *fat* as a label, the tabloids frequently represented the person or people in question in comedic ways but also in ways that made them look silly or which ridiculed them, for example in this headline and subtitle from an article in the *Sun* about a fairground ride in Wales imposing a weight restriction. Note how people with obesity are referred to not just as 'fat people' but also 'fatties'.

> Thrill ban on fatties
> A HOTEL is banning **fat** people from its planned zip wire thrill-ride by imposing a weight limit.
>
> (*Sun*, 22 May 2017)

We did not encounter this kind of jocular tone in the broadsheet samples, where descriptions of people as *fat* instead occurred in more serious contexts, as in this extract from an article in the *Guardian* about the implications of healthcare privatisation for people with obesity.

> This is how capitalism profits from people's desperation. This is how capitalism benefits when we keep lowering the bar for what is considered **fat** – and continue to ignore that dieting has some pretty heinous health risks of its own. So what does this mean for **fat** people? Or even for people who aren't actually **fat**? It means that big business and private investors are both going to profit from people hating themselves.
>
> (*Guardian*, 18 July 2012)

We also noted differences in the representations of *fat* as body tissue. The broadsheets frequently described internal biological processes involving fat tissue. For example, the extract below was taken from an article in the *Guardian* explaining a theory about the relationship between insulin production and obesity and contains three mentions of *fat*, all of which refer to the body's fat tissue.

> Far from being an inert dumping ground for excess calories, **fat** tissue operates as a reserve energy supply for the body. Its calories are called upon when glucose is running low – that is, between meals, or during fasts and famines. **Fat** takes instruction from insulin, the hormone responsible for regulating blood sugar. Refined carbohydrates break down at speed into glucose in the blood, prompting the pancreas to produce insulin. When insulin levels rise, **fat** tissue gets a signal to suck energy out of the blood, and to stop releasing it.
>
> (*Guardian*, 8 April 2016)

On the other hand, the tabloids tended to discuss fat tissue in the context of weight loss, including through diet, exercise and surgical procedures. This includes a propensity to construe this type of *fat* using a fire metaphor as something that is burnt, as in this example from the *Mail*.

MYTH: You must eat regularly to keep blood sugars up FACT: In THE study I mention above, participants lived on water for three days and the researchers measured the volunteers ' blood sugar levels. Although these levels did fall after three days without any food, they remained well within the normal range. At the same time, the levels of **fat** in their blood shot up, showing that their bodies had switched into major **fat** burning mode. Eating lots of small meals simply feeds your hunger.

(*Mail*, 6 March 2016)

Finally, we even found differences between tabloids and broadsheets in uses assigned to the 'other' category. The majority of 'other' uses of *fat* in the broadsheets featured in proper nouns, particularly names of books, films and plays that were being reviewed along with a few references to organisations. For the tabloids, on the other hand, the 'other' category consisted mainly of uses of *fat* in puns and word-play, reflecting a stylistic feature associated with this format.

Fat chance of fairness

(*Morning Star*, 4 January 2013)

BRITAIN'S obesity crisis has caused a big **fat** rise in knee and hip operations.

(*Star*, 21 September 2015)

Despite being a shared keyword, then, *fat* is used in decidedly different ways in the tabloids and the broadsheets. Before concluding this section, it is worth reflecting briefly on frequency. The representations of *fat* discussed in this section are based on analysis of balanced samples (100 uses per sub-corpus). However, it is worth remembering that the tabloids not only constitute a larger proportion of the texts and words in our corpus but also contain relatively more mentions of *fat* (1,550.36 PMW vs. 939.13 PMW in the broadsheets). We should bear in mind, then, that in reality the tabloids' uses of *fat* account for a larger proportion of the press's coverage of obesity overall.

Conclusion

This chapter has considered the shared keywords across four sections of our corpus representing newspapers' formats and political leanings. These shared keywords are used in a variety of ways. However, they all also contribute to a series of shared representations of obesity. First, we noted a proliferation of keywords that denote or are related to medical concepts. Analysing their use, we found that while obesity was framed as a medical problem that could cause other medical problems, its status as a disease was more complex and con-tested, with the word *disease* generally being reserved for other, more established illnesses, where its use in relation to obesity was more likely to feature in articles arguing that obesity is *not* a disease. We also found evidence that all of the newspapers construed obesity as something that was predominantly caused by individuals' lifestyle choices (mainly consuming high calorie and sugary food and drink and not exercising enough) and which could thus be addressed by individuals making different choices and modifying their lifestyles, for instance by dieting and exercising more. We have interpreted these types of representations as instantiating a discourse of personal responsibility around obesity, whereby it is individuals and their actions that are held responsible for both causing obesity in the first place and then addressing it, if and when it occurs. Another set of shared representations surrounded the NHS, which was depicted in all sections of the corpus as being placed under considerable (economic) strain by obesity and people with it.

If we consider what we know about the social and political contexts in which the articles in our corpus were produced, these overlaps in obesity-related discourses are not too surprising, as they all reflect wider social trends in contemporary British society. The prevalence of medical terminology could be viewed as reflecting the broader dominance of the biomedical perspective on the ways that obesity (and an increasing number of other aspects of life) is conceptualised and explained in Western societies. Likewise, the prominence of responsibilising constructions of obesity's causes and solutions can be viewed as an extension of the neoliberal political system which, as we discussed in Chapter 1, governs all aspects of social and political life by placing responsibility and accountability at the feet of individuals; who are accordingly implored to be 'good' citizens by ensuring their own health, wellbeing and economic productivity (as well as that of their family's), rather than having to rely on support from the state. This, in turn, can be linked to the representation of obesity as a burden on the NHS; since the objective of the neoliberal political system is to ensure self-governance to lessen the burden that citizens place on the state, it seems logical that obesity would be considered a burden on the state's healthcare system in this context, particularly given the longer-term, wider societal discourses which posit that the NHS is under increasing strain due to the country's growing and ageing population, as well as government spending cuts on healthcare.

Setting these areas of overlap to one side for a moment, it is important to bear in mind that we also found differences in the ways that some of the shared keywords were used in the contexts of the articles themselves. A good example of this is the shared keyword *fat*. While the broadsheets tended to use this term as a noun, in reference to body tissue and slightly less often to refer to the nutrient found in food and drink, the tabloids tended overwhelmingly to use this word in its adjectival sense, to label and describe people, sometimes in pejorative ways. Although keywords, and the shared keywords approach in particular, proved to be useful for identifying words and concepts that were salient across the press coverage as a whole, these kinds of distinctions in meaning and usage, which only become apparent when we consider how the keywords in question are actually used in context, underscore the importance of supplementing any analysis of abstracted word or keyword lists with more fine-grain, qualitative examination of patterns in-use.

Returning to areas of overlap, we should acknowledge that the newspapers in our data are of course likely to hold differing views about government spending on healthcare and the extent to which it is individuals who are most 'responsible' for developing obesity (and, in turn, for placing extra strain on the NHS), and the analysis in the next chapter will address some of these points of difference. However, it appears that certain discourses, such as the centrality of personal responsibility and concerns about strain on the NHS, appear to be so widely held and potentially normalised that they transcend the division between newspapers according to political leaning and format and instead characterise coverage of obesity in the press as a whole.

As well as representing dominant perspectives on obesity – and, to an extent, health more generally – within society, these discourses also, we would argue, interlock. We can find evidence for this connection not just by looking at the social and political contexts surrounding these newspaper representations but also by looking at the articles themselves. For example, consider this extract from the *Sun*, which provides readers with a link to a website where they can calculate their BMI.

> Research published in the International Journal Of Obesity found that higher intakes of calcium were associated with lower body fat measurements. Check your BMI at thesun.co.uk/health.
>
> (*Sun*, 29 January 2009)

Not only does this passage serve to legitimise the BMI and the biomedical perspective on obesity that sits behind it but by addressing readers directly through the second-person possessive form, *your*, and explicitly directing them to 'check your BMI', this article – and others like it – implore individual readers to monitor their body weight and BMI, presumably with a view to them practising better self-care, which could be linked to the personal responsibility discourse. Likewise, we could interpret some of the shaming uses of the word *fat* as an adjective as an indirect instantiation of the personal responsibility discourse, where such shaming and ridicule of people with obesity can act as a form of social control designed to enjoin its targets to lower their bodyweight while serving as a warning to others about the social perils of developing obesity.

Yet, the discourses identified in this chapter also fit together in more subtle ways. The dominance of the neoliberal, responsibilising perspective could explain why obesity, though presented using biomedical concepts and alongside diseases such as cancer and heart disease, was not quite conferred the status of *disease* in the press. A reason for this could be that the press views the two positions – obesity as a disease and obesity as something over which individuals have responsibility and control – as somewhat incongruous. Indeed, earlier in this chapter we noted cases where *disease* status was constructed as existing in an oppositional relationship with the notion of obesity as being preventable. Of course, in reality these qualities are not mutually exclusive, and many, less contested diseases are also regarded as preventable (like many types of cancers, for example). Such a nuanced perspective is seldom adopted in press debates around obesity, though. Faced with representing obesity as a disease or a choice, the press generally opts for the latter.

So, if obesity is not a disease, then how do we interpret the frequent use of medical terminology that was characteristic of articles across all sections of the press? One explanation could be that this reflects the dominance of medical frameworks over the ways that we conceptualise and communicate about the human body. BMI measurements are a medical tool and are drawn on relatively uncritically by all sections of the print media for the purposes of defining obesity and encouraging readers to monitor their own body weight. If we regard this use of medical terminology more critically, we could also argue that the tendency for the press to frame obesity as a medical issue without quite committing to describing it as a disease allows it to be presented in two, somewhat incongruent, ways. Specifically, it is presented, on the one hand, as threatening human health by contributing to other diseases and placing a burden on healthcare services. Yet on the other hand, the press generally denies the possibility that people with obesity are absolved of responsibility on the grounds that obesity is a disease and something outside of their control. Whatever the case, we can certainly argue that the contested status of obesity as a disease, discussed in the previous chapter, is reflected in the complex of discourses that surround it in the press. The relationship between these discourses – of obesity as a disease and/or as something that can be controlled by the individual – is a theme that looms large over the analysis reported in this book and, like many of the keywords introduced in this chapter, is something that is revisited in the forthcoming chapters.

3 Studying Difference
Comparing Sections of the Press

Introduction

In the previous chapter, we used the keywords technique to explore similarities between the different sections of the press. In the present chapter, we use the keywords procedure again, this time to consider differences. We use what we have previously referred to as the 'remainder method' of keyword analysis (Baker et al. 2019: 29) to carry out a series of corpus-internal comparisons to find out what is lexically distinctive about articles published in different sections of the press. Specifically, we compare each of the sub-corpora representing different sections of the press introduced in the previous chapter against the rest of the data to find out what is characteristic about the language in each one. For example, to find out what is characteristic about the language used in articles in the right-leaning tabloids, we compare the Tabloid Right sub-corpus (containing articles from the *Express*, *Mail*, *Star* and *Sun*) against all of the other sub-corpora (Broadsheet Left, Broadsheet Right and Tabloid Left) combined. This chapter is divided into four parts, each of which addresses a different section of the press, beginning with the right-leaning tabloids.

Tabloid Right

This sub-corpus comprises articles from four newspapers – the *Express*, *Mail*, *Star* and *Sun*. This is by far the largest of our four sub-corpora in terms of both its number of texts (21,356; 48.67 per cent of entire corpus) and words (16,609,707; 46.07 per cent). Table 3.1 shows the top fifty keywords for this sub-corpus, ranked by log-likelihood score. As a reminder, these keywords were obtained by comparing this sub-corpus against the other three sub-corpora combined.

Given that, as in the previous chapter, many of the keywords obtained have large frequencies, in order to gain a sense of how they are used in context, our analyses are based on examining random samples of 100 uses of each keyword, noting how they are typically used in representations of obesity, as well

Table 3.1. *Top 50 Tabloid Right keywords, ranked by log-likelihood (frequencies in brackets)*

weight (44,759), *her* (63,077), *she* (67,559), *cent* (28,561), *risk* (24,926), *blood* (15,785), *per* (33,014), *diabetes* (20,755), *U.S.* (2,365), *study* (22,301), *diet* (22,817), *loss* (10,614), *found* (22,633), *researchers* (11,019), *said* (56,310), *body* (20,229), *heart* (18,346), *Dr* (14,666), *disease* (17,739), *size* (10,479), *revealed* (5,837), *percent* (2,382), *type* (9,540), *fat* (25,640), *ten* (4,927), *cancer* (18,019), *surgery* (9,046), *symptoms* (4,697), *condition* (6,617), *can* (51,813), *after* (29,420), *could* (32,966), *skin* (5,430), *calories* (10,690), *experts* (8,024), *lose* (9,744), *also* (32,537), *brain* (7,471), *help* (17,021), *women* (22,829), *obese* (21,459), *levels* (12,007), *eating* (17,217), *stone* (7,920), *gastric* (3,479), *was* (95,444), *stomach* (4,139), *cells* (4,223), *day* (21,474), *pressure* (7,968)

as describing any interesting minority and counter-discourses where these occur.

The first point to make about Table 3.1 is the presence of keywords which, like many of the shared keywords examined in the previous chapter, denote medical terminology. Again, this includes keywords denoting illnesses and diseases, with the shared keywords *diabetes*, *heart*, *disease* and *cancer* re-emerging as key for this sub-corpus. This suggests that as well as being prevalent in the corpus as a whole (compared to general written British English), these words are especially frequent in the right-leaning tabloids. We can find further evidence in support of this interpretation in some of the other Tabloid Right keywords which are similarly used to frame obesity as a medical problem and a cause of other health problems. This includes the keyword *skin*, which can be used to refer to illnesses like *skin cancer* (195 occurrences), *skin condition[s]* (136) and *skin infection[s]* (31); *type*, which tends to occur as a left-sided collocate of *diabetes* to generate terms like *type 1/one diabetes* (857) and *type 2/two diabetes* (5,716); and *blood* and *pressure* which frequently co-occur in the bigram *blood pressure* (5,828).

Much like the keywords denoting heart disease, cancer and diabetes which we explored in the previous chapter, the right-leaning tabloids mention high blood pressure in ways that contribute to the framing of obesity as a medical problem. In an examination of 100 concordance lines of references to *blood pressure*, we found that the most common pattern (42 per cent of the sample) was to group high blood pressure together with obesity in lists of health problems.

> People with psoriatic arthritis are also more likely to have other prob-
> lems including high **blood pressure**, diabetes, obesity and fatty
> liver disease.
>
> (*Mail*, 2 September 2014)

Almost as frequently (32 per cent), high blood pressure was construed as a cause of obesity.

> The consequences of obesity are far reaching, with it potentially leading to increased health problems such as diabetes, heart disease, high **blood pressure** and joint problems.
>
> *(Mail,* 1 April 2008)

An associated keyword is *condition*, which tends to be used in reference to medical problems (usually diabetes) that obesity is framed as contributing towards. However, in a minority of cases (10 per cent), the word *condition* refers to obesity itself.

> It could lead one day to the production of an anti-obesity drug designed to tackle the **condition** and its related health problems such as diabetes, heart disease and cancer.
>
> *(Express,* 4 January 2014)

Another way in which the articles in this section construed obesity as a medical problem was by offering biological, scientific explanations of it and its causes and consequences. This was indicated by the keywords *brain* and *cells,* as well as in some uses of *body* and *fat.*

> Cancer Research UK has explained how obesity causes cancer. It said: "As people become obese, and more fat **cells** build up in their tissues, specialised immune **cells** are called to the scene, possibly to clear up dead and dying fat **cells**."
>
> *(Express,* 1 June 2016)

> Obese people's brains could be hard-wired to want food in the same way that drug users are addicted to their habit, new research suggests. The revelation that certain parts of the **brain** promote obesity could help manage the condition, scientists say.
>
> *(Mail,* 31 August 2015)

Consistent with this characterisation of obesity as resulting from and contributing towards internal biological processes, these words also featured in articles reporting on trials of biomedical and pharmacological interventions that could be used to 'treat' obesity, as in this example from the *Mail* reporting on a study showing that anti-smoking drugs could reduce 'sugar cravings'.

> Anti-smoking drugs could stub out your sugar cravings:
>
> - Common treatment that targets **brain**'s 'reward pathways' may be used on people who are addicted to sugar
> - Treatment given to smokers could reduce **brain**'s dependence on sugar

- Researchers in Queensland, Australia, found drug can reduce cravings
- Discovery could prove a significant breakthrough in the war on obesity

(Mail, 10 April 2016)

This example brings us to a set of medical keywords which we did *not* encounter in the previous chapter; namely, words denoting medical experts and research. This includes the nouns *study, researchers*, and *experts*, the honorific *Dr*, and the lexical verbs *found* and *revealed*. All these words are used by the newspapers in this section overwhelmingly to present findings from scientific research and public health reports concerned with the prevalence, causes and consequences of obesity. For example, the extract below cites an epidemiological study in the context of an article arguing for a ban on advertising of 'fatty foods' targeted at children.

> ADVERTS flogging fatty foods to kids must be tackled to stamp out childhood obesity, **experts** warned yesterday. The caution comes after a survey **revealed** the number of chubby teens was on the rise, with obesity in boys up 14 per cent and in girls 2 per cent since 1990.
>
> (Sun, 25 January 2008)

Reporting the perspectives of medical researchers and practitioners is one way in which the press can give prominence to medical framings of obesity, with these social actors given a platform that is not afforded – at least to the same extent – to other commentators, such as fat activists. These words occur with a marked frequency in the right-leaning tabloids compared to the rest of the corpus, suggesting that this focus on scientific research and expertise was especially frequent in this section of the press relative to obesity coverage as a whole.

This heightened focus on research and scientific expertise also helps to explain why words denoting statistics and quantification (i.e. *per, cent* and *percent*) were key for this section of the press, as the statistics cited were typically derived from scientific studies and public health reports. Most commonly, in 39 per cent of cases, these keywords were used to report the percentage of the population who either are or are predicted to be affected by obesity. For example, this extract from the *Mail* cites four percentage figures to this effect.

> Some 25 **per cent** adults and 16 **per cent** of children are obese. But experts believe this will rise to 60 **per cent** of adults and 25 **per cent** of children by 2050. Nice claims that the NHS spends 64.2 billion every year treating patients with obesity-related conditions. This is expected to rise to 610 billion by 2050.
>
> (Mail, 6 June 2011)

Aside from prevalence figures, other uses of *per cent* and *percent* involved enumerating the degree of risk that certain behaviours could lead to obesity and the risks of certain health problems that could follow from obesity (31 per cent of cases), as well as to quantify the proportion of a person's body mass that was made up of fat tissue (17 per cent of cases), once again drawing on the BMI metric used by medical practitioners. As well as being a keyword for the right-leaning tabloids, *risk* was also one of the shared keywords we analysed in the previous chapter, where we outlined its uses in this and other sub-corpora, so we will not spend too much time on it here. However, we do note that the citation of statistics, including in discourse around *risk*, can be interpreted as further foregrounding the biomedical research perspective on obesity in this section of the press.

In the previous chapter, we observed how shared keywords around consumption could signal a responsibilising discourse, with obesity represented as something that is caused by individuals' over-consumption of certain types of food and drink, as well as by individuals consuming food and drink in certain ways, particularly in conjunction with physical inactivity. The re-emergence of keywords like *diet*, *calories* and *eating* in Table 3.1 indicates that this focus on consumption is likely to be particularly characteristic of the right-leaning tabloids compared to the rest of the press.

Similarly linked to the concept of risk management, another keyword from this sub-corpus, *day*, could be used to inform readers about how much activity they need to engage in or how much of a certain food or drink they should (or should not) consume each day to reduce their risk of obesity.

> She believes upping our flavonoid intake could be a valuable and easy way to prevent obesity. "We're all told to eat five a **day**, but this new evidence suggests some fruit and vegetables might be better than others, particularly in terms of weight maintenance."
>
> (*Mail*, 29 January 2016)

Another context in which the keyword *day* features is in articles centred on narratives around individuals' weight loss. Such articles usually focus on (female) celebrities but also 'ordinary' women, and in a minority of cases men, who once had obesity but have since reduced their weight, typically through diet and exercise. Such narratives were indicated by a range of the keywords in Table 3.1. In addition to *day*, this includes keywords which explicitly denote weight loss (i.e. *loss*, *lose* and *weight*) and words used to quantify the body and body weight (i.e. *size* and *stone*). These narratives could be written from a first-person perspective, a third-person perspective or a combination of the two. As past-tense accounts of sequentially ordered events, these narratives also help to explain the emergence of keywords like *after* and the past-tense copular, *was*. Narratives of this kind typically span the length of the articles in which they feature, meaning that they can be quite lengthy. For demonstrative purposes, this headline and lead paragraph from the *Mail* contain a number of keywords and provide a conveniently concise illustration of how these are used in this context, as well as of other key features of the weight loss narratives we encountered in this part of the corpus.

My **size** made it painful to walk but I couldn't resist beer or sugary treats: Obese woman loses 4st **after** finally beating urge to raid fridge at night

- Amy, 23, **was** stuck in a vicious circle of failed diets and comfort eating
- **Her weight** crept up to nearly 20st
- **She** overindulged in sugary snacks, beer and raided the fridge late at night
- Hated **her size** but didn't know what to do about it
- Tried diet plan of two shakes and a healthy evening meal a **day** for 90 days
- Helped **her** kick start **her** new lifestyle
- Now **she** eats healthy, exercises and is 4st lighter

(*Mail*, 17 March 2014)

As this extract demonstrates, a key feature of the weight loss narratives published in this section of the press is the theme of redemption. Redemption narratives have been found to be a significant element in self-help discourse (Irvine 1999) as well as in other forms of popular culture, like magazines (McAdams 2006). In the narratives in this section of our corpus, the weight loss – or 'redemption' – is framed as the result of the individual dieting and/or exercising. The subjects of these weight loss narratives are celebrated for enacting par excellence the type of neoliberal ideal of the responsible citizen that we have observed to drive discourses both in this section of the corpus and, in the previous chapter, across the press as a whole. Weight loss narratives will be explored in more detail in Chapter 7, specifically through the lens of gender. For now, we note that such stories constitute a more linguistic-ally creative means for the tabloids to weave discourses around personal responsibility into their coverage of obesity.

Another context in which the articles in this section of the corpus employed a narrative style was in the representation of surgical responses to obesity, as evidenced in uses of the keywords *surgery*, *gastric* and *stomach*. However, unlike diet and exercise, which tended to be represented as not only effective but morally redemptive means of losing weight (see Chapter 6), stories about surgical responses to obesity tended to have a more negative evaluative prosody. These stories typically fall into one of two types. The first are stories about operations resulting in complications, sometimes with patients dying.

> Widower says anyone considering having band 'should think very hard'
> A mother-of-three who was once classified as 'morbidly obese' before losing
> an astonishing 14 stone has died nine days after having a **gastric** band fitted.
>
> (*Mail*, 31 August 2016)

In one study, the mortality rate within thirty days following bariatric surgery
was reported to be 0.3 per cent (based on 6,118 patients) (Smith et al. 2011), so
this is a rare occurrence, and these stories draw on the news values (Galtung
and Ruge 1965) of unexpectedness and negativity. The fact that the newspapers in this section of the press foreground negative stories, rather than
success stories, relating to these operations contributes towards a general
negative evaluative prosody around this method of weight loss.

The second type of story about these operations is concerned with how
much they, and by extension the people who receive them, cost the NHS and
taxpayers. The following example was selected because it represents some of
the features noted in other articles of this type.

> So does someone force a doughnut down your neck? Fury as 35 stone
> man claims the NHS have 'let him down' by refusing him a **gastric** band.
> Unemployed Steve Beer, 46, from Plymouth, says he is 'too fat to work'.
> The married father-of-six has reached his heaviest weight at 35 stone. But
> he says the NHS has 'let him down' after refusing weight loss **surgery**.
> Medics said he would need to lose weight before getting a gastric band.
> But This Morning viewers have blasted him as a 'lazy slob' on Twitter.
>
> (*Mail*, 6 September 2016)

This story from the *Mail* is about a man who appeared on a TV show to talk about
how he felt let down because the NHS refused him gastric band surgery unless he lost
weight first. He is clearly evaluated negatively in this article, the headline of which
asks rhetorically, 'So does someone force a doughnut down your neck?' (where the
use of 'force' constructs his eating habits as a form of self-harm). The article
foregrounds certain aspects of the man's identity which do not appear to be directly
relevant to the story but which help to construe him as a financial burden on the state;
he is described as 'unemployed' and a 'father-of-six'. Further down, the article also
quotes viewers who called him 'lazy slob', without offering any other, perhaps more
sympathetic, perspectives on his circumstances. We examine the relationship
between social class and representations of obesity in Chapter 8 but, for now, let us
move on to examining the next section of the corpus – the right-leaning broadsheets.

Broadsheet Right

Table 3.2 shows the top fifty keywords for the right-leaning broadsheets
(*Telegraph* and *Times*) compared against the rest of the corpus.

Table 3.2. *Top 50 Broadsheet Right keywords, ranked by log-likelihood (frequencies in brackets)*

sir (3,279), *telegraph* (1,174), *that* (91,777), *BBC* (2,164), *the* (372,966), *Britain* (5,552), *billion* (1,413), *its* (10,117), *television* (1,657), *Prof* (1,104), *sport* (2,381), *dear* (582), *America* (1,837), *company* (2,529), *is* (92,824), *book* (2,453), *letters* (925), *learnt* (450), *there* (18,676), *British* (4,778), *he* (33,170), *founded* (428), *French* (1,234), *we* (30,416), *film* (1,883), *you* (36,329), *cycling* (988), *about* (20,423), *novel* (794), *it* (75,096), *Jebb* (134), *London* (4,864), *buyout* (103), *RRP* (141), *his* (21,983), *Mr* (3,764), *sales* (1,253), *books* (1,059), *France* (980), *business* (2,126), *not* (31,555), *of* (203,766), *war* (1,349), *English* (1,041), *FA* (330), *art* (756), *Shriver* (236), *perhaps* (1,750), *great* (3,280), *writes* (607)

Before examining these keywords in detail, it is first worth commenting on the fact that some keywords result from distinctions between newspaper style, with the broadsheets having a more formal style than the tabloids. For example, *dear*, *sir* and *letters* are keywords due to the highly formalised letters pages in the *Telegraph* and *Times*. The honorific *Prof* tends to be used as a stylistic choice in the *Telegraph* as an abbreviation of *Professor*, a term which tends to be much more common in the *Express*, *Mail* and *Independent*. The Broadsheet Right keywords also contain an abundance of terms relating to the arts and media. This includes keywords such as *BBC*, *television*, *book*, *film*, *novel*, *RRP* (referring to recommended book prices), *books*, *art*, *writes* and *Shriver*, which refers to the author, Lionel Shriver, who wrote a novel about her brother who had obesity. These words are key here because, compared to other sections of the corpus, the right-leaning broadsheets contain a large number of review articles.

Another keyword from Table 3.2, but one which reveals something about how obesity is construed, is *billion*. In 64 per cent of cases, this term was used to refer to money as part of passages or longer stories about the purported costs endured by the NHS as a result of high and rising obesity rates, echoing the types of discourse we noted in the previous section on the right-leaning tabloids, as well as in the previous chapter when studying the corpus as a whole. In these cases, obesity is framed as not only a medical problem but also an economic burden on the country's healthcare system and, by extension, its taxpayers.

> Obesity-related disease currently costs the health service 47 **billion** a year, just under half the entire NHS budget.
>
> (*Telegraph*, 14 July 2016)

Less frequently, in 20 per cent of cases, obesity was construed as something that costs industry and taxpayers through related illnesses causing staff to take days off work. The following example from the *Times* focusses on the cost of NHS staff absences.

> The average NHS worker takes almost ten days a year off sick, costing the health service 2.4 **billion**. Tam Fry, of the National Obesity Forum, said fat NHS staff ought to get a "taste of their own medicine" by being weighed to see if they slimmed down, as with overweight children.
>
> *(Times*, 5 March 2016)

A similar discourse surrounded some uses of the keyword *war*, with 3 per cent of its sampled uses framing obesity as something that costs the country more than wars have. Encoded within this comparison is a negative moral evaluation, whereby obesity is equated to war. In the next example, this comparison also extends to forms of crime, specifically terrorism and 'armed violence'.

> The consultancy McKinsey says that obesity costs the UK three per cent of GDP; more than **war**, terror and armed violence.
>
> *(Telegraph*, 16 February 2015)

Other keywords in Table 3.2 centre on the theme of business and industry, with the newspapers in this section more likely to use terms like *company* and *business*, where keywords such as *founded*, *buyout* and *sales* appear when the articles give contextual detail about the background and history of the particular companies being reported on. These terms referred to a wide range of companies, mostly food manufacturers and supermarkets, but also restaurants and gymnasiums (among others). In most cases (62 per cent), these companies are represented as making a positive contribution towards tackling obesity rates, for example in this extract from an article in the *Telegraph* about the supermarket chain, Tesco.

> Tesco chief executive Philip Clarke talks of his **company**'s plan to cut food waste and the problem of obesity.
>
> *(Telegraph*, 18 May 2013)

If the companies being referred to were not evaluated positively, they were more likely not to be evaluated at all (33 per cent), while only 5 per cent of the articles in this sample gave an explicitly negative evaluation of the contribution of these industries to rising obesity rates. This marks an interesting distinction, then, between the right-leaning tabloids and broadsheets; where the former tended to emphasise an individualistic model of obesity, the latter can be characterised in terms of its attention to certain industries in contributing to, but mainly reversing, the country's rising obesity rates. Although such companies tended to be evaluated positively in this coverage, with critical perspectives constituting a minority of the sample, the right-leaning broadsheets were at least engaging in such debates about the role of more powerful institutions in the context of obesity. Consistent with this focus on more powerful institutions, another set of keywords indicate references to sporting organisations; specifically, *sport*, *cycling* and *FA* (short for Football Association). Like the positive evaluation of the aforementioned companies, the focus of these articles was on the positive role that sporting organisations and associations play in helping to reduce rates of obesity.

> The **FA** negotiates sponsorship deals with supermarket chains who build on schools pitches; it happily accepts millions to associate England with alcohol, fast food and sugar-filled drinks and then wonders about national obesity levels. Yet the **FA** also does magnificent grassroots work at home and abroad.
>
> *(Telegraph*, 12 May 2009)

Again, it is notable that although the newspaper acknowledges the role of supermarket chains and certain food and drink industries, the focus of the coverage is not on those industries directly but rather on the role of the FA and its affiliation with them. Even the evaluation of the FA is complex; in the first sentence it is criticised for its sponsorship deals but in the second sentence is praised for its 'magnificent grassroots work'.

In addition to companies and sports institutions, the articles in this section of the corpus also paid greater attention to the role of politicians when discussing responses to obesity. This was signalled by the keywords *Mr*, which was used to refer *inter alia* to politicians (in the next examples, then-London Mayor, Boris Johnson), and *Jebb*, in reference to the Government's obesity adviser, Susan Jebb.

> Lord Coe, the chairman of the London 2012 Olympic organising committee, is known to have lobbied **Mr** Johnson recently for some of his 70million anti-obesity budget, arguing that sport can help to prevent some of the problems that are plaguing the National Health Service.
>
> *(Times*, 6 June 2008)

> Children at Valence Primary School in Dagenham are being provided with water instead throughout the day. The move comes days after Susan **Jebb**, a Government adviser on obesity, said that people should stop drinking orange juice because it contains as much sugar as Coca-Cola.
>
> *(Times*, 16 January 2014)

The keyword *war* is also relevant here. Earlier we saw how some articles in this section of the press framed obesity as being more expensive for the country than the cost of war (among other things). In this context, the keyword *war* was mostly used in reference to the First or Second World Wars. However, a minority pattern (in 5 per cent of cases) constituted the metaphorical use of this keyword to frame the United Kingdom's, and more specifically the UK Government's, response to obesity as a *war*.

> The fizz was taken out of soft drinks companies after the surprise announcement from George Osborne to introduce a sugar levy as part of the government's **war** on obesity, sending shares in the sector lower.
>
> (*Times*, 17 March 2016)

As this extract exemplifies, the war between the Government and obesity tended to focus on taxation of sugar- and calorie-laden products. Again, tellingly, what is foregrounded here is not the roles of those industries in causing obesity but, rather, the role of the Government in preventing obesity. In fact, the stories are sometimes framed from the perspectives of these industries, whereby they are presented as victims of such measures. For example, the previous extract from the *Times* foregrounds the lowering of sector shares as a corollary of higher taxation on sugary drinks.

This notwithstanding, compared to the right-leaning tabloids, the right-leaning broadsheets do at least report on government initiatives and so invoke the sense in which obesity is not (just) the responsibility of the individual but of society more broadly. This sense of societal responsibility was also conveyed through the pronoun keywords *we* and *you*. Mulderrig (2011: 566) describes the collective *we* as 'semantically complex', as '[i]ts meaning can be "inclusive" (including the reader/hearer) or "exclusive" (excluding them)'. When used in this section of the data, this pronoun tends to refer to Britain as a whole, invoking a sense of shared agency for responding to obesity.

> Consultant cardiologist Dr Aseem Malhotra said it was time "for a complete U-turn" in Britain's approach to diet, and demonisation of fat. "The sooner **we** do that the sooner **we** reverse the epidemic in obesity and diabetes and the sooner start improving health."
>
> (*Telegraph*, 29 August 2017)

In the above extract, a quote attributed to a cardiologist constructs 'Britain' as a social actor in possession of an approach to diet (which is represented as being in need of change). This sense of shared agency is then reinforced through the choice of pronouns, whereby this social actor (i.e. Britain) is referred to anaphorically using the collective pronoun 'we', as if to subsume both the author and readers under this social actor label.

On first viewing, the second-person keyword *you* does not have this same inclusive effect. However, analysing how this term was used in context, we found that its use was more complicated. It could be used to address readers directly with weight loss advice (31 per cent). However, it was more likely to be used in a general sense (45 per cent), indicating commonality of experience (see Pearce 2001: 220), typically for rhetorical effect, as in this excerpt taken from an article questioning the ethics of fast food companies

> **You** look at a McDonald's, and **you** wonder, "How do they do that? Grow a cow, kill a cow, mince a cow, cook it, make a bun, put it in a van, build a restaurant, put ads on the telly, find a gherkin, hire all those kids and then smile, for a quid?" Sorry, **you** probably don't want to think about Maccy D's right now.
>
> *(Times,* 8 January 2012)

The final keywords from this section of the data we want to consider are the noun *France* and its corresponding adjective, *French*. While the latter could be used (in a minority of cases) to refer to the actor Dawn French, overall both terms tended to be used in reference to the country for the purposes of comparing the obesity prevalence rates and reduction strategies of France with those of the United Kingdom. This could be a result of the tendency for the broadsheets to give a more international perspective on their stories than the tabloids do (though we also note the keywords relating to the United States in the right-leaning tabloids).

> Although the prevalence of obesity in British adults is more than twice that in **France**, with 25 per cent in Britain compared to 10 per cent in **France**, child obesity is now almost on a par.
>
> *(Telegraph,* 10 April 2008)

To conclude this part of the analysis, a major difference between the right-leaning tabloids and broadsheets is that, while the tabloids tend to focus on the role of individuals in reducing their risk of and reversing obesity, the broadsheets are more inclined than the tabloids to frame obesity from the perspective of societal responsibility, including foregrounding the role of food and drink industries in causing obesity, and politicians, sports organisations and society as a whole in responding to it. In the next section we switch our focus to the left-leaning data, beginning with the broadsheets.

Broadsheet Left

The Broadsheet Left sub-corpus consists of articles from the *Guardian* and the *Independent* (including the *i*). Table 3.3 shows the top fifty keywords from these newspapers compared against the rest of the corpus.

Earlier in this chapter we saw how the right-leaning tabloids tended to locate the causes of and solutions to obesity with and within the individuals affected by it. The keywords from the left-leaning broadsheets, on the other hand, suggest that these newspapers tended to construct obesity as a social rather than strictly medical problem. This theme manifests in a range of keywords,

Table 3.3. *Top 50 Broadsheet Left keywords, ranked by log-likelihood (frequencies in brackets)*

---

the (388,993), *Guardian* (1,469), *government* (8,729), *public* (8,369), *its* (12,001), *we* (33,377), *social* (4,680), *that* (90,356), *of* (209,513), *political* (1,947), *sector* (1,285), *global* (1,997), *policy* (2,373), *tax* (4,031), *services* (2,564), *poverty* (1,224), *local* (3,555), *world* (8,304), *there* (19,745), *climate* (1,009), *society* (2,908), *related* (1,791), *funding* (1,592), *city* (2,724), *inequality* (605), *economic* (1,465), *is* (93,348), *advertising* (1,488), *independent* (1,282), *not* (32,845), *cities* (1,001), *us* (10,303), *health* (21,311), *countries* (2,358), *Cameron* (2,062), *sport* (2,449), *report* (4,608), *what* (15,606), *Observer* (307), *community* (1,671), *companies* (2,072), *media* (1,952), *in* (140,754), *coalition* (757), *politics* (943), *housing* (860), *cuts* (1,456), *Labour* (2,382), *England* (3,941), *UK* (7,418)

---

such as *global, climate, society* and *housing*. Another characteristic feature of the left-leaning broadsheets was that they construed obesity not as a strictly individual issue but, rather, a challenge for the whole of society. For example, the keyword *society* could function as a social actor that represented all people living in the United Kingdom, who were depicted as having to 'face' or 'deal with' obesity.

> **Society** is facing an issue with obesity and obesity in kids.
>
> (*Guardian*, 28 January 2008)

In this sense, we can draw parallels between the left-leaning broadsheets and their right-leaning counterparts, which, as we have seen, could also be characterised as constructing obesity as the responsibility of society as a whole, and not just individuals. Yet in the left-leaning data, obesity was not just restricted to specific societal contexts but, as the keyword *global* indicates, was also framed as a global issue requiring global responses:

> The Romanian experiment is being watched closely by other countries desperate for measures to halt the **global** explosion in obesity.
>
> (*Independent*, 3 April 2010)

The keyword *global* also occurs in the bigram 'global warming' 151 times. Meanwhile, over half (596) of the uses of the keyword *climate* are found in the bigram, 'climate change'. In 29 per cent of a random sample of 100 articles containing one or both of these terms, obesity was likened to a mixture of other pathologised and non-pathologised global issues.

> We live in a time of environmental and health meltdown in terms of **global warming** and obesity.
>
> (*Guardian*, 30 August 2013)

> An all-party commission warns that taxes will have to rise to cope with the financial pressures caused by an ageing population; an increase in chronic diseases such as diabetes and obesity; combating **climate change**; closing the gap between rich and poor; abolishing child poverty and improving skills levels in the workforce.
>
> (*Independent*, 14 September 2010)

A related keyword is *housing*, which includes cases where obesity is grouped together with the United Kingdom's housing crisis as a societal problem.

> Our sluggish, low-pay economy, high levels of poverty, the **housing** crisis, our obesity epidemic and welfare bill are all driven by the UK's extraordinary levels of inequality.
>
> (*Guardian*, 25 January 2014)

In the previous chapter, we saw how articles from all sections of the press construed obesity as a medical issue, if not quite a *disease*, by grouping or listing it with other, arguably less contentious medical conditions like diabetes, heart disease and cancer. It is interesting, therefore, to see this same discursive feature being applied by the left-leaning broadsheets to represent obesity as a social problem, too. Consistent with this definition of obesity as a social problem, the left-leaning broadsheets also attributed obesity to social causes, specifically social inequality. Thus, the words *poverty*, *inequality* and *economic* emerge as key for this section of the data.

> I have just returned from travelling the length of England, and am depressed. The physical fabric – substandard housing and roads – and the social fabric – a collapsing NHS, a divisive education and class system, serious **poverty** and spectacular obesity – all indicate a nation in decline.
>
> (*i*, 13 July 2017)

> According to Arcadis, US destinations are "generally weighed down by a high degree of income **inequality**, high crime, obesity, a lack of affordable housing, and long working hours.
>
> (*Independent*, 15 September 2016)

> As those at the bottom of the socioeconomic ladder are the most likely to suffer from loneliness, might this provide one of the explanations for the strong link between low **economic** status and obesity?
>
> (*Guardian*, 12 October 2016)

Inequality could also be cited as the cause of obesity in more implicit ways. An example of this is the keyword *housing*. As we saw earlier, *housing* could collocate with *crisis* in cases where obesity was given as a social problem alongside the United Kingdom's housing crisis, among other things. Less frequently, *housing* preceded *association* to form the bigram, 'housing association', as well as following the keyword *social* to form the more general expression, 'social housing'. In the United Kingdom, housing associations are non-profit organisations that provide low-cost housing, also referred to as 'social housing', for people in need of a home. All occurrences of each of these bigrams are found in the *Guardian*. When analysed in context, we found that mentions of people living in social housing indexed people from lower income backgrounds.

> It was discovered last week that the world's heaviest man was not in America, the junk food and obesity capital of the world, but in a **housing** association bungalow in Ipswich eating takeaways and playing computer games.
>
> (*Guardian*, 25 October 2009)

On face value, the fact that the man referred to in this article lives in a 'housing association bungalow' has little to do with his weight. However, by mentioning it in this context, this aspect of his identity is implied to be relevant to his obesity, or at the very least is implied to be reportable. Mentions of social housing and housing associations are also frequently accompanied by other markers of lower income, and perhaps working class, identities. For example, in the extract just shown, we also learn that this man enjoys eating takeaways and playing video games. So the fact that he lives in social housing is not presented as the cause of his obesity per se, but it is one of a number of markers of his lower income identity, and we would argue that it is this very social inequality that is positioned as the overall determinant of obesity in these cases.

As well as using abstract terms like *inequality* and *poverty* in their accounts of the causes of obesity, the left-leaning broadsheets also related the causes of inequality – and, in turn, of obesity – to cuts in funding for certain public services implemented by various (mainly Conservative-led) governments across the time span of our corpus. This helps to account for the keyness of words denoting government, politicians and politics generally (i.e. *government*, *political*, *Cameron*, *coalition*, *politics*, *Labour*); the cuts themselves and the policies involved (*policy*, *cuts*); and the targets of those cuts (*public*, *sector*, *services*, *local*, *community*, *funding*). The newspapers in this section tended, perhaps unsurprisingly as left-leaning publications, to be critical of such cuts and the government/individuals who implemented them, as the representative example here demonstrates.

> Hundreds of children's playgrounds have been closed by **local** authorities across England thanks to "unprecedented budget constraints"

introduced by the **Conservative government**. [. . .] And the real figures
are likely to be higher still, with a third of councils still working out their
latest response to years of **funding cuts**. By the end of the decade,
authorities will have faced real-terms **cuts** of up to 30 billion since
2010. [. . .] Since 2010, 285 children's centres have closed or merged
and over the last three years over 82m has been cut from children's
centre budgets, while many other leisure **services** providing exercise and
outdoor air to children have also faced **cuts**. One in five children in their
last year of primary school are now obese, a figure which rises to one in
three if overweight children are included.

(*Independent*, 13 April 2017)

Relatedly, in 62 per cent of cases, the keyword *sport* was used in articles
criticising the lack of sport take-up among schoolchildren, which was linked to
rising rates of obesity and, in some cases, attributed to a lack of government
investment.

Heads fight back to stop cuts in school sports: Top teachers launch
broadside at death knell for the 162m School **Sport** Partnerships
Headteachers will launch a national revolt today against plans to cut
school **sport** as Michael Gove comes under intense pressure from inside
and outside government to rethink his plans.

(*Observer*, 28 November 2010)

Another keyword connected to government funding is *social*. This word is
used in a number of different ways, including in the bigram 'social care' (589).
Most frequently, this phrase occurs as part of proper nouns denoting organisations. However, the second most common pattern, found in 25 per cent of uses,
constituted discussions about the funding of social care in the context of public
health challenges, including obesity.

David Cameron must personally explain the steps he will take to bring
services back up to acceptable standards after taking **social care** support
away from hundreds of thousands of people.

(*Guardian*, 1 July 2015)

Like their right-leaning counterparts, the left-leaning broadsheets also
exhibited keywords denoting companies, such as *companies*, focussing in
particular on the fast food and so-called 'junk' food industries. However,
where food manufacturers tended to be presented positively in the right-
leaning broadsheets, the left-leaning newspapers adopted a more critical
stance, particularly in regard to the role that advertising targeted at children
played in increasing rates of childhood obesity, which is why *advertising* and
media also emerge as keywords for this section of the press.

A qualitative survey carried out by Cancer Research UK suggests that entertaining TV adverts for sweets, crisps and fast food have a real impact on primary school children, reinforcing the calls by health organ- isations for tougher **advertising** curbs in the forthcoming government childhood obesity strategy.

(*Guardian*, 5 July 2016)

This discourse is also evident in combined uses of the keywords *social* and *media* in the bigram 'social media' (501) in particular. This phrase was used in a wide range of senses. However, in 20 per cent of cases, the left-leaning broadsheets were critical about the role of social media advertising of junk food, especially that targeted at children, and supported a ban on this, for example describing the decision as a 'landmark' one in this extract.

Ban on junk food advertising aimed at children extended to online and **social media**; Changes bring print, cinema and online and **social media** into line with television, where strict regulation prohibits the advertising of unhealthy food to children; Junk food advertising is to be banned across all children's media – including online and social – in a landmark decision to help tackle childhood obesity.

(*Independent*, 8 December 2016)

As the previous extracts demonstrate, when the left-leaning broadsheets talk about these industries, they are also focussing – perhaps even more so – on the role of the Government and its perceived failure to properly regulate these types of goods and the ways they are manufactured, advertised and/or taxed. Consistent with this, the aforementioned political keywords also featured in articles which placed responsibility for responding to obesity at the feet of the Government, with the implication, and sometimes explicit imploration, that the Government should cease curbing its spending on public services and impose stricter regulations on the fast food and 'junk' food industries.

Another area of government intervention discussed by both the left- and right-leaning broadsheets was taxation (*tax*), and the 'sugar tax' (1,029) in particular. In 72 per cent of cases, these newspapers presented the sugar tax initiative in positive terms, including imploring the Government, and then- Prime Minister David Cameron in particular, to implement it (while the remaining 28 per cent gave a more balanced picture).

Current policies are ineffective and we urgently require policies that work. Unequivocal evidence from other countries has shown that a sugar **tax** duty on soft drinks will reduce sales of sugar-sweetened soft drinks, particularly among the more socially deprived who are more likely to develop obesity and type 2 diabetes. The **tax** will encourage behavioural change for those who drink sugar-sweetened soft drinks to either change to an artificially sweetened drink (which is lower in calories than sugar-sweetened) or to drink water – an even better option.

(Guardian, 21 January 2016)

Similar to uses of the keyword *sport*, another way in which the Government's role in curbing obesity rates by facilitating increased physical activity was mentioned was in relation to urban planning. In a sample of 100 articles containing the keywords *city* and/or *cities*, 22 per cent of cases attributed obesity to the planning of urban spaces in ways that made them more conducive to driving and using public transport as opposed to cycling or walking.

> This town will drag you down: UK's least healthy **cities**; PLANNING
> Dense housing linked to poor obesity scores.

(i, 30 January 2014)

To summarise, in this section we have seen how the left-leaning broadsheets are comparable to their right-leaning counterparts in the sense that both focus more than the right-leaning tabloids on the role that powerful institutions, such as the Government and certain food industries, play in contributing towards obesity rates, as well as the role that they do (or should) play in responding to these. However, a major difference is that where the right-leaning broadsheets are generally positive about the roles that these institutions play, the left-leaning broadsheets adopt a more critical stance, focussing, among other things, on what they perceive to be the detrimental effect of cuts in government spending on public services and a lack of both sufficient taxation and advertising restrictions on food and drink industries.

The left-leaning broadsheets are thus characterised by their representation of obesity as a social issue. This included grouping it with other social problems and framing it as being caused by social inequality. This in turn was attributed to cuts in spending on the welfare sector by (mainly Conservative-led) governments, who are also criticised for failing to clamp down on the fast food, 'junk' food and sugary drinks industries in terms of regulating their manufacturing and advertising and by imposing a so-called sugar tax. The Government was also responsibilised for rising obesity rates when it was accused of failing to design cities and urban spaces in ways that made them more conducive to cycling and walking rather than driving.

Tabloid Left

In the final part of this chapter, we turn our attention to the remaining section of the press: the left-leaning tabloids. Before proceeding further, we need to note that we carried out the analysis of this sub-corpus in a slightly different way to the previous sections. The Tabloid Left section consists of articles

Table 3.4. *Top 50* Mirror *keywords, ranked by log-likelihood (frequencies in brackets)*

I (27,196), *she* (12,865), *her* (11,889), *stone* (2,866), *mum* (1,529), *my* (7,842), *was* (16,401), *weight* (7,008), *after* (5,640), *Katie* (619), *size* (2,169), *'d* (2,079), *me* (4,100), *n't* (8,650), *your* (5,586), *lost* (1,604), *now* (4,374), *kids* (1,208), *slimming* (540), *incredible* (368), *Hopkins* (311), *sheds* (230), *had* (6,178), *dad* (461), *losing* (824), *crisps* (566), *shed* (574), *started* (1,123), *myself* (881), *amazing* (417), *weighed* (601), *obese* (3,329), *got* (1,531), *so* (5,750), *star* (644), *lose* (1,577), *transformation* (265), *felt* (855), *gastric* (652), *dress* (494), *just* (4,168), *him* (2,086), *10* (1,463), *day* (3,279), *mum-of-two* (87), *'ve* (1,845), *'m* (1,912), *but* (11,204), *get* (3,380), *when* (5,678)

---

published by two newspapers, the *Mirror* and *Morning Star*. However, the overwhelming majority of texts (95.7 per cent) and words (97.2 per cent) in this section are from the *Mirror*. By comparison, other sub-corpora made up of two newspapers are much more evenly balanced. Namely, the Broadsheet Right section (*Telegraph* and *Times*) takes 59 per cent of texts and 55.6 per cent of words from the *Telegraph*, while the Broadsheet Left sub-corpus (*Guardian* and *Independent* (including *i*)) takes 53.6 per cent of its texts and 61.3 per cent of words from the *Guardian*.

This great imbalance in the Tabloid Left section means that the keywords obtained from this corpus are more likely to represent the *Mirror* than the *Morning Star*. Therefore, for this part of the analysis we treated the *Mirror* and the *Morning Star* as separate datasets, comparing each newspaper separately against all of the others in the corpus.

Beginning with the *Mirror*, Table 3.4 shows the top fifty keywords for this newspaper compared against all other newspapers in the corpus (including the *Morning Star*).

Strikingly, most of the keywords from the *Mirror* contribute towards narratives of weight loss, the likes of which we observed in the right-leaning tabloids earlier in this chapter. This includes pronouns indicating both first- and third-person perspectives (i.e. *I, she, her, him, my, myself* and *me*), as well as contractions (*n't,'ve,'d* and*'m*), which also reflect a more informal tabloid style, as well as verbs denoting weight loss (*lost, lose, shed, sheds*), ways of measuring weight loss (*stone, size, dress*) and adverbial keywords which help to sequence the events in the narratives (*after, now*). As in the right-leaning tabloids, these narratives also tended to focus on women, reflected in gender-marked pronoun keywords (*she, her*) and the keywords *mum* and *mum-of-two*, which tend to describe the women at the centre of these narratives (77 per cent of cases). Also similar to the right-leaning tabloids, the individuals at the heart of these narratives are overwhelmingly evaluated positively, which results in weight loss being labelled using the keyword *transformation* and described using keywords like *amazing* and *incredible*.

> An obese single **mum** has revealed her **incredible weight loss** after admitting **she** was struggling to keep up with **her** disabled son and shedding more than nine stone.
>
> (*Mirror*, 25 September 2016)

Over half of the uses of the keyword *slimming* feature in the bigram 'Slimming World' (342), referring to a UK-based weight loss organisation that provides weight loss management programmes to its members. Slimming World tends to be mentioned in one of two ways in the *Mirror*. Most commonly (91 per cent), the organisation functions as a turning point in weight loss narratives, with the act of individuals joining being framed positively as a catalyst for their subsequent weight loss.

> She also confessed that she was a serial yo-yo dieter and that her weight would fluctuate up to 13 stone, meaning she had to pick out a size 18 wedding gown last year. But now, after a year at **Slimming World**, Gemma was able to surprise her loved ones at her wedding this June to fiance James with her new svelte size eight frame.
>
> (*Mirror*, 29 December 2014)

Less frequently, Slimming World employees are quoted as part of advice-giving passages, as in this extract from an article advising about the difficulties of losing weight following pregnancy.

> Lynda Thwaites, a **Slimming World** consultant for 13 years, said that it's better not to gain too much weight in pregnancy because it can prove difficult to lose afterwards.
>
> (*Mirror*, 7 June 2015)

Monaghan (2008) argues that weight loss organisations like Slimming World are underpinned by a neoliberal logic which positions members as rational individuals who act in the interests of preserving their health. By framing positively evaluated weight loss narratives as hinging on the membership of such clubs, and by quoting representatives from these organisations for the purposes of giving weight loss advice, the *Mirror* can be viewed as upholding this responsibilising model of obesity risk management. This is also accomplished through the second-person possessive pronoun keyword *your*, with readers addressed directly with advice about obesity risk management.

> But without the recommended 150 minutes of physical activity every week you increase **your** risk of obesity, depression, heart disease and Type 2 diabetes.
>
> (*Mirror*, 27 December 2016)

As well as denoting readers' risk of obesity, the keyword *your* also directly preceded words denoting children, including *child* (121), *children* (48) and the keyword *kids* (56). In these cases, readers, who are assumed to be parents, were advised on how best to manage their children's risk of developing obesity. In most cases (54 per cent), this manifested in advice on what parents should and should not allow their children to eat, including giving tips on how to wean them off their favourite unhealthy drinks and snacks. The implication underlying such advice-giving passages is that parents are responsible for managing their children's health and that responsible parents will not allow their children to develop obesity (Brookes et al. 2016). However, a corollary of this is that the opposite is also true, and not effectively managing your child's risk of obesity can leave readers open to the accusation that they are irresponsible or 'bad' parents.

> Giving **your** kids a bad diet is a form of child abuse; Alison Phillips is mortified that a five-year-old girl was allowed to balloon in weight to 10st – and says the parents don't deserve her
>
> *(Mirror*, 10 December 2013)

Both weight loss narratives and the intersection of discourses around parenthood (particularly motherhood) and obesity are explored in more detail in Chapter 7. For now, we want to note the parallels between the *Mirror* and the tabloids on the other side of the political spectrum, both of which can be characterised in terms of their emphasis on conveying to readers the sense in which they are personally responsible for managing their obesity risk, with weight loss narratives serving as a rhetorical device through which individuals who have perfected this bodily project by losing weight are positively evaluated and presented to readers almost as role models.

We now turn our attention to the other left-leaning tabloid and the final newspaper analysed in this chapter: the *Morning Star*. The keywords for this newspaper, compared against all the other newspapers in the corpus combined (including the *Mirror*), are presented in Table 3.5.

Similarly to the (particularly left-leaning) broadsheets, the *Morning Star* contained a number of political keywords, specifically *Labour*, *government*, *Tory*, *neoliberal* and *minister*, as well as names of politicians: (Margaret) *Thatcher*, (Liam) *Fox*, (Alan) *Milburn*, (Michael) Gove, (Patricia) *Hewitt* and (Caroline) *Flint*. Analysing samples of articles mentioning these terms, we observed that the *Morning Star* was more explicitly partisan than both the *Mirror* and the left-leaning broadsheets studied earlier. For example, the *Labour* Party was generally represented in a positive way as being proactive in responding to (particularly childhood) obesity, while Conservative(-led) or *Tory* governments were consistently represented as not doing enough in this regard and in some cases as undoing what is perceived to be good work done by previous Labour governments.

Table 3.5. *Top 50 keywords for the* Morning Star, *ranked by log-likelihood (frequencies in brackets)*

Labour (100), *government* (163), *Britain* (138), *Milburn* (19), *Krave* (14), *GMB* (15), *firm* (42), *placement* (20), *Carillion* (11), *gross* (22), *Kellogg* (25), *yesterday* (51), *Hertz* (9), *union* (33), *Tarmac* (13), *the* (3,145), *Flint* (15), *midwives* (28), *Unison* (13), *workers* (41), *secretary* (44), *Tory* (34), *capitalism* (17), *Thatcher* (19), *privatisation* (13), *education* (48), *Dyson* (9), *Fox* (19), *Hewitt* (10), *Gove* (20), *trade* (25), *department* (42), *Afghan* (10), *Bridgepoint* (7), *council* (42), *NHS* (110), *Cuba* (11), *corporations* (14), *health* (243), *academies* (14), *poverty* (27), *Rotherham* (13), *Labute* (8), *cuts* (32), *argued* (19), *neoliberal* (7), *minister* (40), *Solomon* (8), *schools* (51), *food* (190)

> Tories are taking food out of our children's mouths; This is said to be in defiance of initiatives and plans set in place by the **Labour** government [. . .] Yet again the coalition Tory-run government is playing political football when our children's health is in the balance.
>
> (*Morning Star*, 9 July 2012)

The Labour party wasn't always depicted positively, though, and politicians associated with the 'New Labour' movement received more negative evaluation, seemingly for its economically liberal policies, including privatising public services. Such policies were framed as benefiting capitalist institutions and big businesses, thereby running up against the *Morning Star*'s traditional socialist values, and as contributing to social inequality and obesity.

> Those at the "top" of society still take too much of a slice of Britain's wealth. But does this matter? Some in new **Labour** think not. Yet evidence that income inequality affects society is out there. The recent book The Spirit Level by Kate Pickett and Richard Wilkinson showed how very unequal societies damage our physical and mental health, as well as increasing obesity and teenage pregnancies.
>
> (*Morning Star*, 26 February 2010)

This rhetoric was applied not just to the Labour party itself but also to individual MPs who were evaluated negatively for not imposing stringent enough restrictions on big industries, including 'junk' food and sugary drinks manufacturers. This included Caroline *Flint* and Alan *Milburn*.

> **Flint**'s old ministerial brief included grappling with obesity. She had to decide whether junk food firms needed more regulation. In 2006, I sat in a fringe meeting at the Labour Party conference organised by the Smith Institute, a "think tank" which is very close to Gordon Brown. The Food Advertising Unit, "a coalition of food and soft drink advertisers," funded

the meeting. The chairperson gave a grovelling thanks to these junk-food pushers at the start of the meeting.

(Morning Star, 15 February 2008)

This example touches on other themes indicated by the keywords in Table 3.5, including the role of food and drink manufacturers in contributing to rising rates of obesity. The breakfast cereal manufacturer *Kellogg*'s, and in particular one of its products, *Krave*, come in for particular criticism. Consistent with the political keywords, the specific target of this criticism was not the sugar content of these products per se but rather the involvement of this company in New Labour's anti-obesity public health initiatives.

> **Kellogg**'s: a taste of dog farts; Solomon Hughes explains how the government's big anti-obesity drive is being undermined by the involvement of big business **Kellogg**'s is a "partner" in a Department of Health anti-obesity drive. And it is just about to launch a campaign to persuade young people to chomp through **Krave**, one of the most calorific breakfast cereals available. **Kellogg**'s is part of the Department of Health's Change4Life campaign. The cereal firm funds a few breakfast and swimming clubs and puts out the odd advert telling people to "move more."
>
> *(Morning Star*, 19 February 2010)

The keyword *placement* arises through criticism of New Labour for not doing enough to prevent product placement on television and is thus comparable to the left-leaning broadsheets (except that the target of the ire here is not just Conservative-led governments but also New Labour's).

> Product **placement** only helps the big global players, as they are the only ones who can afford the high advertising fees. Because of vociferous opposition by organisations like the British Medical Association as well as by individuals, the government has been forced to backtrack a little and now says it will not be allowing alcoholic drinks, over-the-counter medicines or junk food to be advertised in this way.
>
> *(Morning Star*, 8 February 2010)

Another theme indicated by the keywords is the *Morning Star*'s critical stance on the involvement of private industries in healthcare. Articles using terms like *firm*, *Carillion* and *Tarmac* (where the latter two refer to specific private companies involved in healthcare delivery) consistently construct the interests of these corporations as being in opposition to those of the public's health and the *NHS*, which is another keyword in this newspaper.

> Right now we are hearing a lot about the unreasonable "demands" sick people make on the **NHS** – according to all kinds of "experts" all those

old folk and obese people put too much "pressure" on the **NHS**, so there must be cuts or an end to free services. But the demands of big corporations on the **NHS** are ignored. Since PFI came in the **NHS** has been made to look after the financial health of big corporations as well as patients. **Tarmac** seems much keener on the new financial engineering than old fashioned building engineering.

(Morning Star, 14 March 2013)

Another keyword related to healthcare services is *midwives*. This keyword tends to be used in articles expressing concern about midwives' working conditions. In the example that follows, this is linked to more complex births resulting from mothers having obesity.

General secretary Cathy Warwick said: "As a result of the increase in obesity among pregnant women in the UK, **midwives** are dealing with more complex births – on top of the continuing baby boom. **Midwives** need more time to spend with these women to help and advise them. NHS trusts should be making sure that they have the resources in place to do this."

(Morning Star, 15 November 2010)

This foregrounding of concern about workers is also evident in the keyword *workers* as well as in keywords denoting unions: *GMB, union* and *Unison*. Where other sections of the press published quotes from and interviews with, *inter alia*, scientists, politicians and public health officials, the *Morning Star* can instead be characterised by its dedicating page space to the views of these unions and sometimes even workers themselves, such as in these extracts, which are taken from articles which report on the introduction of schemes focussing on weighing schoolchildren and giving them free school meals. In these cases, the newspaper's respective negative and positive evaluation of these schemes are supported with, and perhaps even derive from, the views of the Unite and GMB unions, as well as school kitchen workers.

Weighing schoolkids a waste of money, warns Unite; Weighing and measuring children when they enter and leave primary school is a waste of public money, as it is not tackling the obesity epidemic in England, the Unite **union** warned yesterday.

(Morning Star, 15 December 2008)

Britain – School kitchen **workers** back 20m free school meals plan; School catering staff welcomed a government pilot scheme to provide free school meals to all primary school children yesterday. General **union** GMB, which represents 100,000 school staff, including most catering **workers**, welcomed the announcement, which will involve a series of regional pilots to evaluate the effectiveness of free school meals for primary school pupils.

(*Morning Star*, 25 September 2008)

Compared side-by-side, the differences in the keywords and attendant representations between the *Mirror* and *Morning Star* justify our decision to approach these newspapers separately. The *Mirror* is characterised by keywords which tend to feature in the context of weight loss narratives, along with second-person pronouns indicating instances of direct audience address, wherein the newspaper advises readers on how to manage their and their children's obesity risk. In these respects, the *Mirror* is similar to the right-leaning tabloids, whose keywords indicated a similar proclivity for narratives and responsibilising, reader-directed health implorations. These features, therefore, appear to be characteristic of tabloid rhetoric and obesity discourse, and seemingly transcend the traditional political dividing lines between newspapers published in this format. The *Morning Star*, on the other hand, is more comparable to the left-leaning broadsheets in its focus on obesity as something that results from the actions (and inaction) of powerful institutions. Similarities here include the criticism of fast food, 'junk' food and sugary drinks manufacturers, as well as the Government for failing to regulate these in terms of curbing or restricting advertising directed at children. However, the *Morning Star* was more openly critical of New Labour, as well as of (healthcare) privatisation and (New Labour) politicians' involvement in large corporations linked to rising obesity rates (e.g. breakfast cereal manufacturers and fast food companies). A further distinction between the *Morning Star* and other newspapers was that it presents issues, including government anti-obesity measures, from the perspective of unions and workers, such as midwives and school kitchen staff, through quotations and interviews which accordingly privilege those perspectives.

Conclusion

Using keywords as its starting point, the analysis in this chapter has explored what is linguistically characteristic about obesity coverage in different sections of the press. Although our analysis was trained mostly on differences, it also uncovered some similarities and overlaps. Moreover, some of the themes we have identified through the keywords echo some of the findings based on the shared keywords studied in the previous chapter, with certain shared themes emerging as particularly prominent in certain newspapers and parts of the press. For example, personal responsibility was a general theme and we found that this was particularly prominent in the tabloids (excluding the *Morning Star*). We also found a new way in which this manifested, namely through the use of weight loss narratives which told positive, even glorifying, stories about people who have lost large amounts of weight through diet while publishing more scornful stories about people who have lost weight through surgical means, particularly if these were taxpayer-funded. Perhaps this is because individuals pursuing surgical weight loss are perceived by these newspapers to represent the antithesis of the 'good' neoliberal subject. Rather than eradicating obesity through diet and exercise, they are instead portrayed as burdening the healthcare system and taxpayers by relying on state-funded operations. These stories therefore constitute another manifestation of the neoliberal model of obesity risk management. In the previous chapter, we argued the emergence of this feature across all sections of the press to be evidence of the pervasiveness of this mentality in UK society as a whole, to the extent that where it was previously associated with the political right, it now seems to transcend traditional political divides (at least in the media). The appearance of weight loss narratives in left- and right-leaning newspapers in this chapter supports this interpretation. However, the genre of the weight loss narrative is particularly common in the tabloids, where it could be viewed as a symptom of the format's more sensationalist style (the people at the centre of these narratives are typically extreme cases), as well as its tendency to focus more than the broadsheets on stories about individuals and particularly celebrities.

In the previous chapter, we saw how obesity and people with it could be framed as a burden on the NHS. The construction of people with obesity as an economic burden occurred across the whole press. However, its marked frequency in the right-leaning press in particular could reflect the individualistic and economically liberal values that are associated with these newspapers. On the other hand, the left-leaning broadsheets can be characterised by their framing of obesity as a social issue by likening it to problems like climate change and the country's housing crisis. For them, obesity is caused not (just) by individuals' lifestyle choices but by broader social issues, like inequality.

A political distinction was also apparent in the newspapers' treatment of powerful institutions that were perceived to have some responsibility for the population's obesity rates. Unlike the tabloids (except the *Morning Star*), the broadsheets were all likely to report on the role and activities of powerful industries, including the Government, food and drink industries and sports organisations like the FA. Consistent with their support for the Conservative party and favourable stance on businesses, the right-leaning newspapers tended to offer more positive representations of these institutions, presenting them as responding proactively to rising obesity rates. The left-leaning publications, on the other hand, adopted a more critical perspective, with obesity levels linked to government spending cuts; weak regulation of food and drink industries; and urban planning that makes driving more convenient than physically active alternatives like walking and cycling. This politicising perspective on obesity was particularly characteristic of the *Morning Star*, which was critical of the economically liberal policies of the Conservatives but also New Labour, whose MPs were negatively evaluated for their ties to private corporations. In the *Morning Star* and the left-leaning broadsheets, then, obesity is presented a form of health inequality which results from a broader kind of social inequality. For the *Morning Star* in particular, this seems to be caused (or at least exacerbated) by what it perceives to be the privileging of corporate capitalist interests over those of public health.

The different representations of obesity offered across these distinct sections of the press are likely the result of coverage being designed for each newspaper's target, 'imagined' readerships. The preceding paragraphs have highlighted some of the ways in which we have interpreted obesity coverage to be shaped by the political values of each newspaper (and thus those of their perceived audiences). The focus on obesity as a cause of certain diseases in the right-leaning tabloids could be intended by these newspapers to grant stories more relevance to their likely older audiences,[1] who are disproportionately affected by these health issues. Meanwhile, on the other side of the political spectrum, the 'imagined' socialist readership of the *Morning Star* will likely be sympathetic towards the newspaper's disdain for corporate capitalist institutions and share in its interest in how obesity-related initiatives affect and are perceived by trade unions and workers. So, the various representations identified in this chapter, both distinct and overlapping, could be explained by the newspapers' political leanings and formats but also their values and those which they attribute to their perceived readers. If the media does indeed have the power to shape health-related attitudes, beliefs and behaviours, then the differences across the various sections of the press identified in this chapter could result in the different audiences that each section (and newspaper) reaches accessing different perspectives on obesity. It is beyond the scope of this book to explore empirically how individuals' beliefs and actions could be shaped by the press's obesity discourses (though we do begin to consider this question through our analysis of readers' comments in Chapter 9). However, the marked presence of neoliberal, responsibilising discourses around obesity across most of the tabloids relative to the remainder of the press could be problematic when we bear in mind their generally lower-income readerships (see Chapter 8). Research suggests that individualised approaches to addressing health problems are likely to be less successful with low-income individuals because the emphasis on personal behaviour usually fails to grasp that, when people engage in activities that might be perceived as damaging towards

---

[1] www.inter-media.co.uk/uk-newspapers-reveal-readership-demographics/

their health, it is not necessarily due to lack of awareness but usually has more to do with the fact that the constraints of their life experiences and environments render them *unable* to change those behaviours (Anthony et al. 2004). Given that such nuance appears to be absent from obesity coverage in most of the tabloids, as well as other sections of the press, then we could argue that the perpetuation of such discourses is unlikely to motivate positive health behaviours in readers but, rather, is more likely contribute to the shaming and stigmatisation of an already relatively disempowered group within society. We will explore potentially shaming and stigmatising discourses in Chapter 5 and discuss their ramifications in detail in Chapter 10.

4   Change over Time

Introduction

The corpus of news articles we collected spans a ten-year period, from the start of 2008 to the end of 2017. These start and end dates were somewhat opportunistic. We could only collect articles up until the point at which our research began (2017) and the decision to go back ten years involved covering a period which would allow us to identify a meaningful picture of change or stability over time while not taking on an unmanageable amount of work. Furthermore, the online news archive we were using had somewhat patchier coverage for some newspapers when we tried to obtain articles from the 1990s, so we could not go too far back in any case. The choice of 2008 could thus be seen as rather arbitrary, simply allowing us to say we collected a decade's worth of data. However, there are two other important reasons why this date was chosen, one political and the other statistical.

The political reason relates to the start date being linked to a major economic event which precipitated UK Government policy for the following decade. During 2007–2008, a global financial crisis occurred. It started with the subprime mortgage market in the United States and resulted in the collapse of investment banks such as Lehman Brothers which had taken excessive financial risks. The crisis spread to Asian and European markets, triggering a global economic downturn which was subsequently referred to as the Great Recession. In the United Kingdom, Gross Domestic Product saw negative growth for the last three quarters of 2008 (a recession is normally defined as two successive quarters of negative growth). The Royal Bank of Scotland, Lloyds TSB and HBOS had to be bailed out by the Government, using taxpayers' money. Two years following the recession, the new Conservative–Liberal Democrat coalition government adopted a controversial policy of austerity, intended to decrease the government budget deficit by reducing the role of the welfare state in people's lives. The austerity programme was upheld until well after 2017.

The statistical reason for our 2008 start date relates to how the proportion of people in the United Kingdom who are defined as overweight or obese has changed over time. Data tends to be made available separately for England, Scotland, Wales and Northern Ireland, and although there are slight differences between them, they follow a similar pattern. In 1993, 15 per cent of adults in England were classed as having obesity. This figure had risen to 26 per cent by 2016, although, at the time of writing, it has remained at a similar level since 2010 (National Statistics 2018: 2). Data from the Health Survey for England found that, in fact, between 2006 and 2016 there was actually little change in the proportion of adults in England who could be diagnosed either as over-weight or as having obesity (Baker 2019: 4), comprising 64.3 per cent of people in a 2017 survey. Self-reported data from the National Survey for Wales gave 59 per cent of people as overweight or having obesity in 2018/19 (*ibid.*: 14). A Scottish health survey in 2017 put 65 per cent of people as overweight or having obesity, with the most notable recent change being a 3 per cent rise between 2003 and 2008 (Scottish Government 2017: 4), while a similar survey for Northern Ireland put this figure at 62 per cent in 2018/19 (Corrigan and Scarlett 2020: 6). The data points to an increase in terms of numbers of people who can be classed as being overweight or having obesity between 1993 and 2006–2008 but this figure has levelled off since that point. Thus, the period we analyse (2008–2017) is one of relative stability in terms of numbers of people with obesity and overweight across the United Kingdom, as well as one characterised by economic austerity and governments seeking to reduce spending on welfare.

In this chapter, we take two perspectives on change over time, one which is perhaps more obvious than the other. We begin by considering year-on-year change across the whole corpus, identifying keywords that are distinctive of each year, grouping them into thematic categories and then noting which categories have risen or fallen over time. This is a necessarily broad-brush approach, lending us an overview on the changing linguistic contexts in which obesity has been discussed over time. Following the analysis in the previous two chapters, we are most interested in considering the discourses used to frame obesity in terms of explanatory models (i.e. in terms of personal responsibility, a bio-medical model or as a result of societal factors).

The second perspective on change over time relates to the sense of the annual news cycle, considering how, month-by-month, the same events occur each year (e.g. Christmas is always in December) and how this cycle of events influences how obesity is reported on a month-by-month basis. Here, news values such as meaningfulness and consonance can come into play, with newspapers keying into familiar, predictable events and filtering their stories about obesity through these. While the month-by-month comparison shows less overall variation than the year-by-year comparison, it does indicate an additional level of variation which potentially complicates the overall picture. We begin, though, by looking at changes year-on-year.

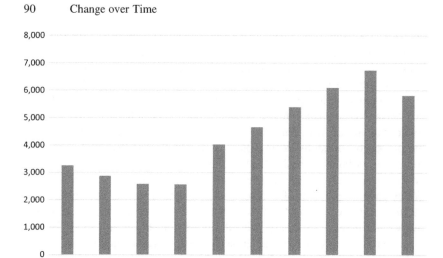

Figure 4.1 Number of articles published about obesity per year

Changing Keywords over Time

Figure 4.1 shows the number of articles containing the words *obese* and/or *obesity* that were published in the British national press in each year between 2008 and 2017. While the topic appears to have slightly decreased in importance between 2008 and 2011, there is then a sharper rise from that point, with more than double the number of articles on obesity being published in 2016 compared to 2011. Considering that rates of overweight and obesity remained pretty stable in the United Kingdom during the period we consider, the marked rise in stories about this topic between 2011 and 2016 is worth noting. There is a dip between 2016 and 2017, making it unclear whether interest in the topic has peaked or whether this is a brief blip in the upward trend. It is certainly the case that the latter half of our corpus contains more data than the first half. The period 2008–2012 produced 12,003,951 words of articles about obesity, while there was double this amount, 24,049,235 words, in the period 2013–2017. This is an important point to consider over the entire book, as it means that language use occurring in the second half of our corpus is twice as likely as that in the first half to influence the general patterns reported.

The rise in the number of articles is likely to indicate that obesity has increasingly been viewed as a newsworthy topic for the British press (at least between 2011 and 2016). For this reason, it is likely that if we simply compare word frequencies across different periods, we will find that most words will have increased over time too. For example, in 2008 the British press used the phrase *obesity epidemic* 200 times, although this had increased to 335 cases by 2017. However, it is useful to take into account proportional frequencies, asking, of the amount of discussion around obesity in a given year, how much space was devoted to the concept of an obesity epidemic? The year 2008 saw 2.4 million words written about obesity, while there were 4.8 million words in 2017. Proportionally, then, *obesity epidemic* occurred 82.21 times per million words (PMW) in 2008 and 69.03 times PWM in 2017. Thus, the phrase *obesity epidemic* may have occurred more often in 2017 but in terms of the scale of the focus, compared to other ways of thinking about obesity, it was not as common as in 2008.

So, we begin the analysis in this chapter by considering how the language used in the articles in our corpus changed over time, in terms of the proportion of the discussion. To do this, we derived a list of keywords for the whole corpus and then examined how their relative frequencies changed over time. We could compare our obesity news corpus against a larger reference corpus such as the 100 million-word BNC, as we did in Chapter 2. However, since most of the articles in our corpus were published from 2013 onwards, the language appearing in these later texts would be disproportionately represented, while words that were only common in the earlier parts of the corpus would be unlikely to appear as keywords. For the purpose of analysing change in language over time, this is not ideal. Therefore, we tried another approach, which was to identify sets of keywords for each year of the corpus separately by comparing each year against the remaining years in the news corpus (the remainder method discussed in the previous chapter). For example, we first obtained keywords for 2008 by using years 2009–2017 as the reference corpus, then we acquired the keywords for 2009 by using 2008 plus 2010–2017 as the reference corpus, and so on. We initially considered every keyword produced by *CQPweb* but found that, due to the differing sizes of the annual sub-corpora, the later years produced more keywords than the earlier ones. In order not to give undue priority to the later period, we took 100 keywords from each annual sub-corpus. Experimenting with ordering the keywords according to different measures (e.g. log-likelihood, log-ratio) resulted in some cases where very low frequency keywords were prioritised. To focus on what were the largest amounts of change over time, we ordered the keywords in terms of frequency and removed grammatical items such as *the* and *of*. This resulted in 1,000 keywords (i.e. 100 for each year), although some were repeated, being key in two or three years. We only counted repeated cases of keywords once, meaning we removed 255 words from the list, resulting in 745 keywords.

These keywords were then grouped according to the themes or concepts that they referred to. This was done by the analysts in a bottom-up way, rather than beginning with a pre-defined set of categories or using a pre-existing categorisation set such as those provided by semantic taggers (e.g. the USAS tagger built into *Wmatrix* (Rayson 2008)). Automatic taggers tend to categorise words based on their surface meanings and do not always fully take into account the context that a word occurs in. For example, one category we created was ILLNESS, to which we assigned keywords such as *cancer, diabetes* and *inflammation*. However, we also included words such as *heart* and *liver* in this category because, even though they appear to be words that refer to body parts, when we examined how they were used in the context of articles about obesity we found that they tended to refer to how obesity can cause illnesses such as heart and liver disease (as we have seen in Chapters 2 and 3). However, we did not class the word *epidemic* as ILLNESS, even though it would appear to refer to this topic, because it was almost always used metaphorically to refer to the 'obesity epidemic', used in reference to increases in rates of obesity. For this reason, we assigned *epidemic* to the category PROBLEM, alongside words such as *risk, crisis* and *problem*.

Classifying the keywords involved examining 100 random cases of each and identifying their most typical uses. Not all words could be easily categorised in this way and so we discarded 131 keywords, either because they had several meanings, with none that stood out as especially frequent, or because to include them would have resulted in the creation of a category containing only one or two words, which would result in an unhelpful proliferation of categories. To account for the different amounts of data for each year, we compare relative frequencies based on occurrences PMW. And to narrow our focus further, we decided to only consider categories where the keywords within them collectively appeared at least 1,000 times PMW in at least one year of the dataset, resulting in the removal of a further 306 keywords. This resulted in a total of 439 keywords spread across a set of twenty-seven categories, shown in Table 4.1.

Table 4.1 shows some quite large differences in the overall frequencies of the keywords in each category. For example, keywords referring to FOOD occur 448,536 times across the whole corpus, while those relating to SOCIAL appear only 28,283 times. As Table 4.1 stands, this gives us a sense of how some ways of discussing obesity are more common in the press than others, with discussion of food, measurement and scientific research being highly frequent, and mentions of places outside the United Kingdom, collective efforts to reduce obesity and social issues being much less frequent. These patterns are consistent with what we have seen in Chapters 2 and 3. However, we can take this analysis further and examine the extent to which these categories change in relative frequency over time.

Figure 4.2 takes the relative frequencies (PMW) of the keywords belonging to the most common category, FOOD, plotted as a bar chart for each year.

Table 4.1. *Main categories of language use in news articles about obesity*

Category	Relation to obesity	Keywords	Total frequency
FOOD	Eating practices that can raise or reduce levels of obesity	*added, allowance, beer, beverages, binge, biscuits, bottles, breakfast, caffeine, cereal, chocolate, Coca-Cola, consumption, corn, diet, diets, dinner, drink, drinks, Dukan, eat, fasting, fizzy, fish, foie, food, foods, fructose, fruit, gras, honey, intake, juice, juices, junk, lunch, lunches, meals, milk, nutrition, oil, pies, processed, products, protein, soda, soft, soya, Stevia, sugar, sugars, sugary, takeaway, takeaways, teaspoons, trans, unhealthy, water*	448,536
MEASUREMENT	Ways of measuring weight	*19st, 1st, 4lb, amount, BMI, calories, high, higher, increase, increased, less, levels, low, lower, size, stone, weighed, weight,*	304,866
RESEARCH	Scientific research relating to obesity	*according, AstraZeneca, claims, data, evidence, experts, findings, found, professor, published, report, research, researchers, science, scientists, studies, study, university, Warwick*	261,555
ILLNESS	Health issues which result in obesity or are caused by obesity	*anorexia, apnoea, breast, cancer, condition, death, decay, dementia, diabetes, die, disease, flu, gallstones, gout, heart, hip, inflammation, liver, migraines, osteoarthritis, rickets, swine, symptoms, type, virus*	202,263
WEIGHT	Labels relating to weight	*fat, fattest, obese, obesity, overweight, plump, plus-size, thin*	180,570
QUOTATIVES	Statements made by relevant social actors relating to obesity	*said, says, told*	169,959
PLACES (UK)	The context of obesity in the UK	*Britain, British, country, English, Glasgow, Hull, Jersey, Leeds, London, nation, north, Scotland, Scots, Scottish, town, U.K., UK, west*	118,710

Table 4.1. *(cont.)*

Category	Relation to obesity	Keywords	Total frequency
CHILDREN	Stories focussing on childhood obesity	*child, childhood, children, kids, paediatric, puberty, teenage, teenager, youngsters*	101,980
HEALTHCARE	The role of healthcare in reducing obesity	*consultant, Dr, GPs, hospital, NHS, nurse, patients, PCT, PHE, trusts,*	94,031
BIOLOGY	Describes potential causes of obesity	*brain, blood, body, cells, cholesterol, genes, genetic, genetics, genome, knee, leptin, skin, oestrogen, telomeres, testosterone, uric*	92,273
SPORT	How physical exercise can reduce obesity	*athletes, athletics, ball, competitive, cricket, cycling, cyclists, dance, dancing, exercise, FA, fitness, football, game, games, medal, medals, Olympic, Olympics, PE, players, playing, rugby, sport, sporting, sports, stadium, swimming, team, teams, yoga*	91,107
WOMEN	How obesity specifically relates to women	*Dame, daughter, girls, lady, mum, Mrs, Ms, sister, woman, women*	84,987
POLITICS (UK)	The effect of politics on obesity levels	*budget, coalition, council, cuts, department, government, Labour, Liberal, minister, ministers, MPs, parties, party, political, secretary, ruling, tax, Tory, UKIP*	90,438
PROBLEM	Obesity represented as bad	*epidemic, crisis, inadequate, problem, risk, wrong*	72,275
WEIGHT LOSS	Losing weight	*anti-obesity, goal, lose, losing, loss, lost, reduce, watchers, weight-loss*	69,439
TV, FILM & ARTS	Representations of obesity in the media	*Aladdin, art, BBC, BBC2, Bloomburg, Bond, book, bookshop, channel, character, comedy, drama, DVD, film, films, gallery, magazine, movie, music, novel, paintings, programme, RRP, Sky, talent, television, tv*	63,950

Table 4.1. *(cont.)*

Category	Relation to obesity	Keywords	Total frequency
ECONOMICS	The financial aspects of obesity	*annuity, credit, cut, debt, deficit, economic, Euro, funding, GB, GBP, money, pounds, prices, recession, sales, saving, spending*	55,175
EDUCATION	The role of education in raising or reducing levels of obesity	*academies, class, curriculum, education, pupils, school, schools, secondary, teacher, teachers*	52,949
PLACES (NON-UK)	The context of obesity outside the UK	*Africa, America, Angeles, Australian, countries, Denmark, EU, Europe, Eurozone, France, French, Georgia, Ireland, Irish, Los, Mexico, Pakistan, Samoa, States, U.S., Washington, York*	48,934
HELP	Advice and help to lose weight	*advice, guidance, guidelines, help*	42,509
BUSINESS	The potential influence of business in causing obesity	*Amazon, Boots, commercial, company, customers, Disney, firm, Ford, industry, Kellogg, market, placement, private, profits, sponsors, sponsorship, Subway, Tesco*	36,703
RESPONSE	Collective efforts to reduce obesity	*action, campaign, change, counter, labels, nudge, recommendations, reforms, strategy*	35,716
MEDICINE	The effect of medicine on obesity	*antibiotics, Aspirin, drug, drugs, pill, pills, statins, treatment*	34,207
LIFESTYLE	Non-food related behavioural choices related to weight	*behaviour, gardening, lifestyle, meditation, sleep, tobacco*	33,078
CAUSES	General words indicating causes	*associated, cause, linked, related*	30,106
SOCIAL	How social issues impact on obesity levels	*benefits, crime, culture, discrimination, inequality, middle-class, poverty, societies, society, unemployment*	28,283
MATERNITY	The impact of obesity on having a baby	*babies, baby, birth, caesarean, childbirth, maternity, midwife, midwives, stillbirth*	24,611

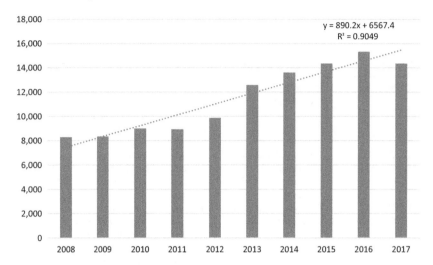

Figure 4.2 Relative frequencies (PMW) and trend line for the FOOD category over time

Generally, the relative frequencies rise over time. The straight line, which represents the trend line, shows this more clearly. The trend line is a line which best fits all the data points at once. It can be represented as the equation $y = mx + b$ for which m is the slope or gradient, b is the y intercept, x is any x value and y is any y value. In Figure 4.2, the formula is $y = 890.2x + 6\,567.4$, meaning that the slope is 890.2. The further away the number is from 0, the steeper the slope. An R^2 value is also provided for each trend line. This is a number between 0 and 1 which measures the amount of difference between the actual values and the line that was fitted to them. A low R^2 value (close to 0) indicates that the measurements do not fall in a straight line, while a high R^2 value (close to 1) indicates that they do. The R^2 value thus gives an indication of the reliability of the trend line.

We plotted trend lines for each of the twenty-seven categories in Table 4.1, the equations of which are shown in Table 4.2. Sixteen categories had a positive gradient, which indicates that these sets of keywords increased in relative frequency over time. However, eleven categories had a negative gradient, indicating a relative decrease in frequency over time. Table 4.2 also shows the R^2 values for each category, giving an indication of the goodness-to-fit of each trend line associated with a particular set of keywords.

We have ordered the keyword categories in Table 4.2 in terms of how steep their gradient, i.e. their rise or fall, is. The categories towards the bottom of the

Table 4.2. *Trend lines indicating rises and falls over time for keyword categories*

Increasing over time			Decreasing over time		
Category	Gradient	R^2	Category	Gradient	R^2
FOOD	890.20	0.90	PLACES (UK)	−134.00	0.88
RESEARCH	513.68	0.84	SPORT	−128.93	0.41
MEASUREMENT	477.89	0.95	TV, FILM & ARTS	−117.35	0.70
BIOLOGY	458.53	0.94	EDUCATION	−98.16	0.65
ILLNESS	394.36	0.79	POLITICAL (UK)	−94.03	0.35
WEIGHT LOSS	141.63	0.90	ECONOMICS	−63.27	0.64
QUOTATIVES	144.12	0.74	BUSINESS	−43.96	0.72
HEALTHCARE	112.08	0.62	SOCIAL	−33.03	0.76
WEIGHT	107.62	0.43	CHILDREN	−25.83	0.08
PROBLEM	72.96	0.65	PLACES (NON-UK)	−24.84	0.17
CAUSE	72.72	0.90	MEDICINE	−17.53	0.35
HELP	56.72	0.85			
LIFESTYLE	55.01	0.69			
WOMEN	23.10	0.15			
RESPONSE	6.97	0.04			
MATERNITY	1.37	0.00			

table show relatively low amounts of change over time and appear almost like horizontal lines when their relative frequencies are plotted onto a bar chart. Particularly for RESPONSE and MATERNITY, we note the low R^2 values. So the picture for these categories is more one of fluctuation.

Table 4.2 indicates a complex pattern of change around discussion of obesity between 2008 and 2017, which involves increased problematisation of obesity (PROBLEM) along with a focus on its link to health problems (ILLNESS) and effects on healthcare provision (HEALTHCARE).

> Obesity **crisis** threatens to increase strokes and **heart disease**. Obesity rates rising faster in UK than the US. **NHS** says obese patients will not get surgery until they lose weight.
>
> (*Independent*, 5 December 2017)

The increasing problematisation of obesity over time is notable, particularly considering the research mentioned at the start of this chapter, which indicated that in fact there has not been a lot of change in rates of obesity between 2006 and 2016. Despite this, collectively, the relative frequencies of keywords such as *epidemic*, *risk*, *crisis*, *problem* and *wrong* have increased in articles about obesity over time.

We also see more discussion around weight loss and how this can be enabled (WEIGHT LOSS, HELP).

> So, on the **advice** of her family and friends, Lucy joined Slimming World in July 2012. She says: "I immediately felt welcome and this gave me the confidence and motivation to **lose** weight."
>
> *(Sun*, 31 March 2014)

Along with this is increased scientific framing of obesity (RESEARCH) and focus on the reasons why obesity occurs (CAUSES).

> Obesity awareness may be **causing** overeating, finds international **study**.
>
> *(Guardian*, 15 September 2015)

Such causes appear to be related to several areas of increased mention, what people eat (FOOD), other factors relating to personal choice (LIFESTYLE) and the way one's body works (BIOLOGY).

> Further findings showed participants who skipped breakfast were more likely to have an overall unhealthy **lifestyle**, including poor **diet**, frequent alcohol consumption and **smoking**.
>
> *(Express*, 2 October 2017)

> The desire for **food** in obese people is associated with **brain** activity that 'rewards' their behaviour, in a similar manner to substance addicts, the research suggests.
>
> *(Mirror*, August 2015)

On the other hand, discussion of the role of food manufacturers has taken up less space in debates around obesity over time (BUSINESS), as has consideration of other economic and social factors that relate to obesity such as poverty and inequality (SOCIAL, ECONOMIC), all of which exhibit a decrease in relative frequency over time.

> The link between **inequality** and obesity is stark around the world: among developed nations, America is the most unequal **society** and the fattest, with Britain and Australia next on both scores.
>
> *(Guardian*, 18 August 2016)

> The WHO report, 'Fiscal Policies for Diet and Prevention of Noncommunicable Diseases', did acknowledge that fat and salt also fuel obesity. However, it concluded thoughtless habit of including sodas in a standard diet is one of the most dangerous – yet preventable – activities. The global soft drink **market** is worth nearly $870 billion in annual **sales**.
>
> *(Mail*, 8 November 2016)

Over time, obesity appears to be have been discussed proportionally less as a political issue (POLITICS UK), suggesting that the role of the Government and its policies are perhaps viewed by the press as less important to obesity than was previously the case.

> A leaked draft revealed that the **government** had dropped a target to halve childhood obesity in ten years along with more stringent incentives to make the food industry act.
>
> *(Times*, 18 August 2017)

Childhood obesity has also become less central to discussion of obesity (CHILDREN), along with consideration of the roles that schools and teachers play in preventing obesity in children (EDUCATION).

> **Schools** are there to educate, not to act as social workers, health visitors, therapists, nutrition experts or to take on a parent's role. **Children** have one meal at school and every time **teachers** check a child's lunchbox and removes an unhealthy snack, the press blames them for being heavy-handed.
>
> *(Times*, 4 July 2010)

Related to this is a relative decrease in reference to physical exercise (SPORT) in relation to obesity.

> My children would rather be watching TV than jumping on a trampoline outside. We know less **sport** contributes to obesity. My sons play **football** and swim in the week. My husband takes them **swimming** some weekends, but it's expensive – about 10 for less than an hour.
>
> *(Independent*, 3 June 2012)

The overall picture, then, is one which, on the one hand, indicates large increases relating to discussion of the personal responsibility discourse around food consumption and other lifestyle choices such as smoking and alcohol but, on the other hand, points to decreased discussion of the role of exercise. Thus, over time, the causes of obesity are being framed more at the level of the individual as opposed to society, which can sometimes mean that personal responsibility is seen as central. However, this is not always the case, as the biomedical model of obesity, which arguably foregrounds factors that are to an extent beyond the control of individuals, such as those relating to the brain, bacteria and hormones, appears to have increased over time.

We should not view each of these categories as occupying equal amounts of attention. Table 4.1 indicated that, in terms of the frequencies of the keywords in each category, words relating to FOOD, MEASUREMENT and RESEARCH were extremely frequent across the corpus as a whole, whereas words belonging to the categories SOCIAL, RESPONSE and PLACES

(NON-UK) were much less frequent. FOOD, MEASUREMENT and RESEARCH also show the steepest rises over time and have very high R^2 scores. This indicates that these three ways of situating obesity were already common in the early part of the dataset and have also showed the greatest and most consistent rises over time. The categories SOCIAL, RESPONSE and PLACES (NON-UK) show less impressive and less consistent changes over time and were not especially frequent in any year. The single strongest pattern of change over time, then, is the increased focus on diet; the types and amounts of food that people eat and how these relate to obesity. However, this rise does not seem to have resulted in an increase in discussion around government regulation of, or policies relating to, food manufacturers or advertisers.

What emerges from the British press, then, is a somewhat conflicted picture of obesity. However, one thing that seems consistent is that obesity is viewed increasingly as a problem, and what the representations of it as a biomedical problem and matter of personal responsibility have in common is that they locate this problem within individuals, as opposed to wider social, political and environmental factors. In fact, the frequencies of categories indicating a focus on such factors, such as EDUCATION, POLITICS, ECONOMICS, BUSINESS and SOCIAL, actually decreased over time. Thus, the focus of the causes and responses to obesity is placed on the will and actions of individuals much more than those of more powerful institutions, such as the Government and food and drinks manufacturers and marketers. These complementary patterns can be viewed as symptoms of the wider neoliberal rationality which presently governs almost all aspects of social life in the United Kingdom (and more countries besides) (Brown and Baker 2012), not least those pertaining to health (Lupton 1995), and which we have observed in our more general analyses over the previous two chapters.

The reasons for these temporal trends are difficult to account for, although we could perhaps begin by considering the political backdrop and changes in government over the period under examination. Between 2008 and 2010, the United Kingdom had a Labour Government led by Gordon Brown. However, he was replaced in mid-2010 by a Conservative–Liberal Democrat alliance led by David Cameron, signifying a switch in government policy, with another Conservative, Theresa May, assuming power in 2016 and remaining in position beyond the end of our analysis period. Conservative and coalition policies between 2010 and 2017 could, as noted, be characterised by fiscal austerity and welfare and social service cuts, which, along with a growing and ageing population, have placed increased strain on the NHS. Conservative values tend to emphasise self-sufficiency, entrepreneurship, concerns of individuals over communities and business owners over workers, thus usually being more benign towards the rich and powerful. The British press is independent of the Government, though, so does not necessarily echo the viewpoints of the

Government of the time. With that said, there tends to be a correlation between the success of a political party in elections and the number of national newspapers who declare support for it. It is not surprising, then, that the changing pattern of discourse around obesity in our corpus also matches the values of the dominant political party in the United Kingdom during most of the time period we analysed, particularly considering that 70 per cent of the articles in our corpus were published by newspapers right-of-centre on the political spectrum.

An interesting question to ask, then, is if we only consider the left-of-centre newspapers (*Independent, i, Guardian, Mirror* and *Morning Star*), do we see similar patterns of change to the overall picture, or a polarising picture in which these newspapers show increasing focus on topics such as SOCIAL, BUSINESS and ECONOMICS, which we noted to be characteristic of them (particularly the broadsheets and *Morning Star*) in the previous chapter. To answer this question, analysis of categories was carried out again, just for the left-leaning newspapers. This resulted in an extraordinarily similar picture to the patterns of change over time for the entire corpus. Of the twenty-seven categories, all but two showed the same general slope direction, although the actual gradients of the slope differed slightly. For example, the most frequent category of keywords, FOOD, had an upwards gradient of +890.2 when the whole corpus was considered. When just the left-leaning newspapers were examined, the slope still had an upwards gradient, although it was somewhat steeper, at +949.7. The two categories which showed contradictory patterns were CHILDREN, which sloped downwards over time for the whole corpus (−25.83) yet went up slightly for the left-leaning newspapers (+4.48). However, the difference here is negligible, with very low R^2 values in both cases (0.08 and 0.0016, respectively), indicating a pattern of fluctuation over time. The same is true for the other contradictory category, MEDICINE, which had a slight downwards slope for the whole corpus (−17.53) and an even slighter upwards slope for the left-of-centre newspapers (+2.92), with low R^2 values for both cases (0.35 and 0.02).

Some of the differences in gradient of the slopes are slightly more dramatic. For example, the category BIOLOGY has one of the steepest slopes for the whole corpus (+458.53) and a high R^2 value (0.94), indicating a consistent increase over time. This is the fourth steepest slope of all the categories (see Table 4.2). However, for the left-leaning newspapers, it is the ninth-steepest slope, with a gradient of +137.13 (although the R^2 value is still reasonably high at 0.81). But this is the exception, and in other cases the left-leaning gradients are very similar to those found for the entire corpus. It is perhaps surprising to see that newspapers such as the *Guardian* and *Independent* are writing about obesity less in terms of its relationship to wider socio-political factors as well as moving away from discussing the role of business,

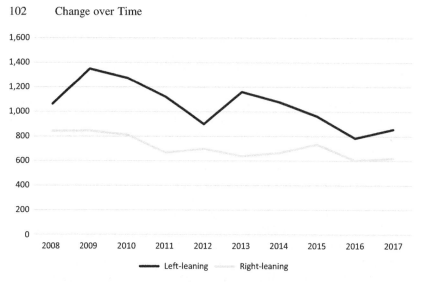

Figure 4.3 Relative frequencies (PMW) of the SOCIAL category for left- and right-leaning newspapers over time

economics and education in relationship to obesity, as we might expect that such newspapers want to present an alternative picture to the more neoliberal discourses of personal responsibility proffered by the right-leaning newspapers, whose views are more congruent with the ruling political class.

That is not to say that the amount of space devoted to particular representations of obesity is equal for both left- and right-leaning newspapers. Figure 4.3 shows occurrences PMW for keywords which we classed as SOCIAL (words such as *inequality*, *poverty* and *unemployment*). The darker line shows the relative frequencies for the left-leaning newspapers, while the lighter line shows the same figures for the right-leaning data. At every point of measurement, the left-leaning newspapers refer proportionally more often to these SOCIAL keywords in articles about obesity, as we would perhaps expect. However, what the figure also shows is that both lines slope downwards. In fact, the frequency for the left-leaning newspapers in 2017 (855.74) is remarkably similar to that for the right-leaning newspapers in 2008 (845.26). One way this could be interpreted is as a kind of 'follow-my-leader' pattern (Mair 2002: 109–112), where the right-leaning newspapers are leading the change, and the left-leaning newspapers are following in the same direction, although they are some way behind.

Looking at the trend line equations can give us a sense of whether the left-leaning newspapers are following in the same direction, doing something different or appearing to lead the way compared to what is happening across the press as a whole. For the categories where these newspapers are increasing over time, all but one have lower intercepts in their trend lines compared to when all newspapers are taken into account. The intercept is important because it tells us the starting point – the first point on the trend line. So, for increasing categories, in 2008 the left-leaning newspapers almost always have fewer references to keywords in that category compared against all newspapers. The outlier category is RESPONSE, although this actually only shows a very small increase over time and has a low R^2 score, so conclusions about patterns there are negligible.

For the majority of the keyword categories that are decreasing over time in the left-leaning press, the intercept is higher compared to the intercept for all newspapers. Again, the left-of-centre press is appearing to follow a trend, rather than leading it. There may be a range of different reasons for the rising sets of keywords. A set of related keywords may rise in relative frequency over time but that does not necessarily mean that there is agreement around the way that the category is discussed – it may, for example, indicate that the topic has become increasingly controversial and that there are numerous ways of pre-senting it. So, we cannot take a rising category in Table 4.2 such as FOOD as simply meaning that there is a single, increasing way of relating obesity to food. It could be the case that some journalists write about food to stress how it is an individual's own fault if they gain weight because they eat too much. However, others may write about food in order to be critical of this position. What we can conclude from the left-hand side of Table 4.2 is that, overall, categories such as FOOD, RESEARCH and MEASUREMENT are increas-ingly referred to in relation to obesity. However, for the categories that are decreasing over time, such as ECONOMICS, BUSINESS and SOCIAL, the interpretation we can make is that these concepts are simply viewed as being less relevant to the central concept or news story (in this case, obesity). The falls in these categories, then, suggest a slow but sure shift over time in the ways that obesity is understood and written about, with even the newspapers that we would expect to offer more socially and politically oriented discourses beginning to show signs of abandoning these positions in favour of those relating to individualistic models. Depending on our own point of view, this may be worrying or reassuring.

Seasonal Changes

In this section, we consider change not by year but by month. Although each year is different from others, they all follow the same procession from January to December with various events occurring at the same pre-determined points each year. To an extent, what is considered newsworthy depends on these repeating events that are tied to specific months. A question arises, then, regarding how, if at all, this impacts on representations of obesity. It should

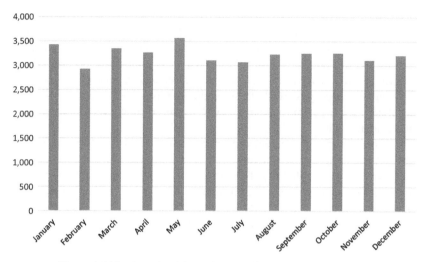

Figure 4.4 Number of articles published about obesity per month

be noted, for example, that stories about obesity are not equally distributed across each month (see Figure 4.4). There was a total of 3,568 articles published in the month of May across all years in the corpus, compared to only 2,924 articles in the month of February. In order to check that this was not due to a particularly large spike in a single year, we examined frequencies of articles for each of the 120 months in the corpus. May had either the most or second-most articles in four years (2012, 2013, 2016 and 2017), suggesting its high frequency was not due to a single outlier year. Similarly, the month of February contained the lowest or second-lowest number of articles in four years (2010, 2012, 2015 and 2016), again indicating that this is a reasonably regular occurrence and not due to the idiosyncrasy of any single year.

To explore linguistic variation across the months, we examined the frequencies of words in the twenty-seven keyword categories outlined in Table 4.1. Plotting the frequencies as trend lines across the months was not productive, as patterns tended to fluctuate more widely rather than showing a straightforward up or downwards tendency, as was the case when we examined annual change across the ten-year period. Instead, to see which keyword categories fluctuated most and least from month to month, we used a measure called the Coefficient of Variation (CV), which indicates the amount of variation over a set of points. Higher CVs indicate that points are widely distributed, which suggests more variation between months, as opposed to keyword categories with lower CVs. To calculate the CV, we take the standard deviation of a set of values and

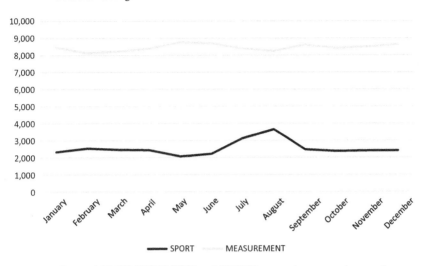

Figure 4.5 MEASUREMENT and SPORT categories across the months (frequencies PMW)

divide it by the mean of that set of values (this helps to cancel out the potential skewing effect of overall frequency size). We then multiply that figure by 100, which normally produces a number between 0 and 100.

Unlike the trend line patterns found for change across the years, which indicated some fairly substantial changes in the relative frequencies of keyword categories over the decade, for the months the CVs for all keyword categories were fairly low, ranging from 2.3 (MEASUREMENT) to 17.1 (SPORT). Figure 4.5 shows the patterns of fluctuation for these two categories, which represent the most and least amount of change over the months.

While the line for the category MEASUREMENT remains fairly flat, indicating little change month-by-month, the line for SPORT shows a small but notable peak, beginning in July and continuing through to August before falling back to June levels. Our analysis in this section, then, is based on less substantial changes than those we observed in our year-by-year analysis in the first half of this chapter.

We have noted which months show particularly strong peaks of each keyword category but decided to supplement this with a focus on individual keywords by carrying out a keyword analysis similar to that which we carried out in our analysis of year-by-year variation, this time comparing word frequencies for each month against the remaining months in turn. However, the top 100 keywords for each month tended to be relatively infrequent. For example, forty-one of the top one hundred keywords for December occurred fifty times or less. Many of these keywords were also proper nouns (e.g. thirty-nine of the hundred keywords for December), and closer analysis revealed that the dominance of a particular news story in one year of a single month could be enough to result in words connected to that story being key for that month when the whole corpus was considered. We were more interested in more generalisable keywords that were associated across the same month in different years. Therefore, we set the minimum frequency for a word to be considered as a keyword to be 100 within that month across all years. Additionally, we removed all monthly keywords where over half of their uses occurred in a single year. Putting these keywords aside, what do the more generalisable keywords tell us about variation around obesity reporting across months? Table 4.3 shows the keywords for each month, many of which relate directly to the categories we identified in Table 4.1.

The appearance of pronouns in this table might indicate a focus on different 'imagined' readers, or at least an intention by newspapers to construct a different relationship with their readers, during different months in the year. January contains more direct address to the reader (i.e. *you* and *your*), while May and June contain more third-person pronouns – *she* and *her* – indicating greater emphasis on women and girls, potentially suggesting a high frequency of stories aimed more at female readers. October has the male-marked pronoun keyword, *he*, while *I* is key in August, suggesting either more articles on obesity written from a personal perspective (e.g. opinion columns) and/or more use of the types of first-person narratives we saw in the previous chapter.

Table 4.3 also indicates that certain discourses appear to come into sharper focus at particular points. For example, January witnesses greater emphasis on diet and exercise in order to lose weight, which is often described as being caused by excessive calorie intake over Christmas. Foods viewed as causing weight gain, such as *sugar*, *alcohol* and *cake*, are contrasted with foods that are perceived as 'healthy', such as *carrots*, *berries* and *salad*, and it is common to find articles describing new diets or recipes

> The **diet** has **you** eat **foods** that the medical literature suggests are good for the brain. These **foods** fall into 10 categories, including: green leafy vegetables, nuts, **berries**, fish, beans, whole grains, and olive oil.
>
> (*Independent*, 6 January 2016)

The categories FOOD and WEIGHT LOSS are most frequent in January, as is the category TV, FILM & ARTS, which is perhaps because January is one of the coldest and darkest months in the United Kingdom, resulting in people being more likely to participate in indoor pursuits. The January sub-corpus also contains references to TV chefs, weight loss DVDs and warnings about the dangers of sedentary activities. There is an emphasis on *fitness* and joining a *gym*, although this is not always viewed with enthusiasm.

Table 4.3. *Keywords for each month of the corpus*

Month	Keywords
January	*sugar, you, diet, resolutions, cubes, weight, eat, lose, food, calories, plump, cereals, foods, fat, campaign, your, wine, pill, year, loss, it, alcohol, new, avocado, fruit, juice, dog, cold, cake, diets, days, so, drink, fitness, salad, berries, carrots, classes, easy, gym, fructose, units, campaigns, sugar-free, breakfast, stick, here, do, film, us*
February	*yoga, insomnia, sleep, asthma, profits, pollution, ambulance, alcohol, butter, welfare, cancer, PE, blame, midwives, asleep*
March	*sugar, chocolate, sleep, liver, announced, teaspoons, anorexia, sugary, price, gout, egg, fizzy, Pepsi, Coca-Cola, Cola*
April	*eggs, egg, dementia, underweight, gardening, BMI, teachers, teacher, chocolate, running, marathon*
May	*obesity, overweight, bacteria, gut, she, her, eating, vegan, study, salt, food, glass, risk, babies, maternal, breast, stroke, Watchers*
June	*diabetes, babies, milk, corn, her, syrup, she, traffic, broccoli, girls, glucose, low-fat, premature, fathers, disease, cure, malnutrition*
July	*dementia, school, fertility, coconut, meals, pupils, sweeteners, pasta, society, park, parks, sausages, dinners, their, food, water, pepper*
August	*sport, sports, sporting, antibiotics, I, cycling, brain, drugs, PE, swimming, bikini, risk, girlfriend, cricket, playing, photo, cancer*
September	*school, your, uniform, pupils, risk, cook, link, diabetes, she, sleep, skin, sweeteners*
October	*NHS, report, he, conference, health, patients, minister, care*
November	*walking, stress, funding, men, midwives, tax, birth, sleep, vitamin, soda, Coca-Cola, Coke*
December	*sales, mince, resolutions, turkey, pies, pudding, alcohol, discrimination, dementia, obese, men, drinking, children, women*

All this **gym** nonsense reaches its climax in January, as people resolve to become healthier in the new year. The tendency has been made worse of late by the no-**alcohol** fad, Dry January. Who thought up that particular incarnation of Orwellian nightmarishness?

(*Telegraph*, 30 January 2016)

Similarly, the January keyword *stick* acknowledges the difficulty in maintaining weight-loss programmes.

By incorporating more slow-release foods into your normal eating plan, you will cut calories without feeling that you're on a diet – and that's a weight loss regime you CAN **stick** to.

(*Sun*, 29 January 2009)

Personal responsibility discourses abate somewhat in February, as references to gyms decrease (one physical activity keyword in February is the somewhat more restrained *yoga*, while another refers to *PE* classes as a means of reducing childhood obesity). If anything, there is a focus on how lack of activity can reduce obesity, illustrated by the keywords *sleep*, *asleep* and *insomnia*.

One in eight Brits **sleep** for less than six hours and **insomnia** has been linked to obesity, heart disease and cancer.

(*Sun*, 26 February 2013)

Discussion of 'healthy' food is much reduced in February, with *butter* being the only food keyword for this month. After the calls for culinary restraint in January, discussions in February suggest a desire for comfort eating, with butter viewed alternatively as a source of fear and delight.

Whilst most people get cravings for chocolate or crisps, I couldn't wait to tuck into a spud! My favourite was a jacket potato with loads of **butter** – even thinking about one made my mouth water.

(*Mail*, 26 February 2015)

Dietary advice to cut out **butter** and full-cream milk is outdated and misguided, new research suggests.

(*Times*, 14 February 2015)

Eating two pieces of toast with **butter** can double diabetes risk, experts have said

(*Express* 18 February 2017)

After the dieting and exercise frenzy of January, news reporting around obesity in February feels cosier and slower, perhaps with a sense of resolutions already falling by the wayside. The discourse shifts somewhat during March with the Government's annual budget, placing focus on political intervention in terms of its ability (or not) to affect the collective weight of the nation. The keyword categories ECONOMICS and POLITICAL are most common in this month as well as individual keywords relating to 'unhealthy' items such as *fizzy drinks*.

> This week the chancellor, George Osborne, **announced** a 25p-a-litre **sugar** tax on **fizzy** drinks that will be enforced from 2018. It comes not a moment too soon for a nation of **sugar** addicts who consume far more of it than we need – on average 238 **teaspoons** each a week.
>
> (*Times*, 19 March 2016)

Because the exact date of Easter changes each year, there is discussion around *chocolate eggs* in both March and April.

> We as a society are addicted to sugar, and food companies know it. With my own four-year-old daughter, I have already weakened in the face of pressure from her for **chocolate** – she eats more **Chocolate** Mini Rolls than I would like her to. This Easter weekend I will indulge her with **chocolate eggs**.
>
> (*i*, 1 April 2015)

The improving weather usually marks April as the start of *marathon* season in the United Kingdom, which results in brief emphasis on the benefits of *running* for weight loss.

> Snooker? As mesmerising as the World Championship may be, it's not going to solve the obesity crisis. The BBC athletics coverage, and the London **Marathon** in particular, however, is an absolute winner.
>
> (*Independent*, 24 April 2017)

However, other articles suggest less vigorous ways to lose weight, as in this example which recommends *gardening*, coming out of the annual National Union of Teachers' conference that is timed to coincide with Easter weekend (helping to explain the keywords *teacher* and *teachers* for April).

> Put **gardening** on the curriculum to combat obesity, say **teachers**
>
> (*Independent*, 6 April 2016)

As mentioned earlier, May is the month when the most articles about obesity are published, on average (the words *obesity* and *overweight* are keywords for this month), and it is also the month that makes most use of the keyword categories WEIGHT and WEIGHT LOSS. Individual keywords for this month include female pronouns (*she*, *her*) and a range of words relating to other categories such as biology (*bacteria*, *gut*), food (*eating*, *food*, *glass*), illness (*breast*, *stroke*), research (*study*), maternity (*maternal*, *babies*) and diet (*Watchers*, which relates to the dieting organisation Weight-*Watchers*).

Weight loss redemption narratives involving female protagonists (introduced in Chapter 2 and discussed more in Chapter 7) appear to be particularly common in May. Perhaps this is due to such articles playing on readers' anxieties about the prospect of summer holidays where they may have to display their bodies at the beach or in hotel swimming pools.

> Incredible transformation of 23st mother who lost HALF **her** body weight after being denied life insurance due to **her** size
>
> • Sarah, 33, dropped an incredible eight sizes, from a 28 to a 12
> • **She** lost 12 stone over three years using Weight **Watchers**
> • Sarah had **her** wake-up call after being refused life insurance.
>
> *(Mail,* 28 May 2015)

The focus on women continues into June, which also has *she* and *her* as keywords, along with *girls, babies, milk* and *premature* (referring to childbirth).

> Findings could help improve IVF treatments and reveal new insights into how a mother's diet can effect obesity and **diabetes** in a child's later life A mother's **milk** provides the valuable nourishment a baby needs during its first months of life, but it seems women also provide a form of **milk** for their child while they are still in the womb.
>
> *(Mail,* 5 May 2015)

Stories about *corn syrup* peak in June, perhaps due to warmer weather resulting in higher sales of cold fizzy drinks.

> And the particular villain is high fructose **corn syrup**, used in sweet, fizzy drinks and processed foods.
>
> *(Guardian,* 14 June 2011)

June also sees more reference to the keyword category CAUSES, which, considering the collocates of keywords in this category such as *cause, linked, related* and *associated*, indicates that they refer to health problems caused by obesity such as *cancer* and other forms of *disease*.

The period during the latter half of the summer is sometimes referred to as the 'slow news' or 'silly' season, this second term dating back to 1861 when it was used in the 13th July edition of the *The Saturday Review* to refer to an alleged reduction in the quality of the editorial content of the *Times*. Perhaps unexpectedly, then, July contains more reference to two relatively 'sensible' keyword categories: EDUCATION and SOCIAL, suggesting that this period, half-way through the year, is when societal aspects relating to obesity are most likely to be discussed by the press. Despite being a month when schools close for summer, keywords relate to *pupils* and *school meals/dinners*, perhaps because journalists expect that parent-readers will be spending more time with their children. July is normally the month with the warmest weather in the United Kingdom, which helps to explain why there are more references to the weight-loss perks of visiting *parks* in this month. Part of the reason for the higher discussion of SOCIAL words in July relates to speeches made by David Cameron in July across various years. In July 2008, he gave a speech about Britain's 'broken society', which was characterised as individuals lacking responsibility for their actions or those of others.

> Society stayed silent on issues such as crime or obesity for fear of causing offence, with damaging consequences, Mr Cameron warned.
>
> (*Mail*, 8 July 2008)

In July 2010, after Cameron came to power as leader of the Coalition Conservative–Liberal Democrat Government, he launched an initiative called the Big Society, an idea which proposed integrating the free market with a theory of social solidarity based on hierarchy and voluntarism. Left-leaning newspapers were not impressed

> In their Big Society – which casts everything as personal responsibility – social injustice, like obesity, is indeed a moral failure, but only on the part of those who suffer it.
>
> (*Guardian*, 9 July 2010)

The greater attention to societal aspects of obesity, then, appears to be a somewhat coincidental consequence of two of Cameron's July speeches. And the way Cameron relates obesity to social causes, in fact, links more to the personal responsibility discourse. He does not adopt a typical 'social causes' view of obesity, that it results from factors such as structural inequality, poverty and aggressive food and drink advertising, but instead presents the view of it as resulting from uncaring, selfish or misguided individualism – the fear of upsetting others by speaking out, or that people with obesity refuse to accept that they need help to lose weight. The larger point to make here is that a set of keywords based around a certain topic or concept do not necessarily indicate that the topic is discussed in a single or straightforward way. Sometimes when the SOCIAL keywords are mentioned, it is to argue against the idea of social causes, or to try to redefine what social causes actually are.

August seems to be a particularly anxious time of the year with the keyword categories PROBLEMS and ILLNESS being most frequent during this month. Individual keywords include *cancer* and *risk*, indicating more focus on health problems linked to obesity. The continued good weather and holiday season partly explain the presence of keywords such as *playing, sport, sports, cycling, swimming* and *cricket*. The Ashes (a series of Test cricket matches) takes place in August, while the London Olympics occurred in July and August of 2012, and although there is definitely a peak in the SPORTS category for 2012, this alone does not account for the higher frequency of such keywords in August generally. Many references to sports within the context of articles relating to obesity involve quotes from professional sportspeople, aimed at inspiring others (particularly children) to join in, such as the following quote from Holly Lam-Moores, who competed in the 2012 Olympics.

> Everyone wants to keep fit and healthy, but we have this culture of thinking of exercise being a chore. **Sports** like handball are fun, easy, cheap and social. If we can encourage children to do more **sport** at school, it will help them realise **playing sport** is fun, not boring.
>
> (*The Sun*, 7 August 2012)

With most schools closed for the entirety of August, this month is the period when many people in the United Kingdom go on holiday. This explains keywords such as *photo* and *bikini*, which tend to relate to fear and shame about women's bodies being exposed while on holiday and can form part of the redemptive weight loss narratives we saw in the previous chapter.

- Lisa Brady, 44, was 17 stone and size 24 during Goan holiday
- Gained weight after drinking four bottles of rosé wine a week
- Shrunk to size 10–12 after she saw **photo** and "felt sorry for the elephant"

> A 17-stone mother did not realise she was overweight until she saw holiday pictures of herself sat on an elephant in a **bikini** – and felt sorry for the animal carrying her weight.
>
> (*Mail*, 11 August 2015)

The keyword *I* indicates that August is a month in which news coverage of obesity is likely to be characterised in terms of first-person perspectives, including weight loss narratives.

> "**I** hated taking them swimming because **I** looked fat in my swimsuit," says Fran, a housing officer. "When I got on the trampoline **I** worried people were laughing and thinking **I**'d burst it."
>
> (*Mirror*, 25 August 2014)

September sees an end to school holidays, accounting for keywords such as *uniform*, *pupils* and *school* which are linked to renewed focus on child obesity.

> Child obesity is causing a rise in demand for super-size **school uniforms**, according to retailers.
>
> (*Telegraph*, 14 August 2012)

On the other hand, BIOLOGY is the most frequent keyword category in September, indicating that this is a period of the year in which biomedical discourse around obesity is likely to be prominent. The September keyword *your* collocates most strongly with *body*, indicating a plethora of informational articles that directly address readers with regard to understanding their bodies' relationship with weight. For example, this *Times* article asks readers to eat a cream cracker and time how long it takes for its taste to change from bland to sweet.

> More than 30 seconds **Your** carb type is Restricted.
> **Your** body finds carbs hard to process.
> This means you should have no more than 25 per cent of **your** calories coming from carbs, 35 per cent from protein and 40 per cent from fats.
> We require different diets tailored to our own genes.
> *(Times*, 3 September 2016).

October has a focus on reported research relating to obesity, with keywords such as *report* and *conference*, as well as having most frequent use of keyword categories such as RESEARCH and QUOTATIVES.

> The new **report** shows a widening gender gap in childhood obesity, and a gulf between different sections of society.
> *(Telegraph*, 11 October 2016)

> Diamond, who is writing a book about the global obesity epidemic, chaired a discussion at the National Obesity Forum's annual **conference** in London yesterday.
> *(Telegraph*, 8 October 2008)

The political party conference season takes place between September and October while the House of Commons is in recess, which helps to explain the high frequency of *conference* in October.

> Tories blasted for railing against child obesity at party **conference** sponsored by a sugar firm
> *(Mirror*, October 2017)

With other keywords such as *NHS*, *care* and *minister*, October, like March, indicates a more politicised discourse around the topic of obesity, at least compared to other months.

> The number of people needing hospital **care** for obesity shot up tenfold in the past decade, the **NHS** Information Centre's figures also showed.
> *(Mail*, 29 October 2010)

> MPs and peers have called on PM David Cameron to appoint a **Minister** for Children to tackle obesity in youngsters.
>
> (*Star*, 21 October 2014)

The October keyword *he* suggests that this is one of the few times of the year when men and male perspectives are foregrounded in obesity coverage. In October, *he* collocates strongly with quotatives such as *said*, *says*, *added* and *told*, and tends to appear in articles with a political or scientific focus, so it is likely that its use is linked to both the greater prevalence of men in positions of authority and the likelihood that male views will be sought during a month where political and scientific reporting are at the forefront.

> Lansley himself acknowledged the nannying nature of trying to deal with obese children, when **he** said they needed more of a Mary Poppins than a Miss Trunchbull, the fearsome headteacher created by Roald Dahl.
>
> (*Guardian*, 2 October 2008)

Political discourse around obesity continues into November as a result of autumn budget statements, helping to explain keywords such as *funding* which are also related to the NHS, and *tax* which involves debates around taxes on products such as *Coca-Cola*,

> **Tax** soft drinks to cut obesity, say researchers
> A 20% tax on **Coca-Cola**, Pepsi, Fanta and other sugar-sweetened drinks would cut the number of adults who are obese or overweight, researchers claim.
>
> (*Guardian*, 1 November 2013)

However, November also sees a renewed focus on women, with keywords in the categories MATERNITY and WOMEN being more frequent in this month, along with keywords such as *midwives* and *birth*. *Men* is also a November keyword, although its strongest collocate is *women* and the two words tend to co-occur in articles which compare rates of obesity (and related illnesses) among men and women.

> On its own, being overweight was responsible for almost twice as many cancers as diabetes – 544,300 versus 280,100 cases. Cancers linked to the two conditions were also nearly twice as common in **women** than in **men**.
>
> (*Independent*, 29 November 2017)

Darker nights and inclement weather mean that during November people are more likely to stay indoors rather than go outside. Lack of sunshine can result in vitamin D deficiency, resulting in the November keyword *vitamin*, which tends to occur in articles linking lack of exercise to both obesity and vitamin D deficiency.

Vitamin D deficiency affects as many as 40 per cent of adult Americans, according to the Centers for Disease Control and Prevention. Risk factors for the deficiency include being obese or overweight, limited outdoor activity, having darker skin and suffering from certain inflammatory conditions, such as diabetes and inflammatory bowel disease.

(*Mail*, 16 November 2015)

Compared to sunnier months, during which the newspapers extolled the virtues of highly active sports or physical activities, the bar is lowered somewhat in November, with *walking* being the activity keyword of choice.

I was thin when I started (in my late twenties, single-digit dress size, one of the lower ones) but now in my forties, for as long as I've been **walking**, my weight hasn't fluctuated by so much as a couple of pounds, even during my cake-iest periods.

(*Telegraph*, 8 November 2015)

Finally, December encompasses the Christmas holiday period, a time normally associated with staying indoors and celebrating with friends and family members, particularly with food and sometimes alcohol. The keyword category CHILDREN is most frequent during this month (again, perhaps because children are not in school and likely to be spending more time with their parents), with journalists making frequent reference to the responsibility that parents have towards ensuring that their children maintain a healthy weight.

Head of the NHS Simon Stevens is right to warn parents of obese **children** that they must show "tough love" and stop them consuming sugar-packed fizzy drinks and junk food.

(*Express*, 27 December 2016)

Other December keywords include *mince pies*, *turkey*, *pudding*, *drinking* and *alcohol*, and there are numerous stories relating Christmas indulgences to obesity.

How many **mince pies** and glasses of mulled wine can you refuse without feeling like a party pooper? How much calorie and carb calculation can your brain take before it addles? Obesity is a serious issue, I know. But an equally serious problem is the despair so many women feel because they yearn to be thinner and thinner and still thinner and are trapped in demented and permanent dieting. Stuff that I say.

(*Independent*, 15 December 2008)

There is a somewhat rueful sense in the press that this holiday period does not do much to help people stick to a consistent diet, and that the period of excess will be followed by new year *resolutions* to lose weight.

The last two weeks of the year must be the "fattest" period on the calendar. New Year **resolutions** for exercise and weight loss are around the corner, but if a nationwide weigh-in was carried out, I'm sure there would be a national peak around the last week of December. It's just too easy to over-indulge, with drinks parties and the temptation of high calorie finger food, not to mention the full feast of Christmas dinner.

(*Telegraph*, 22 December 2008)

However, the December period also contains acknowledgements that many resolutions will be broken, as in the following article, which is addressed to an assumed reader who is implied to have tried and failed to keep resolutions in previous years,

Yes, we know many **resolutions** bite the dust before the end of January, but at least we start thinking about possible health improvements after Christmas. According to a survey last year, the most popular New Year pledges were to "do more exercise" followed by "lose weight" and to "eat more healthily". And there are a few tips to increase your chances of success

(*Mirror*, 19 December 2013)

And so the news cycle begins again in January, when the press go back to stories about starting diets and joining gyms.

Conclusion

The month-by-month analysis shows how UK reporting around obesity fluctuates according to religious traditions and holidays, the political calendar and weather. For someone aiming to maintain a consistent weight, the monthly variation in terms of expected eating and activity-based behaviours is perhaps less than ideal. Journalists are aware of the annual cycle, acknowledging that some points of the year will be characterised by brief bouts of dieting and exercise and others by reduced activity and higher-than-usual consumption of food. The mild yet changeable British climate plays a strong role in expectations about activity – staying indoors to work out in a gym is the goal for January, whereas journalists focus on running in April but also gardening for those who would rather not get involved in marathons. August has a surfeit of stories about cycling, swimming and cricket, while by November the best that can be hoped for is a commitment to walking. While the main trend we found was for journalists to reinforce expectations around these pre-determined cycles of eating, dieting, exercise or repose, there were also cases where the typical behaviours were discouraged or warnings were given, for example about over-indulging at Christmas.

While we could make a stronger case for the year-on-year change in terms of representations of obesity being somewhat politically or at least ideologically charged, it is more difficult to apply similar explanations to the month-by-month changes. Instead, the changes in reporting across a single year seem to be a less ideologically motivated attempt to represent obesity according to the relevant seasonal contexts. News values such as consonance, personification and mean-ingfulness come into play here; readers will likely expect certain types of stories around Christmas, New Year, Easter, the budget, the school holidays and the party conference season, and it is likely not to be just articles about obesity that are affected by the month they appear in but other topics, too (e.g. clothing, relationships, travel). Even inadvertently, the annual cycle we have identified indicates another dimension of instability around representations of obesity. As well as presenting readers with a complicated set of competing explanations for obesity, the time of year introduces yet further variation in terms of how readers are directed to think about obesity, with the result being further inconsistency and conflicting messages. Moving from month to month, we had a sense of readers being pulled around – start a new diet and join a gym in January, hibernate in February, eat chocolate in March and April, worry about being overweight in May, play sport in August, go for a walk in November, then over-indulge in December. Such messages do not merely come from newspapers but are likely to be transmitted via other media and through interactions with family and friends. In this context, the newspapers act as a form of reinforcement, largely normalising the stages of the annual cycle.

Ultimately, though, the monthly fluctuations identified in the latter half of this chapter are less significant than the overall patterns of change we observed in our analysis of year-by-year change across the whole decade. Here we see a sobering picture – a clear shift in the discourse around obesity. Not only has there been increased focus on the topic over time, but ways of representing obesity have increasingly prioritised individual factors, notably discussion of people's food intake or an innate disposition to gain weight, while at the same time de-emphasising wider political and societal factors relating to obesity. While this trend might be expected of the right-leaning, conservative newspapers, it was also visible in the left-leaning newspapers, which appear to follow rather than set such trends. We only examined a decade of articles, and it is not wise to extrapolate beyond this point, for example by predicting that the current direction of travel is irreversible. However, for the period under study, there is a clear movement, by the press, towards situating obesity as mostly personal rather than political. Bearing in mind that this period co-occurs with one of government austerity and policies aimed at reducing spending on welfare payments, housing subsidies and social services, the message that 'if something bad happens it is your own fault' in stories about obesity feels congruent with the dominant political ideology of the time.

For this reason, the following two chapters focus on two specific themes which are directly related to individualising discourses around obesity. In Chapter 5, we consider how newspapers engage in shaming people with obesity, before examining more closely language used by journalists around the topic of losing weight in Chapter 6.

5   Shaming and Reclaiming

Introduction

This chapter examines the stigmatisation and shaming of people with obesity, focussing on linguistic patterns around their representation. Some of the earliest work on stigma was carried out by sociologist Émile Durkheim (1895), who viewed stigma as both unavoidable and relative, envisaging that even in a perfect society with no crime, 'venial faults' would create scandals and that if such societies were able to judge and punish, they would define such acts as criminal. Falk (2001) argues that stigmatisation occurs because it helps to create group solidarity, helping in turn to distinguish between insiders and outsiders. While people possess a multitude of identity variables, it is the stigmatised ones which tend to be noticed first (Becker 1963: 33–34). Epstein (1998: 145) claims that stigmatised identities are thus likely to subsume other aspects of identity so that the behaviour of a stigmatised person is likely to be attributed to aspects of their identity that are stigmatised.

People are sometimes able to conceal aspects of their identity that are stigmatised. For example, in homophobic societies, gay men and lesbians might claim to be heterosexual. However, it is more difficult to conceal obesity. Therefore, a person with obesity is almost always visibly stigmatised and thus discredited. The propensity of society to stigmatise people with obesity is well-documented (Farrell 2011; Lupton 2018), and seen as rising (Brewis et al. 2011), with the term *fat shaming* used as a way of critically highlighting stigmatising language and social practices around obesity and larger bodies.

Nath (2019: 2) writes, 'we regard fatness as bad by labelling some people as fat, by casting that label in negative terms, and by taking that ascription to, at least in part, define a person's social identity (the sort of person she is perceived to be in the eyes of others). We treat fatness as bad by allowing fat people to endure numerous disadvantages in virtue of their size being regarded a bad thing.' In this chapter, we focus on how language is used to stigmatise people with obesity by identifying repeated linguistic patterns across the corpus. However, to provide a counterbalance, we also consider the extent to which newspapers report or put forward alternative positions such as one that is critical of fat shaming or which embraces fat positivity.

The word forms and their associated excerpts analysed in this chapter were identified through somewhat different means to the analyses in previous chapters. We began by examining keywords from individual newspapers by comparing each newspaper against the rest, noting that some contained several words that appeared to refer to obesity using euphemistic and/or pejorative language. For example, the nouns *fatties* and *flab* and adjectives *tubby* and *lardy* were key in the *Star* compared against the other newspapers in the corpus. An examination of the collocates of the words *obese* and *obesity* across different newspapers found negatively loaded terms such as *unfit* and *illiterate*, as well as verbs such as *branded*, in articles where someone was described as being 'branded obese by a doctor'. We focus in this chapter on the ways that people with obesity are stigmatised, paying particular attention to similar cases that are frequent enough to collectively indicate patterns. Through initial collocation and concordance analysis of the terms just mentioned, we identified further terms. Our analysis in this chapter was not therefore based on thinking of potential words that could be used to stigmatise people with obesity but on identifying initial cases through exploratory analysis and then searching for grammatically related forms (e.g. for the verb *branded*, we also considered *brand*, *brands* and *branding*). In many cases, we used what Hunston (2002: 62) refers to as 'probes' in order to identify additional terms contributing towards a representation. For example, through concordance analysis of *obese* we noted the verb phrase *gobbling chips*. To find other verbs used in a similar way, we searched for all verbs preceding *chips* and identified additional terms such as *scoffing* and *shovelling*. Additionally, searching all verb forms of *scoff*, *shovel* and *gobble* identified other kinds of foods that people with obesity were described as eating (e.g. *cakes*, *chocolate*, *junk food*), with further searches of references to those food terms identifying other verbs denoting eating. This process can be likened to snowball sampling, a term commonly associated with sociology, where existing study subjects recruit future subjects from among their acquaintances (Goodman 1961).

Our analysis followed some of the central aspects of Reisigl and Wodak's (2001) Discourse-Historical Approach, in that it involved considering referential/nomination and predicational strategies. The former relates to how people are named and referred to, while the latter relates to how they are described and what qualities or characteristics are attributed to them. A nomination strategy would therefore involve using a noun such as *fatty*, while a predicational strategy could involve the use of adjectives, such as *illiterate*, or verbs which describe people as engaging in certain actions (e.g. *gobbling* chips) or being the recipient of actions (e.g. *branded* as fat). Another aspect of Reisigl and

Wodak's framework that we draw on here is consideration of legitimation or ways that social actors justify a course of action. As we are dealing mainly with cases of negative representation, we were interested in identifying how journalists were able to justify their negative language use and the stigmatising representations these invoked.

Another framework we have drawn on in this analysis is van Leeuwen's (1996) social actor representation, which provides a categorisation system for identifying 'the ways that social actors can be represented in English discourse' (*ibid.*: 32). For example, a term such as *the obese* is a form of *physical identification* which 'represents social actors in terms of physical characteristics which uniquely identify them in a given context' (*ibid.*: 57). This framework helps to identify how references to people with obesity can include or exclude, personalise or impersonalise, assimilate or differentiate.

Our analysis first considers nouns used to refer to people with obesity, then moves on to adjectives and verbs. The final section focusses on a particular kind of stigmatising article we encountered: one which links obesity and criminality. We then conclude the chapter by reflecting on the potential effects that shaming representations of people with obesity might have in a wider societal context.

Nouns: Naming Strategies and Labels

Naming strategies, or nominations, are important as they can shape our understanding of a social group, encouraging us to conceptualise that group in a certain way by focussing on some aspects of its identity while backgrounding others. In terms of how people with obesity are named by the press, a key distinction can be drawn between whether a person's weight is assigned as a modifier to their identity (e.g. *obese people*) or actually constitutes their entire identity (*the obese*). In the former term, *obese* is an adjective which, while indicating that obesity is the aspect of identity under focus, discursively allows for the possibility of the person being referred to as having other traits. On the other hand, referring to a set of people as *the obese* arguably reduces their identity to a single trait – their weight. There are 38,781 occurrences of the word *obese* in the corpus, so we employed a search heuristic to obtain a sense of the proportions of times that the word was used in its adjectival or noun forms when referring to groups of people. The term *the obese* (*obese* as a noun) occurs 891 times, while *obese people* (*obese* as an adjective) occurs 2,842 times. Taking the smaller frequency and dividing it by the sum of both together (i.e. 891 / (891+ 2842)) gives 0.23. Therefore, 23 per cent – so roughly a quarter – of such cases are the noun version. As Table 5.1 indicates, there is variation between newspapers, with the *Mirror* having the fewest cases of *the obese* relative to *obese people* (0.17) and the *Times* having the most

Table 5.1. *Proportions of* the obese *vs* obese people *across newspapers*

	the obese	*obese people*	**Proportion of cases** of *the obese* vs *obese people*
Times	104	182	0.36
Guardian	96	260	0.26
Telegraph	117	348	0.25
Mail	317	1029	0.23
Star	41	135	0.23
Express	97	335	0.22
Morning Star	1	4	0.20
Independent	70	292	0.19
Sun	13	55	0.19
Mirror	35	202	0.14
Total	891	2842	0.23

(0.36), as well as other broadsheets, the *Guardian* and *Telegraph*, having relatively more uses of *the obese*. It could therefore be argued that this is related to broadsheet style, although we note that the *Independent* is an outlier, as its usage more closely resembles the tabloids.

A similar, though less frequent pattern is found for the word *overweight*, with 327 cases of *the overweight* and 1,259 of *overweight people* (expressed proportionally as 0.20). Again, *the Times* has the highest proportion of nouning (0.37), while this time *the Sun* has the least (0.08).

Nouning can have both distancing and separating effects, whereby the social group in question is positioned as a distinct category, different from everyone else and similar to one another, as in the following example in which there is a sense that *the obese* are seen as a class or even a kind of species.

> This month the Conservative leader suggested in Glasgow that **the obese** should take more responsibility for their lifestyles
>
> (*Times*, 24 July 2008)

Use of this term suggests a formal tone which tends to be more typical of broadsheet style. While this style of writing may appear neutral, when used in reference to human groups, it can seem somewhat cold and detached, and is suggestive of a subtle form of stigmatisation.

Another form of nouning involves using more informal terms that refer to weight in less neutral-sounding or clinical ways. Weight-focussed research journals have more recently begun using person-first language, such as *person with obesity* (Kyle and Puhl 2014). However, we have found that there was little take-up of this form in the press (71 uses in total of *person/people with obesity*) compared to *the obese* (891 cases) or *obese person/people* (3,096 cases). While the terms *obese* and *obesity* are largely accepted in the medical community and are used by authorities such as the World Health Organisation (although researchers such as Meadows and Daníelsdóttir (2016: 3) advocate use of neutral terms such as *higher weight*[1]), there are other words which have more strongly negative connotations. The nouns *fatties* and *fatsos* could be viewed as reductive in a similar way to a term such as *the obese* but instead of using 'neutral' technical terminology, they clearly have a more explicitly negative evaluative tone. A similar set of words involve forms of the word *lard – lardy*, *lard-bucket* and *lard-arse*. In these cases, the referents are depicted as being composed of fat in its food sense, with the implication being that they eat large amounts of food with high fat content. Such labels could be viewed as dehumanising, especially *lard-bucket*, which metaphorically represents the human body as a repository for fat. The third term, *lard-arse*, is an example of assonance (rhyming of vowel sounds), which constitutes one of the numerous stylistic devices employed, particularly by the tabloids, to make articles and headlines more memorable and entertaining.

Other metaphorical noun labels represent humans as other animals and particularly pigs: *pigs, porkers, porkies* and *hogs* – drawing a comparison between people with obesity and pigs – an animal that is culturally associated with greed and undiscerning food preferences. The term *blob*, meanwhile, references shape, while *slob* is suggestive of laziness, and *gut-bucket* is similar to *lard-bucket*, although it uses assonance and somatisation (described by van Dijk (1991: 60) as a 'form of objectivation in which social actors are represented by means of reference to a part of their body') by metonymically representing the whole person in terms of the body part where fat is stored (i.e. the stomach, or 'gut'). Collectively, these terms are used as nouns (singular and plural) 1,155 times across the corpus, with *fatty/fatties* used most often (707 occurrences). Proportionally speaking, these terms are used most often by the *Sun* (18.10 times per 100,000 words).

In reducing people with obesity to a particular trait or body part, or by characterising them as pigs, these labels certainly provide support for Farrell's (2011) point that 'fat people are often treated as *not quite human,* entities to whom the normal standards of polite and respectful behaviour do not seem to apply' (6–7). However, although these terms arguably perform a negative evaluative function in and of themselves, they are not always used with negative intent. For example, of the twenty-nine cases of *lardies*, only four occur in explicitly negative articles which represent people with obesity as causing harm, for example,

---

[1] The term *higher weight* was only used as synonymous with *overweight* or *obese* seven times in the corpus.

DOLE FOR **LARDIES** TOO FAT TO WORK; Fury as obese leech cash; OBESE scroungers are living on handouts because they claim they are too fat to work.

(*Star*, 6 March 2009)

This article uses the term *obese* as a noun as well as metaphorically construing people with obesity as blood-sucking worms by 'leech[ing]' money from the state. The concept of the 'undeserving poor' is regularly employed in conservative tabloids (Shilliam 2018). In terms of perspectivisation, the verb *claim* expresses distance or perhaps incredulity that people with obesity are unable to work due to their weight.

The other twenty-five cases of *lardies* use the term in a way which, while negative in itself, makes less of an explicitly negative value judgement on the people being represented, other than the perspective that these people ought to lose weight.

BRITAIN is a nation of fatties – we've got the wobbliest waists in Europe and face an obesity epidemic. But former fatty Steve Miller is on a crusade to get **lardies** to lose weight.

(*Star*, 22 October 2010)

We did not find any cases of *lardies* being used critically, such as in cases where use of the term itself is queried. On the other hand, if we take the term *pig*, which is used to refer to people with obesity seventeen times in the *Independent*, none of the cases are used in a straightforwardly negative sense. Three cases refer to the title of a Broadway Play, *Fat Pig*, while the others use the fact that someone has called someone a *pig* as the basis of a news story, framing the use of the word as insulting.

Trump called actress Rosie O'Donnell a "fat **pig**" and said she has a "fat, ugly face."

(*Independent*, 29 September 2016)

While this article is critical of Donald Trump for his insults towards women, noting that many female voters find him offensive and unacceptable, it ends by noting that 'Trump . . . boasts about his unhealthy eating habits, dining regularly on McDonald's hamburgers and buckets of KFC fried chicken on his private jet.' Thus, the article appears to be more critical of Trump's implied hypocrisy for fat-shaming, as opposed to the practice of fat-shaming itself.

One legitimation strategy found in the corpus was that shaming language is for people's own good.

We bullied and nagged smokers, made adverts that said they smelt so awful they were unkissable and finally, with the smoking ban, we literally turned them into shivering outsiders – all because we knew it was for their own good. You have to be cruel to be kind and pretending that obesity is groovy is not being kind to anybody … Let's go back to **fatty** baiting – they might get upset but they'll have ten extra years to get over it.

(Times, 20 March 2009)

Citing the health risks of obesity, this 'tough love' argument was found in the right-leaning newspapers and seems to disregard research demonstrating that such stigmatisation can be ineffective (Vartanian and Porter 2016).

Another common way in which offensive nominalisations are legitimated is through quotes from individuals who identify as being people with obesity either now or in the past. For example, of the forty-two uses of *blob* referring to people with obesity, half are used in self-reference, either in interview quotes or because the article is written by a person who self-identifies as having had obesity. These forms of perspectivisation help to legitimate the use of such terms.

She said: "I felt so sad and I realised I was too ashamed to be in pictures because I was such a fat **blob**. I am 28 and I felt 65. I was puffing and panting everywhere."

(Mail, 1 October 2013)

A different perspective is given in the *Telegraph*, where a journalist who self-identifies as a person with obesity accepts shaming labels such as *porker* as she is not ashamed of being fat. Instead, her concern centres on cases where such words are used with the intent to hurt (thereby implying the possibility of non-hurtful uses).

Last week, in a column about online abuse, I mentioned that strangers call me fat every day. I should clarify now that I don't mind being called fat – what I mind is people throwing it out there with the express purpose of belittling (ha!) me. I am not ashamed of being fat, not one bit. Call me chubby, pudgy, a **porker**, whatever – I will simply take it as a sign that my body looks like one that has been loved and lived in, rather than loathed.

(Telegraph, 10 June 2014)

Compared to shaming, the perspective of fat acceptance or pride is relatively rare in the corpus. The term *fat pride* occurs only fourteen times across six articles and is mostly used to criticise this stance, as in the following article where fat pride is personified as a stereotypical person with obesity and cast in opposition to 'us'.

Believe me, **Fat Pride** is coming to get us, moving slowly and deliberately, eating and swigging fizzy drinks as it makes its way towards us. My advice to you is run – if you can without blacking out.

(Mail, 12 November 2008)

References to *fat positivity* are even less frequent (four occurrences), although *fat acceptance* is more common (sixty-two occurrences). Meadows and Daníelsdóttir (2016:2) note how '[fat] is the preferred term within the fat acceptance movement, whose reclamation of the word as a neutral descriptor aims to counter the negative stereotypes that have become associated with it, and normalize the existence of fat bodies'. While *fat positivity* and *fat acceptance* terms do not attract the same level of ridicule as *fat pride* in the corpus, they still tend to be framed as problematic concepts. In the following extract, *fat positivity* is discussed as part of a description of a television debate where a plus-size blogger is interviewed alongside a woman who was quoted as saying she didn't want her children to go to a nursery where overweight staff worked. The article describes the mother as 'provoking controversy', foregrounding her views by placing them in the first four paragraphs of the article.

> 'A lot of the **fat positivity** movement is all about, we're big we're beautiful. All I'm trying to say is it's more beautiful to be healthy. I just want people to be healthy and not celebrate obesity because it's making people ill'
>
> *(Mail*, 21 September 2017)

The views of the plus-size blogger are given later in the article, 'I come from a health at every size viewpoint. I think you can't make snap judgements on people's health just by looking at them.' The article also quotes tweets from people who are supportive of the blogger and those who are supportive of the mother, helping to frame the concept of fat positivity as something that provokes conflict and is thus newsworthy.

As well as words used to label people with obesity, another set of nouns refer to body parts in less-than-favourable terms. These include general terms referring to fat itself, such as *flab* (580 occurrences), *bulk* (208) and *blubber* (120), and rarer terms involving blends, such as *flobber* (1) and *flubber* (3). Other blended words combine references to specific body parts: *moobs* (blending *man* and *boobs*; 175) and *cankle(s)* (blending *calf* and *ankle*; 23).

Additionally, alliteration is used with *beer belly/bellies* (177) and *thunder thighs* (21), while rhyming occurs in *bingo wings* (109). Finally, *muffin top(s)* (132) offers a visual metaphor of a bulging stomach that represents a muffin. These stylistic flourishes suggest a sense of playfulness which is in keeping with some of the newspapers' attitude towards obesity as amusing. Collectively, these disparaging body part terms occur 1,549 times across the corpus, with the *Mail* containing the most (471 occurrences) and the *Star* having the most proportionally (22.9 occurrences per 100,000 words). Some of the terms imply behaviours or activities which suggest how those body parts have accumulated fat. For example, *muffin top* could also imply that someone eats too many muffins, *beer belly* almost certainly implies that someone drinks too much beer and *bingo wings* conjures up a picture of a woman whose hobby is sedentary (playing bingo) as opposed to involving physical activity. One article provides a detailed classification of six types of bingo wing (all of which develop the use of rhymes for 'amusing' labels).

> A fitness expert has identified six types of bingo wing – and come up with specific strategies to combat each kind. Personal trainer Rich Jones lists variants including 'Jabba Flab', 'Double Chubble' and 'Rump Lump', and has identified celebrities who suffer from each different kind. **Bingo wings** are the flaps of skin that hang down from the triceps – particularly visible on an out-of-shape bingo player waving an arm.
>
> (*Mail*, 13 July 2012)

As seen in the use of the noun 'gut bucket' earlier, somatisation sometimes occurs with these words.

> The hippo-sized American in front of me at the airport coffee shop ordered "a large mochaccino with extra cream, hazelnut syrup … and two sachets of zero-cal sweetener". Did this lump of **blubber** really believe having sweetener instead of sugar was going to make any difference to the calorie bomb he was about to ingest?
>
> (*Times*, 1 April 2012)

These labels for fat body parts or fat itself draw attention to and perpetuate a sense of disgust at the overweight body. As a legitimation strategy, this disgust is depersonalised in the sense that it is directed towards the body part or the fat, rather than the human being. The following article describes positive qualities (the family who genuinely love each other and want to change) as 'underneath all that blubber'.

> They have been called the real-life Teletubbies, received death threats and been assaulted. But underneath all that **blubber** there is a family who genuinely love each other and who say they want to change.
>
> (*Sun*, 29 August 2009)

The onus, then, is on 'getting rid of' these parts of our bodies, viewing them as separate from our true, 'good' selves (a point we examine in our analysis of the word *body* in the next chapter). It is no wonder, then, that they comprise some of the most openly derogatory instances of shaming language in the corpus. However, and contrary to such depersonalising language, we cannot really disassociate ourselves from our bodies, meaning that hatred of those features is easily conflated with hatred for the persona and can even become internalised as shame or hatred of the self.

Adjectives: Synonyms and Collocates

Moving on, we now consider the use of adjectives to describe people with obesity. There are two types of adjective we can consider. The first involves labels that directly relate to obesity and are of a similar type to the noun labels used to describe persons with obesity considered in the previous section. The second type involves other adjectives that do not reference obesity directly but frequently occur in descriptions of people with obesity, nonetheless. Both types are revealing, in different ways, about representations of obesity. We will take the obese labels first, as these are more frequent.

The three most commonly used adjectives referring to people of higher weight in our corpus are *obese* (18,174 occurrences), *overweight* (16,031) and *fat* (8,092).[2] While all newspapers use *obese* most often, the *Sun* stands out as the only newspaper to prefer *fat* to *overweight*. We will consider the language around these three words later in this chapter but for now we want to instead note the sheer number of additional adjectives in the corpus that are used to describe such people. Indeed, some of the articles we examined provide them in lists. The excerpt below argues that such euphemisms are unhelpful.

> "Curvy, big-boned, hefty, full-figured, fluffy, chubby. Those are words designed to make people feel better about themselves. That wasn't helpful to me" Star Jones. Still, that doesn't mean black women reject the need to become healthier.
>
> (*Mail*, 10 December 2012)

Over-lexicalisation is a term used by Halliday (1978) to refer to the dense wording of a particular domain. It can reveal topics that are of particular importance or fascination to a society or group, as well as indicating ideological perspectives. One use of over-lexicalisation involves attempts to positively reframe a stigmatised concept or social group. However, this practice is not always successful. Some adjectives used to refer to obesity do have euphemistic uses and are sometimes referred to in articles containing discussions about appropriate terms, particularly over whether euphemisms are useful. Smith et al. (2007), while noting that terms such as *overweight, obese* and *heavy* are often used interchangeably, describe a study they carried out in which a fictional woman placed a personal advert describing her weight in different conditions by using positive (e.g. *full-figured*), negative (*fat*) or objective (*197 pounds*) language. She was rated differently in terms of her attractiveness, friendliness and intelligence depending on which terms were

---

[2] To calculate these frequencies we only considered cases where the words *obese, overweight* and *fat* were used as adjectives and referred directly to people in constructions such as *is obese* or *obese man.*

used, although she was always rated more positively when no description of weight was given. Word choice clearly matters to an extent, then, and it is worth considering how adjectives describing large size are used in the corpus.

Such adjectives range from terms that tended to be used in relatively positive or euphemistic ways, such as *cuddly* (47), *roly-poly* (54), *big-boned* (49), *solid* (15), *full-figured* (19) and *plus-size(d)* (1702), to those which suggest extra weight but do not usually hold an explicitly negative evaluation, such as *expansive* (9), *hefty* (129), *fleshy* (59), *meaty* (5), *portly* (139), *tubby* (261) and *chubby* (664), to those which have more explicitly negative, even insulting connotations, such as *porky* (103), *lardy* (116), *flabby* (198), *blobby* (16), *blubbery* (33) and *gargantuan* (40). Some terms tend to mostly describe men and can sometimes imply that the weight is due to muscle rather than fat (or a combination of the two), for example *beefy* (20), *stocky* (37) and *burly* (62), while others are used more for women, such as *curvy* (415), *voluptuous* (90) and *dumpy* (18). Apart from the latter, these gendered terms tend to have positive connotations, suggesting physical attractiveness.

> There's something that makes your heart flutter when this big, **beefy** man strides across a bar to claim you when he sees you talking to another man.
>
> (*Mail*, 26 November 2014)

> The manager from Hampstead, north west London, believes a healthy appetite equals a healthy bank balance – and also goes towards creating an utterly gorgeous, **curvy** body.
>
> (*Sun*, 5 April 2016)

A number of these adjectives index meat products, for example *beefy*, *porky* and *meaty*, while *roly-poly* references a type of pudding, jam roly-poly, which traditionally contains beef suet. The implication, then, is that such people have either become overweight due to excessive consumption of meat products or that they somehow resemble or even consist of these products.

Collectively, these terms are used to refer to people with obesity or who are overweight a total of 4,762 times across the corpus, with the *Mail* again exhibiting the most uses (1,645 cases) and the *Star* having the most proportionally (52.04 occurrences per 100,000 words). This does not include numerous cases where the meanings or impacts of such words are discussed in articles about obesity. Nor does it account for incidences of adjectives which do not directly modify people, as in the following two cases.

> **PLUMP** MY RIDE – THE CARS FIT FOR FATTIES; The rise of obesity is a **meaty** challenge for vehicle designers.
>
> (*Times*, 23 October 2011)

Last week, the World Health Organisation published some **hefty**, earth-shaking figures which publically body-shamed the UK as having one of the highest obesity rates in Europe and suggesting that by 2030 a whopping 74 per cent of British men and 64 per cent of women will be overweight or obese.

(*Telegraph*, 15 May 2015)

Articles such as this take advantage of the fact that words from the semantic domain of weight gain can be applied not only to people but to other phenomena, too. Thus, articles about obesity often contain words that could refer to weight gain or size but are scattered through the text to refer to other things in terms of their amount. So, when the *Times* describes the challenge for vehicle designers as *meaty* in the previous extract, we are supposed to understand that this will be a difficult challenge but also that the journalist is using language somewhat archly because *meaty* is also a word used euphemistically to describe people with obesity.

There is variation across newspapers, with the *Times* most likely to use *porky* and *blubbery*, the *Sun* to use *tubby* and the *Star* having most uses of *lardy*. There is not always consensus over the exact meanings of these words. In the following extract, the *Mirror* uses *cuddly* and *chubby* in a way that suggests they are at a less problematic end of a continuum.

Because this child wasn't just **chubby** or **cuddly**, she was grotesquely, life-threateningly fat.

(*Mirror*, 11 December 2013)

On the other hand, the following extract, from a reader's letter to the *Star*'s 'Just Jane' problem page, suggests that someone's self-labelling of *cuddly* is euphemistically obscuring a serious weight problem.

Every time I beg her to stop stuffing and start dieting, she chants that she's fit, fab and sexy. She insists that she loves being big and **cuddly**. But she's fooling no-one but herself. I can see the struggle she has getting out of bed.

(*Star*, 11 March 2008)

And in this *Express* article, *cuddly* is implied to be an untruthful, if kinder, alternative to *overweight*, which is viewed as contributing towards our 'confused idea of political correctness'.

Words such as "**cuddly**" are replacing the more brutal (and truthful) "overweight", with even the porky James Corden of Gavin & Stacey lauded for his sex appeal.

(*Express*, 5 July 2009)

These euphemistic terms are often used to refer to animals, particularly pets, as in the following from the *Mail*.

> KitKat-thieving **chunky** chihuahua and Puff the **podgy** puss head to slimming bootcamp to shift the pounds
>
> (*Mail*, 28 April 2016)

The word choices here often appear to be led by tabloid style, which favours alliteration. Of the 125 references to *porky*, 63 (50.4 per cent) are followed by another word beginning with *p* (e.g. *pooch, pets, PCs, pupils*, etc.). Similar alliterative patterns are found with the other euphemistic adjectives, e.g. *chubby children, tubby toddlers, lardy lags, hefty hounds, flabby felines, voluptuous vixens*. A weight-loss narrative story in the *Express* (7 January 2014) begins with, 'I went from a roly poly on the rollercoaster to slimline fan of scuba diving.' Punning is also a common feature of articles containing these adjectives, for example, an article in *The Sun* about obesity rates in commuters is titled, 'The jam roly poly' (8 May 2012).

The second set of adjectives we focus on do not act as synonyms for words such as *obese, overweight* or *fat* but instead collocate with them, investing the referents of these terms with additional characteristics. Collocations help to establish associations between concepts, so if two concepts are frequently connected, the mention of one can trigger thoughts of the other in the minds of readers/hearers (Durrant and Doherty 2010). The first set of collocates describe people labelled as *obese, overweight* or *fat* in terms of not being physically attractive: *ugly, unattractive, frumpy* and *disgusting* (158 occurrences collectively). It is also important to consider how these concepts are linked together. An analysis of the 101 cases where *ugly* collocates with *obese, overweight* or *fat* found a rather mixed picture. Thirty-five cases were used to describe someone as *fat* and/or ugly in a fairly uncritical way, as in this example.

> A staggering 65 per cent of British singletons now turn to the internet looking for love. But everyone who's ever dated online knows personal profiles can be a minefield – too often a tall, dark, handsome millionaire turns out to be a short, **fat, ugly** geek.
>
> (*Mail*, 1 October 2008)

Another twenty-six cases occurred in weight loss narratives, where someone is described as initially feeling *fat* and *ugly* or is labelled as such by someone else.

> Woman called 'ugly piece of fat garbage' by her boyfriend – ditches him and loses 10 stone; Alvina Rayne's bullying ex called her an "**ugly** piece of **fat** piece of garbage" who "no one would want" when she reached 20 stone
>
> (*Mirror*, 22 November 2016)

In these narratives, the reader is prompted to feel pity for the person with obesity and the person calling them names is not framed positively (in the example just shown, referred to as a *bullying ex*). However, the outcome of the narrative is that success is framed as losing weight so that the labels of *ugly* and *fat* no longer apply. In this sense, the labelling, although implied to be cruel, often acts as part of the inspiration for the protagonist to lose weight. This brings to mind Evans's (2006: 262) discussion of a House of Commons report on obesity which refers to 'the psychological impacts of stigma associated with obesity, where the cause of the problem is implied to be the individuals' body size rather than the stigma' (the logical solution therefore being that the individual concerned loses weight, rather than others ceasing stigmatising practices such as bullying and name-calling).

A further thirty cases involve criticisms of people who label others as obese and/or ugly, as in this article about a man who handed people insulting cards on public transport.

> The card went on: "We also object to that the beatiful (sic) pig is used as an insult. You are not a pig. You are a **fat**, ugly human." Ms Florish, from Southend-on-Sea, Essex, said the action was "hateful and cowardly and could potentially upset people struggling with confidence".
>
> (*Independent*, 1 December 2015)

Such cases view 'poking fun' at people with obesity as problematic in as much as it is presented as being unkind but does not intrinsically criticise the view that high weight equates to unattractiveness per se. However, a smaller number of cases (ten) do question such representations.

> No public health campaign could begin to compete with the message sent out every day in every way that thin is beautiful, and **fat** is **ugly**, undesirable and a sign of moral uselessness. That's not a nudge, it's a daily knock on the head with a cudgel.
>
> (*Guardian*, 18 August 2016)

When terms such as *fat* and *ugly* collocate with one another, it is not always the case, then, that they are used uncritically and to stigmatising effect. And such 'critical' cases adopt one of two stances: (i) that such labels are a form of bullying (implicitly accepting that *fat* and *ugly* are linked), or (ii) that high weight does not necessarily equate with unattractiveness. However, the critical cases need to draw on the prevalent discourse first in order to present a different perspective, and as such instances are in the minority, they are likely to be recognised by readers as a less commonly held view.

Other adjectives which collocate with *fat*, *overweight* or *obese* include those which indicate that such people are in poor health (*ill*, *unfit*, *unhealthy*: 384 cases), inactive (*lazy*, *sedentary*: 150 cases), unhappy (*unhappy*, *miserable*, *depressed, desperate*: 122 cases), unintelligent (*stupid, thick, illiterate*: 72 cases) or describe other (arguably negative) attributes: *bald* (27), *drunk* (26), *greedy* (22) and *ashamed* (17). The use of these words supports Flint et al.'s (2016: 24) finding of 'evidence of promotion of Protestant ethic values in newspaper portrayals of obesity, presenting obese people as immoral, slothful, and gluttonous, and expressing the view that obesity is akin to deviant and immoral behaviors'.

Considering the above finding, it is perhaps surprising to find a number of (usually) positively loaded adjectives collocating with *fat, obese* and *overweight*: *happy, funny, jolly, beautiful, attractive* and *proud* (261 cases in total). These adjectives are not always used straightforwardly, though, and are often negated in our corpus. For example, with the collocation of *fat, obese* or *overweight* with *happy*, seventy-one cases associate the two qualities together as in the example that follows.

> I'm not trying to stand up and say that every obese person has some tragic event in their past which they're trying to cover up by way of inhaling multipacks of crisps, some people really do just love food, have no problem with being **overweight** and are **happy** with that, which is fine.
>
> (*Independent*, 19 October 2012)

However, there are almost as many cases (68) where this link is disparaged.

> Katie, who believes there is no such thing as a **happy fat** person – they're simply in denial – was appalled to discover recently that some British mothers were feeding their offspring liquidised Chinese and Indian takeaways.
>
> (*Telegraph*, 8 January 2015)

The adjectives *funny* and *jolly* tend to be used in reference to stereotypes around obesity, implying that obesity is humorous in itself but also that people with obesity can gain a small amount of social capital by making others laugh. The terms often occur as part of the kinds of weight loss narratives described earlier.

> Mr Meola is to speak at a weight loss seminar on December 10 about going from a '246kg **funny fat** guy' to a '120kg personal trainer'.
>
> (*Mail*, 30 November 2016)

As with *happy* seen in the *Telegraph* extract, it is also suggested that people appearing to hold these qualities are masking an inner sadness.

> The old picture of a **jolly fat** person couldn't be further from the truth. Although some fat people might indeed be jolly, the majority don't enjoy their condition and wish they were slim.
>
> (*Mail*, 15 May 2008)

Verbs: Actions

Verbs denote actions and are interesting to examine because they can indicate ways of representing people based on what they do or what is being done to them. One salient category of verbs that people with obesity are linked to in our corpus denotes eating. These include *guzzle, gorge, scoff, feast on* and *devour*. Some verbs imply that the amounts of food being consumed are vast: *cram, shovel, shove, stuff*, and the construction *fill* [possessive pronoun] *face*, while others imply that food is eaten (too) quickly: *wolf, pig out, gobble, gulp, swig, bolt, scoff*. The terms *wolf* and *pig out* construct the referent in animalistic terms, associating their eating behaviour with animals who eat voraciously, indiscriminately or quickly. Additionally, the verb *swill* conjures up images of pigs due to its use within the term *pig swill*. Collectively, the verbs listed in this paragraph are used to refer to the ways that people with obesity eat or drink 3,261 times across the corpus, with the *Mail* once again having the most uses (1,077), and the *Star* containing the most uses proportionally (34 occurrences per 100,000 words). Unlike some of the categories of words noted previously, these verbs tend to be used to straightforwardly insult or shame as opposed to debating the appropriacy or kindness of such language. These verbs suggest disgust at a lack of self-control and place responsibility for obesity with the individual engaging in an eating behaviour.

> Last weekend in Cornwall I stopped at a deli in Tintagel to eat a pasty, and gawped at the procession of fatties, waddling along the main street licking ice creams and **gobbling** chips, their thighs chafing with every tiny step.
>
> (*Independent*, 13 September 2014)

Perhaps because such verbs paint such a strongly negative picture there are numerous legitimating strategies associated with their use. For example, the verbs can be linked to consequences for health.

> Is there no one to tell this profoundly stupid woman that she might be eating her way into the record books but she is also **guzzling** towards an early grave?
>
> (*Sun*, 20 August 2011)

Additionally, they can be used in first-person quotes as part of weight loss narratives.

> He'd since slowly piled on the pounds and now, 12 years later, weighed nearly 20st. 'I coped with problems in my life by eating too much, **shovelling** in ice-cream, stopping on the way home from work to have a Big Mac with extra chips before dinner,' says the civil servant, now 38.
>
> (*Mail*, 15 March 2010)

In this example, *shovelling* appears in quoted speech for a man who once had obesity but now does not, with the potential cruelty of its use ameliorated somewhat by being a self-attributed description of past behaviour.

As with some of the terms discussed earlier, verbs relating to eating are also often found in articles about obesity but in metaphorical contexts that do not refer to the actions of people with obesity directly. A typical use involves stories about the strain that people with obesity place on the NHS.

> Diabetes now **gobbles** up more than 10% of the NHS budget, with that percentage set to rise steeply in the coming years.
>
> (*Guardian*, 13 July 2017)

As a left-leaning newspaper, the *Guardian* is perhaps less likely than other newspapers to directly attribute blame for taking up health budgets on people with obesity, instead using abstraction (van Leeuwen 1996: 59) by referring to the concept of diabetes as doing the gobbling (as opposed to *people* with diabetes). However, in the following excerpt, the metaphorical action of gobbling is attributed to people with obesity, again to focus on their cost to the NHS.

> ... the obese are **gobbling** up limited NHS services and costing taxpayers more than 55 million a year. How can we change this worrying trend?
>
> (*Telegraph*, 23 June 2014)

People with obesity are not just represented as greedy in terms of food consumption, then, but their greed is shown to extend to other contexts, such as their use of healthcare services.

> Young people who take up regular sport are unlikely to become the heavy smokers and binge-drinkers who **devour** a disproportionate slice of NHS funds.
>
> (*Mail*, 11 August 2012)

However, more typically, these consumption verbs tend to refer to certain types of food, including regular mentions of sweet food (*chocolate, cakes, doughnuts*), fast-food or 'junk' food (*burgers, fry-ups, kebabs, chips, pies, crisps, KFC, McDonalds pizza, chicken vindaloo*) or alcohol (*beer* and *booze*). Additionally, portion sizes of meals consumed by people with obesity are often described as large, with typical references including *a three-course meal*, a *giant bottle of fizzy pop, banquet after banquet* and *a gargantuan pork chop*. Like other types of words discussed in this chapter, references to foods consumed by people with obesity are often scattered throughout articles, with the *Sun* in particular employing them in puns.

> Look into my **pies**; FAT PATIENTS HYPNOTISED TO THINK THIN
>
> (*Sun*, 23 July 2010)

In the next extract, people with obesity are construed as not just choosing to eat unhealthy foods but also as placing strain on the NHS, with the author characterising them as selfish and expecting others to pay their medical bills. People with obesity are discursively excluded from the intended audience through use of the inclusive *us* in collective reference to the journalist and readers *other than* those with obesity.

> The NHS spends billions on optional lifestyle surgery, while the annual bill soars for treating obese people who choose a **McDonald**'s fast-food lifestyle, then expect us to pay for its consequences.
>
> (*Mail*, 21 March 2012)

Other verbs denote the movement of people with obesity. These relate to walking (*waddle* 269 occurrences, *haul* 51, *heave* 26, *lumber* 20, *shift* 8) or describe the movement of the body (*wobble* 148, *jiggle* 42). In the following example, a combination of othering techniques is used to represent people with obesity. Along with the verb *waddling*, they are referred to collectively (*a nation*). The nomination strategy employed here, collectivisation, is a technique which depersonalises and de-emphasises individual differences, while abstraction is used to represent them as *health crises*. Additionally, reference to their clothing (*XXL tracksuits*) emphasises their large size and, since tracksuits represent leisurewear, implies that they are unlikely to be found in employment.

> If it's a choice between a nation of **waddling** health crises in XXL tracksuits, or a few size zero models on billboards, it's time to think seriously about which image is really the most damaging.
>
> (*Express*, 5 July 2009)

Just as consumption verbs such as *gobble* and *devour* are used metaphorically, the movement verbs also have metaphorical uses, as in the following cases where collectivisation again appears (*nation, country*) and the metaphor is concerned with representing obesity itself.

> WE are a country **lumbering** towards an epidemic of obesity, with six out of ten adults classed as clinically overweight.
>
> (*Mail*, 1 June 2013)

> The change would allow more time after work for outdoor pursuits such as jogging, football, tennis – not unhelpful for a nation **waddling** its way through an obesity crisis.
>
> (*Times*, 26 October 2016)

As seen previously, the lexis associated with being obese is employed in other contexts – related to obesity but not attributed to the actions of people with obesity themselves.

> After all, every high street is crammed with takeaway food outlets and supermarkets **heaving** with junk food.
>
> *(Mail, 1 October 2016)*

The verbs *haul, heave* and *shift* are of interest because, unlike *waddle* and *lumber*, they are frequently used to denote actions of which a person with obesity is the grammatical patient as opposed to the agent. Such cases typically occur in articles about extreme cases of obesity.

> Britain's fattest teenager had to be **hauled** out of her home and into hospital after being unable to stand
>
> *(Mail, 28 May 2012)*

The dehumanising tone of such articles is emphasised by their use of verbs such as *haul* and *shift* which are more typically associated with the movement of inanimate objects such as furniture. Other verbs associated with movement represent the bodies of people with obesity as undergoing strain: *sweat* (20 cases), *wheeze* (10), *pant* (33) and *puff* (15), further associating obesity with ill-health and unattractiveness. The following excerpt presents such people in terms of spectacle, positioning them as being watched and gawped at.

> We've all seen them and gawped. I'm talking about the obese parents, chain munching chips as they hand their chubby children chocolate bars. We've watched infants waddling like Weebles, thighs chafing as they **puff** and **pant** their way down the street.
>
> *(Express, 6 September 2011)*

In the following excerpt, obesity is used as a general insult with the metaphor of an 'obese, wheezing child' being applied to the state of the Labour Government. The article shows how, even when writing about topics that are unrelated to obesity, the concept provides a widely and easily applied way of evaluating something negatively.

> Roll on the election! A fatigued Labour government has left Britain dishonoured and diminished, its treasury empty and its credit exhausted. Having spent years engorging the public sector, it now finds its obese, **wheezing** child turning on it in a spoilt rage. Strike follows strike.
>
> *(Telegraph, 3 April 2010)*

Another set of verbs are used describe people with obesity as being too large for their environment: *fit* (173), *squeeze* (171), *wedge* (51), *cram* (9), *cramp* (6) and *clog* (3). These verbs often occur in two contexts. First, they appear in stories designed to highlight the 'obesity epidemic' and involve descriptions of everyday objects that are being redesigned to accommodate people with obesity.

> In a new twist, Dr Christian Jessen visits America where, in the city of Evansville, coffins are the size of boats and ambulances have to be redesigned to **fit** the super-obese.
>
> (*Sun*, 25 February 2012)

Other cases involve weight loss narratives where the 'wake-up call' involves a person with obesity having difficulty fitting into a particular space.

> A once morbidly obese man has transformed his life by dramatically losing 10st after he couldn't **fit** on a fairground ride seat with his son.
>
> (*Mail*, 22 January 2013)

Other objects which people with obesity are described as having difficulty fitting in to or through include mortuary doors, mortuary fridges, coffins, plane seats, cars, baths, CT scanners, clothes, tanks, showers, tents, elevators, mobility scooters and polling booths.

While the majority of such stories are reported with a reasonable amount of sensitivity, with readers encouraged to have empathy for the person undergoing the experience, this is not always the case, and in the following excerpt, the reference to people with obesity in general terms as opposed to naming a specific person serves to legitimate the use of dehumanising language.

> Too often I have been stuck in economy class **wedged** half underneath some morbidly obese, sweating flobber; after six hours of this sideways moist pressure, the lard-bucket's flesh fuses with your own and you need a scalpel to extricate yourself and take refuge in the toilets for a cigarette.
>
> (*Times*, 26 April 2009)

So far, we have considered verbs used mostly to position people with obesity as agents. However, a smaller set of verbs are used with people with obesity as the grammatical patient: *dub*, *shame* and *brand* (264 occurrences in total). These verbs tend to be used critically of those who describe people as *obese*, *fat* or *overweight* and such cases are viewed as newsworthy enough to have articles built around them, particularly relating to a set of commonly found narratives. For example, of the thirty-eight cases of people being *branded* as fat, twenty-one relate to narratives about a person with obesity being bullied, sometimes with tragic consequences.

> She was **branded** a 'big **fat** donkey' by cruel tormentors who would physically assault her – leading her to try and take her own life.
>
> (*Mail*, 16 January 2015)

Only one story indicates how a person *branded* as obese responds in a way which indicates pride in their weight.

> Plus-size model Iskra Lawrence shuts down haters by posing on bed of CRISP PACKETS; The size 14 stunner retaliated in amazing fashion after she was **branded** a 'fat cow' by a nasty troll
>
> (*Mirror*, 6 April 2016)

This article positively evaluates Iskra as a 'stunner', while describing her retaliation as 'amazing' and describing her critics as 'haters' and 'a nasty troll'. While this article could be seen as body-positive, we note that what is considered newsworthy is inspired by comments about a woman's body and that the article contributes to evaluation, especially of women, as an everyday social practice. Clearly, the woman in question is a model and the fact she posed on a bed of crisp packets indicates a desire to create a newsworthy story. She is unlikely to complain about the article, especially as it presents her in a positive light. However, we note that throughout the corpus, evaluation of bodies is so common that it becomes banal and almost goes unnoticed. An alternative discourse might be simply not to frame evaluation of bodies as kind or unkind, as in the aforementioned article, but to question whether such (and so much) evaluation is needed in the first place.

The article about Iskra Lawrence is unusual as being one of the few where a supposed 'fat' person shows pride in their body after being bullied. However, nine of the other twenty-one bullying stories that describe how people are *branded* as fat resemble the types of weight loss narratives seen earlier, where the branding serves as inspiration for the protagonist of the story to lose weight.

> Tubby teen to trolley dolly: Junk food addict **branded** "**fat** friend" on girls' holiday sheds 6st and lands job as air stewardess
>
> (*Mirror*, 29 March 2017)

Finally, a further seventeen cases involve stories where someone is described as being incorrectly branded as fat or overweight.

> Harriet Jackson's parents say they were furious after receiving a letter warning that their 'slim and happy' daughter was 'overweight'. Parents have spoken of their outrage after their 'sporty and slim' five-year-old daughter was **branded** too **fat** by NHS children's chiefs.
>
> (*Mirror*, 19 March 2016)

These stories mainly relate to the use of the controversial BMI measure. As noted in Chapter 1, the BMI has received criticism for not accounting for certain body types (particularly shorter but muscular bodies), as well as for being used to diagnose illness. We note, though, that for these kinds of articles the issue is one pertaining to incorrect or unfair labelling, as opposed to whether terms such as 'too fat' are ever appropriate.

A final set of verbs describe weight gain. There are a range of ways that we can describe weight gain. Mostly common in the corpus is the use of the verb *gain* as in *gaining weight, pounds, fat* or *kilos* (7,287 cases). However, other, less common wordings involve the verb *become* (as in *becoming, becomes* or *became obese, overweight* or *fat* – 2,958 cases). Less common still, people can be described as *getting obese, overweight* or *fat* (1,663 cases), *putting on weight/ pounds/fat/kilos* (1,656 cases), or perhaps more negatively, *piling on weight, pounds* etc. (1,660 cases). A particularly negative use involves the verb *balloon* (370 cases), which functions as a metaphor. While *balloon* is normally reserved for cases where weight gain is indicated to be severe, there are exceptions, such as the next excerpt, where a gain of three stones is described as 'balloon[ing]'.

> A FORMER model and fitness trainer is sticking to his New Year's resolution – to pile on more than SEVEN STONE. Paul James, 32, said he wants to understand his fat gym clients. His Adonis-like 12st frame has **ballooned** to 15st – on the way to his target of 20st.
>
> (*Sun*, 25 February 2009)

Obesity and Criminality

In this section, we consider how obesity is made relevant in stories about notorious people, particularly criminals and dictators. Such people are considered newsworthy because of actions they have carried out in the past and their names present a recognisable draw for the public. In the following two articles, the *Star* comments on weight gains of two men who are in prison for committing multiple murders, Ian Huntley and Peter Sutcliffe.

> BEHIND BARS; Evil Huntley clinically obese after guzzling chocolates. SOHAM killer Ian Huntley has ballooned to almost 18 stone after bingeing on Wispa and Toffee Crisp chocolate bars in his cell. The 35-year-old monster is now clinically obese and is nicknamed "Blobby" by fellow lags.
>
> (*Star*, 31 May 2009)

> FAT RIPPER GETS GBP 350 Wii FIT. AND YOU PAY. Broadmoor bosses have blown £350 on a Wii Fit games console for obese Peter Sutcliffe to help the mass murderer stay alive. Doctors say the Yorkshire Ripper, 63, is eating himself into an early grave on a junk food diet of burgers, pies and chocolate. His weight has ballooned to 20st and he faces having his feet amputated after chronic diabetes clogged his arteries. The fiend – jailed in 1981 for murdering 13 women – has refused to follow medical advice to go on a crash diet and start exercising.
>
> (*Star*, 15 August 2009)

The first article simply notes that Huntley has gained weight, an item of information which is thus cast as worthy of public attention in itself. There is something of a sense of glee in the reporting of his weight gain, which, in the context of the general consensus in the press relating to weight gain, could be read as a fitting punishment (the *Star* refers to Huntley as *evil* and a *monster*). The second article uses similar language, referring to Sutcliffe as a *fiend*. Both men are positioned as being responsible for their weight gains through descriptions of their diets, and Sutcliffe is described as refusing to follow a medical diet. Additionally, the purchase of a £350 Wii Fit games console to help Sutcliffe lose weight is described as being paid for by readers (presumably through tax contributions) in a way designed to provoke outrage. Such articles, which position readers as taxpayers, are a common staple of right-leaning tabloid news (See Baker et al. 2013).

In the *Mirror*, quite a lengthy amount of space is given to describing the weight of would-be terrorist, Irfan Naseer.

> Irfan Naseer, 31, is facing life behind bars after being convicted of planning a bomb blitz that would even have rivalled the 9/11 attacks in the US, which killed almost 3,000. The 23 stone fanatic aimed to plant eight rucksack nail bombs in crowded places around the country and was the ringleader of a gang who wanted to turn Britain into "a war zone". He even tried to recruit suicide bombers to join his cause. But despite his secret ambitions, school pals described him as a "joker" and "class idiot" who performed rap songs in the playground. And his own mother called him a "mummy's boy". He was known as Chubs at school and one ex-classmate, who did not want to be named, said: "Irfan was your average Western teenager. He'd spend ages playing Fifa on PlayStation. He was a massive Liverpool fan. Despite his size he was a decent footballer." He was nicknamed Razor because he was about the same size as Neil Ruddock. Irfan loved food. He was always going back for seconds at the canteen if there was any left. He didn't seem bothered about being fat.
>
> (*Mirror*, 25 February 2013)

As with Huntley, we are told about Nasser's nicknames (*Chubs*, *Razor*) and in a quote he is described as a 'decent footballer ... despite his size', implying that people with larger bodies are unlikely to be good at football. His weight is firmly positioned as being due to his love of food, with a description of him as 'always going back for seconds' and, most interestingly, not seeming bothered about his size. In the context of a detailed discussion of the behaviour and motivations of a terrorist, it is notable that Irfan is described as not caring about his weight, a trait which is designed to mark him as unusual and as perhaps contributing towards a wider pattern of social deviance.

Articles about the notorious leader of North Korea, Kim Jong-un, also focus on his weight. In this extract he is alliteratively labelled 'tubby tyrant' and described as 'gorging' on fast food. This behaviour is marked as particularly selfish (again, associating obesity to gluttony as seen in the earlier articles in this section), as the article creates an opposition between this and the fact that millions of people in his country are starving.

> TUBBY tyrant Kim Jong-un is gorging himself on McDonald's, KFC and Pizza Hut flown in from takeaways 100 miles away in China. Many of North Korea's 27 million people live in abject poverty, but the fat dictator spends thousands having food delivered by his personal pilot.
>
> (*Star*, 31 January 2015)

While these articles feature people who are infamous for aspects of their behaviour that are not related to their weight, a set of related articles in the *Mail* also describe the criminal behaviour of more ordinary people with obesity.

> Obese woman who went on TV to complain that she was too fat to get a job caught stealing cakes just hours after This Morning appearance
>
> (*Mail*, 29 March 2013)

> Forty-STONE fraudster who used stolen credit card to order 120 of Domino's pizza fails to attend court 'because he's too fat to get out of his house'
>
> (*Mail*, 4 October 2013)

> Bentley-driving Stephen Sussams, 59, fraudulently claimed nearly £615,000 in housing and council tax benefit but argued he should not be sent to prison because he is obese.
>
> (*Mail*, 18 January 2013)

The first example frames obesity as leading to criminality, with a description of an 'obese woman' caught stealing cakes, while the second also describes food theft. Here, the man's obesity is also described as the reason for him not attending court. The third example involves a man who fraudulently claims welfare benefit but uses obesity as an excuse not to be sent to prison. These stories contribute towards a sense in which people with obesity are bungling, petty criminals with negative qualities such as greed and laziness implied to be linked to their weight. These stories contribute towards representations of people with obesity as flawed comedy characters. However, they form part of a continuum, at the other end of which sit people such as Sutcliffe and Nasser, whose crimes are not viewed as funny, although stories about their weight gain paint them in a more trivial light. While such stories are not as common as the weight loss narratives described elsewhere in this chapter, there are enough of them to constitute a pattern, and the linking of crime with obesity arguably presents one of the most negative types of representation in the corpus.

Conclusion

At the start of this chapter we noted how commentators on stigmatisation have taken an almost fatalistic view of it, seeing it as inevitable in societies – a way that we demonstrate that we belong by identifying those who do not. One way that the stigmatisation of people with obesity in the press occurs is through the connection of obesity with characteristics that are viewed as immoral: laziness, greed, lack of self-control and criminality. Obesity and high weight are equated with unattractiveness, unhealthiness and unhappiness, with the solution almost always being individuals losing weight – something which is framed as a matter of personal responsibility and choice. While, in modern society, stigmatisation is generally viewed as at least unkind and at worst immoral, journalists are able to legitimate their stigmatising practices relating to obesity by relying on the argument that such practices are carried out for the good of people with it. In other words, journalists will argue that they have to be cruel to be kind. This argument naturally extends to the view that if stigma is the solution to obesity, then a society which does not engage in it is actually morally deficient.

However, despite the voices of some more right-wing commentators in the press who claim that obesity is exacerbated by political correctness and that *more* shaming is needed, we found that, in fact, there was a great deal of shaming in the press as a whole. Some newspapers were more openly cruel than others, with certain tabloids using the kind of name-calling we would perhaps associate with schoolyard bullying while others engaged in more subtly distancing language. Others indirectly contributed to the discourse by presenting a sympathetic stance towards people who were bullied because of obesity while leaving the bullying itself unchallenged, except in cases where it was felt to be unwarranted (e.g. cases of people inaccurately being labelled as 'obese' or 'fat'). If shaming is seriously intended to encourage people to lose weight, then it seems ironic that during the period under consideration, average BMI scores did not fall, and instead newspapers are increasingly reporting on the UK's 'obesity epidemic'. Shaming, in other words, does not seem to be having the intended effect.

As with the sly uses of the lexis of obesity – terms such as *meaty*, *hefty* and *gobbles*, which often occur in articles about people with obesity but do not directly refer to them – the use of alliteration and punning indicates that much of the press utilises comedic discourse, drawing on a language style that is commonly associated with humour (Nash 1985). The effect of this kind of discourse is complex. First, readers are encouraged to view obesity as a source of humour, with people with obesity as potential targets. Moreover, the content of the articles tended to indicate that these targets were to be laughed *at*, rather than laughed *with*. To be laughed at is to be a source of entertainment, not to be taken seriously. People with obesity are thus viewed as inherently humorous in terms of how their bodies look, the way they move, their interactions with their environments, their apparently uncontrolled predilection for certain foods that they know are bad for them and the enthusiastic or hurried way in which they consume them, sometimes even causing them to commit crime over their love of food.

A joke, when directed towards a social group or identity trait, can be a way of inoculating a negative representation against criticism – another type of legitimation strategy. Detractors can be accused of having 'no sense of humour' or of being overly sensitive or 'politically correct', as the joke appears to be framed as amusing rather than critical of a social group. Rather than constituting strikingly negative representations, then, the overall tone of the linguistic choices examined in this chapter is one which views people with obesity as clownish figures of fun, deserving of laughter due to their gluttony and lack of self-control. It is, however, a representation that lacks empathy, trivialises, and ultimately shames.

Additionally, making jokes about obesity feels jarring when in other parts of the press a common message is about its dangers to people's health and well-being. For example, there are references in the corpus to people digging their grave with a knife and fork or their teeth – a darkly humorous way of referencing the potential for obesity to have fatal consequences. We wonder whether the same kind of language would be seen as appropriate around other groups of people who are, at the same time, construed as facing significant health risks.

Shaming, of any kind, is likely to result in lower self-esteem of the group that is being targeted. Indeed, a House of Commons (2004: 20–21) report noted that 'Psychological damage caused by overweight and obesity is a huge health burden . . . rates of anxiety and depression are three to four times higher among obese individuals [and] obese women are around 37% more likely to commit suicide . . . Excess weight is also likely to lead to prejudice in the workplace, lower self-esteem and reduced job opportunities' [sic]. A potential consequence of shaming is that it will result in people having an increasingly complicated relationship with their bodies and the food they eat, with binge eating and night eating associated with temporary relief but contributing towards further weight gain (Faulconbridge and Bechtel 2014). Shaming acts as a form of social control. The implicit message behind shaming is that it is not just people with obesity who are urged to monitor their weight but the discourse applies to everyone who encounters it – a social practice which brings to mind the notion of Foucault's panoptical surveillance (Foucault 1979; Couch et al. 2015). We all become the judges and the judged, and fear of gaining weight is likely to result in anxiety, over-preoccupation and harmful behaviours. These points are to be borne in mind as we move to the next chapter, which considers how efforts to lose weight and what counts as *healthy* are represented in the corpus.

6   Healthy Body
Diet and Exercise

Introduction

In previous chapters, we have seen how a discourse of personal responsibility
has tended to take precedence in UK press reporting around obesity. In fact,
the analysis in Chapter 4 indicated that the personal responsibility discourse
has increased in frequency over time, seemingly becoming an increasingly
accepted way of understanding and conceptualising obesity in this context.
In this chapter, we focus on a number of aspects relating to how the
personal responsibility discourse is substantiated, considering four words in
detail: *diet*, *body*, *healthy* and *exercise*. These words are all reasonably frequent and distinctive in our corpus, appearing among the sixty most frequent
content words (lexical nouns, adjectives, verbs and adverbs) and the top forty
keywords compared against the written section of the British National Corpus
(see Table 6.1).

Diet is the most frequent of these words, occurring 38,111 times. We briefly
considered collocates of *diet* in Chapter 2, where it was reported that right-
leaning tabloids featured more use of this word, particularly in weight loss
narratives. Chapter 4 showed how the thematic category FOOD (which contained the word *diet*) comprised the most frequently occurring set of keywords
in the corpus, as well as being the category which increased in frequency the
most over time. So, although we have considered the word *diet* briefly in other
chapters, we use it as a springboard for the focus of this chapter, which is
concerned with how newspapers write about the efforts of individuals to lose
weight. After considering *diet*, we examine the word *body*, chiefly in terms of
the metaphors the press use when constructing the relationship between individuals and their bodies. We then look at the adjective *healthy*, especially in
regard to how the relationship between health and weight is construed. Finally,
we consider *exercise*, which constitutes another component of the 'personal
responsibility discourse, as well as being one of the top ten strongest collocates
of *diet* (using MI^3), with both words regularly occurring together to refer to
either comparable or complementary ways of losing or maintaining weight.

Table 6.1. *Profiles of* diet, body, healthy *and* exercise

	Frequency in Corpus	Content words rank	Keyness position (ranked by LL)
diet	38,111	21	9
body	33,563	25	35
healthy	27,897	35	15
exercise	21,538	58	32

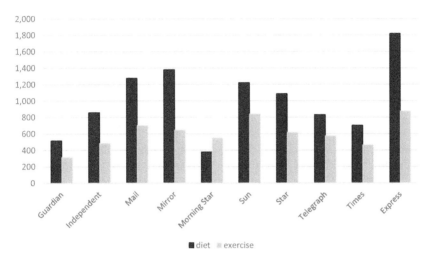

Figure 6.1 Relative frequencies (PMW) of *diet* and *exercise* across different newspapers

There is some variation across newspapers regarding preference for writing about *diet* or *exercise* in articles about obesity, with all but the *Morning Star* exhibiting more use of *diet*, although this pattern is strongest in the *Express*, *Mail* and *Mirror* (see Figure 6.1). Additionally, the *Express* contains the highest relative frequency of both *diet* and *exercise*, while the *Morning Star* mentions *diet* the least and the *Guardian* mentions *exercise* the least, relatively speaking. While Chapter 2 showed that *diet* and *exercise* are top keywords across the whole corpus, Chapter 3 indicated that the frequency of *diet* is particularly pronounced in the right-leaning tabloids relative to other sections of the press, although *exercise* does not appear to be strongly associated with any type of newspaper in particular.

Additionally, Figure 6.2 shows that while use of *diet* is clearly increasing over time, references to *exercise* have remained reasonably stable. The trend

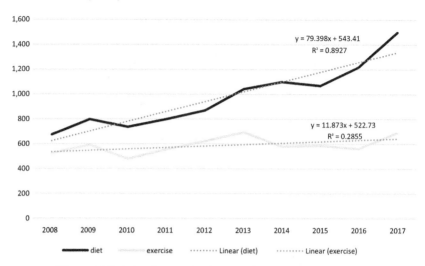

Figure 6.2 Relative frequencies (PMW) of *diet* and *exercise* over time

line for *diet* shows a slope of 79.39 and an R^2 of 0.89, while for *exercise* the trend line slope is lower at 11.87, showing a small upwards trend, and a lower R^2 of 0.28 (see Chapter 4 for explanations of how trend lines are calculated). The relative frequencies of the two words are quite similar in 2008 but by 2017, *diet* is over twice as frequent as *exercise*.

Considering that both words have strong potential to be employed as part of personal responsibility discourses, one of the aims of this chapter is to consider why references to *diet* have gone up over time while *exercise* has remained relatively stable by exploring the wider linguistic patterns around these two words.

Diet

Our analysis begins with a consideration of the strongest collocates of *diet*. Table 6.2 shows its strongest 100 collocates, ranked by MI^3 (span: +/− 3). We have manually grouped these collocates into thematic categories. To avoid proliferation of categories, we specified that each category must contain at least three collocates. Otherwise, we placed the collocates in the 'Others' category. As noted previously, *exercise* was a collocate of *diet*, and that mostly accounted for the presence of the collocate *and*, due to the frequent appearance of phrases such as *diet and exercise*. In terms of the positions in which the two words appear when co-occurring, *diet* is more than seven times as likely to appear before *exercise* than after it, indicating that, discursively, *diet* is

Table 6.2. *Collocates of* diet

Category	Collocates
Grammatical words	*a, the, and, on, of, to, in, is, your, their, with, 's, that, her, for, can, or, as, his, my, by, but, this, from, our, an, which, was, has, you, before, through, it, I, not*
Supplements	*Coke, drinks, pills*
Types of diet	*balanced, Mediterranean, healthy, high-fat, poor, strict, low-fat, 5:2, low-carb, Atkins, high, rich, Dukan, Paleo, low, low-calorie, vegan, plant-based, fat, high-protein, western, unhealthy, vegetarian, crash, varied, daily, calorie-controlled, Mediterranean-style, low-carbohydrate, calorie, Nordic, fad, ketogenic, regular, sugar, fast*
Punctuation	*, . : " - ' ?*
Others	*exercise, plan, lifestyle, eating, breakfast, weight, fed, loss, regime, eat, following, changes, follow, food, change, nutrition, help*

normally given preference over exercise in terms of its 'firstness' (Freebody and Baker 1987: 98).

Five grammatical collocates, *my*, *your*, *their*, *his* and *her* are possessive pronouns used either to address readers directly or to talk about people who want to lose weight more generally (though readers could be indirectly included in this group). For example,

> If people incorporate almonds into **their diet**, they should expect multiple benefits, including ones that can improve heart health.
>
> (*Express*, 13 August 2017)

> BHF dietary advice also includes reducing the amount of salt in **your diet** and making sure you eat five portions of fruit and vegetables a day, and two to three portions of oily fish a week.
>
> (*Telegraph*, 18 February 2011)

In these examples, *diet* refers simply to the food a person generally eats, whether they are aiming to lose weight or not. This meaning of *diet* encapsulates permanent eating habits and does not necessarily imply healthy eating or weight loss.

> Mum-of-three Bella Vrondos, 33, said she weighed 18st at her heaviest as she lived off **a diet including burgers and fries, chocolate and pies**
>
> (*Mirror*, 11 July 2017)

However, *diet* can also refer more specifically to eating-related behaviours that are intended to induce weight loss. The prepositional collocate *on* is used most frequently to denote the state of dieting to lose weight, e.g. being *on a diet*, which occurs in 8.29 per cent of instances where *a* and *diet* co-occur. Being 'on a diet' is implied to be a temporary state, either because it ends once a target weight is reached, or because it is too difficult to maintain.

> True to her word Joanne went **on a diet** and lost nine and a half stone going from a size 30 to a size 12 weighing 12 stone 7lbs.
>
> (*Mail*, 15 October 2013)

> About 28% of young people embark **on a diet** each month and 45% give up after a week.
>
> (*Mirror*, 5 November 2012)

Some of the adjective collocates of *diet* in Table 6.2, such as *healthy* and *varied*, can be used to imply either a time-limited diet to lose weight or general eating habits. Compare the two uses of the bigram *healthy diet* in the following extracts. The first suggests that *healthy diet* involves a sudden change in eating habits designed to facilitate weight loss, while the second indicates eating behaviour from birth.

> Keano was in agony just going for a walk around a park because he was obese. "It was really sad to see so I decided to put him on a **healthy diet** and give him the exercise he wasn't getting before." Cutting out the calories and going for daily walks paid off.
>
> (*Express*, 5 March 2009)

> Children need to start on a **healthy diet** from the day they are born.
>
> (*Guardian*, 21 March 2009)

The multiple and overlapping meanings of *diet* are potentially confusing – does a diet involve losing weight, maintaining a healthy weight or gaining weight? Does a diet require certain foods to be eaten regularly, heavily restricted or omitted altogether? Is a diet meant to last forever or for a set period of time until weight loss goals are achieved? The word *Coke* (which collocates with *diet* 87 per cent of the time in the bigram, *Diet Coke*) illustrates the ambiguity of meaning around *diet*. Marketers brand soft drinks such as Coke as 'diet' to present them as not fattening and even healthy (Chrysochu 2010). However, whether such products constitute 'diet' aids, or should be consumed more widely, is unclear. While some newspapers appear to advocate Diet Coke as a weight loss aid or quote dieters who drink it, others are critical of the brand and claim that it does not aid weight loss.

> I learned how to make better eating choices, I swapped cider for vodka and **Diet Coke** when I wanted a drink.
>
> (*Express*, 13 April 2012)

Is **Diet Coke** making you fat? People who drink at least one can a day
have larger waist measurements

(Mail, 8 April 2015)

There is another reason why the collocate *a* occurs so much with *diet* (apart
from in the phrase *on a diet*) and this is due to the two words appearing in
descriptions of different types of diets, often involving some form of evaluation. This takes us to the third group of collocates in Table 6.2, which lists
different types of diet. A number of these collocates appear in the variable slot,
a [something] *diet*. The words occurring most commonly in the central slot
are adjectives which evaluate the healthiness of the diet *(healthy, poor,
unhealthy)*, its variation *(balanced, varied)*, the foods or nutrients it entails
(low-fat, vegan, low-carbohydrate, plant-based, high-protein), its severity
(strict) or its length *(crash)*.

However, several collocates of *diet* do not appear in this slot but instead
occur in another, related slot: *the* [something] *diet*. *The* is the most frequent
collocate of *diet* overall and, as with *a*, tends to appear with *diet* in the L2
position (two places to the left), indicating that there is often some kind of
modifying or specifying word between *a/the* and *diet*. Proper nouns tend to
occur in the pattern *the* [something] *diet* (e.g. *Atkins, Mediterranean, Dukan,
Paleo, Nordic)*, indicating reference to a specific (sometimes trade-marked)
diet involving specific eating practices.

The Atkins diet is a low-carb, high-protein weight loss programme.
You start with a low-carb diet designed for rapid weight loss. This lasts
at least two weeks, depending on your weight loss goal. During this
phase, you're on a protein, fat and very low-carb diet, including meat,
seafood, eggs, cheese, some veg, butter and oils. During the next three
phases, the weight loss is likely to be more gradual, and regular exercise
is encouraged.

(Mirror, 1 January 2015)

This example, from a New Year's Resolutions article, indicates that some of
the general collocates of *diet* related to food or nutrients, such as *low-carb* and
high-protein, actually give details about specific named diets but, generally, a
distinction can be made between *a* [something] *diet*, which tends to be more
general or evaluative, and *the* [something] *diet*, which indicates a specific
named diet. These are both very productive patterns in the corpus – there are
638 different phrases which fit the pattern *a* [something] *diet* and 618 different
phrases fit the pattern *the* [something] *diet*. The latter pattern includes some
rather strange instances, including *the urine diet, the twinkie diet, the walnut-
enriched diet, the werewolf diet, the tapeworm diet, the steak-and-grapefruit
diet, the pie diet, the raw-meat diet* and *the milkshake diet*. This proliferation of

named diets is sometimes parodied, as in this example, which invents a fictional *sunshine diet*, described as involving the NHS sending people with obesity on holiday and is designed to criticise an actual suggested policy of paying people to lose weight.

> Try **the sunshine diet**
> Latest ploy from the National Institute for Health and Care Excellence to prise fatties away from their triple helpings of curry and chips is to pay them to lose weight. It comes as a report claims warm weather can help the obese fight the flab. How long before the NHS offers free sunshine breaks to Majorca to help these poor victims?
>
> (*Mail*, 25 October 2014)

New and unusual diets are frequently presented as newsworthy, as in the following example, which reports on a new diet craze involving intermittent fasting, known as the 5:2 diet. The text is from an article entitled, '"The SPEED diet" First of a two-part Daily Star guide to kick-starting your fight against the flab', and goes on to note 'today is the day to start your diet'. The reader is directly addressed throughout through use of the second person pronouns *you* and *your*, with the article functioning not merely as a description of the diet but rather as an invitation to readers to imagine themselves on it.

> INTERMITTENT fasting is the new diet craze that involves slashing the number of calories you eat but only on some days of the week, known as fast days. The idea is that you'll reduce your overall calorie intake by around 25%, and start to lose weight without having to deprive yourself every day. You also train your body to crave less food. The most popular version is **the 5:2 Diet** where you fast for two days but eat normally on the other five days of the week.
>
> (*Star*, 15 January 2014)

Elsewhere in this article, intermittent fasting is described as 'the diet frenzy that's sweeping the world', while 'loads of celebrities have got their bodies buff by following the most popular waist-whittling plan the 5:2 Diet'. This association of *the* [something] *diet* with the glamour of celebrities or other well-known people is fairly common.

> I went on **the popcorn diet** that **Madonna** had reportedly used to get back in shape after having a baby.
>
> (*Express*, 30 November 2011)

> **The keto diet** is favored by celebrities such as **Mick Jagger** and **Kim Kardashian**.
>
> (*Mail*, 5 September 2017)

The Dukan diet boasts a host of celebrity followers, including **Jennifer Lopez**, supermodel **Gisele Bundchen**, and Welsh singer **Katherine Jenkins**.

(*Mail*, 9 July 2013)

Hugh Grant has done **the low-sugar 'Clean and Lean' diet**.

(*Independent*, 12 July 2014)

Chancellor **George Osborne** has been on **the celebrity 5:2 diet**.

(*Mirror*, 6 December 2014)

Such diets can form part of the weight loss narratives described in Chapter 3, as this example demonstrates.

Daniel Boulton from Derby lost seven stone on the **Harcombe diet**. He was forced into action when he could no longer weigh himself. He also took up running and is now training for the London Marathon.

(*Mail*, 12 February 2015)

People who have lost weight through dieting are usually positively evaluated in the press. We examined references to weight loss in the articles, identifying three 'productive' phrases which contained evaluative adjectives. These were [ADJECTIVE] *weight loss*, LOSE/SHED *a/an* [ADJECTIVE], and [ADJECTIVE] *transformation*. Within these phrases, the most common adjective was *incredible*, occurring 412 times. This was followed by *dramatic* (241 occurrences), *staggering* (169), *amazing* (157), *whopping* (156), *impressive* (121), *astonishing* (58), *massive* (55), *remarkable* (50) and *huge* (31). The adjectives either emphasise a large amount or impressiveness of the weight loss, with these two qualities often equated with one another.

Obese mother unveils her **incredible transformation** after an unflattering Facebook photo shocked her into losing HALF her body weight

(*Mail*, 3 May 2016)

Slowly but surely, his weight fell away until he had **lost a staggering 32st** through his diet, exercise and mental awareness regime.

(*Express*, 27 November 2014)

A small number of descriptions of the effects of such diets do not follow the usual narrative.

17st BRIDE DIES ON **500 CALORIE WEDDING DIET**; SAM LOST 3st IN 11 WEEKS BRIDE-TO-BE Samantha Clowe died after losing three stone in 11 weeks so she wouldn't be fat for her wedding.

(*Sun*, 9 September 2009)

Jenni Murray told in the Mail how she had lost 5st on the **Dukan Diet**, only to put it all back on again just as quickly.

(*Mail*, 18 July 2013)

Analysis of 100 articles taken at random containing the phrase LOSE a/an [ADJECTIVE] [NUMBER] (e.g. *lost a staggering 48 stone*) found five cases of articles being about dieters left with excess skin and needing an operation to remove it, although all the articles stressed how the weight loss had generally improved the dieter's life and none involved narratives about dieters putting weight back on again or having health problems, so the two examples just shown are rare.

A third way that diets can be assigned credibility is via their association with science – what van Leeuwen (2008) refers to as the authority of expertise – where social actors such as *researchers*, *scientists* or the more informal *boffins* are described as making new findings which can translate into advice regarding the best foods to consume for weight loss.

WEIGHT LOSS is best achieved through good diet and exercise, but **researchers** say they have found the best food to help people lose belly fat fast – protein.

(*Express*, 22 October 2017)

Weight loss diet: THIS tea can help you shed pounds FAST. **Researchers** say a daily cup of tea changes the way body breaks down fat

(*Express*, 6 October 2017)

New research by **boffins** at the University of Surrey reveals cooking then chilling pasta changes the structure, so the body absorbs fewer calories from it.

(*Sun*, 16 November 2014)

Researchers have found a calorie-rich diet packed with 'good' fats such as those in olive oil saw people lose slightly more weight than those who strictly controlled their calories. The findings will fuel the dispute about decades-old guidelines that maintain that eating too much fat is linked to obesity and cardiovascular disease.

(*Mail*, 7 June 2016)

Wine drinkers' diet: now **scientists** say a glass a day may help weight loss DRINKING just a glass of wine a day may actually help people to lose weight, **researchers** now believe.

(*Telegraph*, 18 August 2011)

The last two excerpts both rely on the news value of unexpectedness, in this case that what was previously believed to be true, or 'received wisdom', is now regarded as incorrect, with the opposite being the case. A consequence is that readers who use such stories to inform their weight loss behaviours may find it difficult to stick to a consistent diet, with the information they encounter in the press (and elsewhere) changing over time and exhibiting inconsistency across publications.

While journalists regularly provide details of new diets and explicitly or implicitly encourage readers to follow them, they also acknowledge that diets are often ultimately counter-productive, hence another collocate of *diet*: *fad*, which tends to be negatively evaluated.

> Most people who lose weight by dieting do not keep the weight off over the long term. They try the latest **fad diet**, stick to it for a few weeks or months and drop some pounds, but sooner or later they return to their old eating habits. They regain the weight – possibly adding on even more – and when the next "miracle" diet comes along they try the whole disheartening process again.
>
> (*Times*, 3 September 2016)

Indeed, research on dieting has indicated that short-term diets designed to induce weight loss are usually not successful in the long-term. Mann et al.'s (2007) review study of the long-term effects of dieting found that between one- to two-thirds of dieters regained more weight than they had lost. Part of the reason for this is that calorie-restricted diets can alter metabolic rates and levels of preoccupation with food thoughts, even six years after the diet has ended (Fothergill et al. 2016).

All newspapers refer to *fad diet(s)*, reporting on the dangers of engaging in this kind of weight loss activity, but such references are relatively infrequent – *fad* is the 231st most frequent collocate of *diet* (118 co-occurrences) in the whole corpus, while collocates relating to particular types of diets occur more frequently, e.g. *Atkins* (247 co-occurrences with *diet*) , *low-carb* (239), *5:2* (231), *Dukan* (216) and *Paleo* (165). Some articles which refer disparagingly to fad diets go on to sing the praises of new ways of losing weight, which could also be described as fads. For example, an article in the *Mail* (17 May 2015) begins with the words 'Forget fad diets' but later notes that, 'The popular 5:2 (or Fast) diet whereby you semi-fast for two days a week also seems to be effective.' The article also advises that 'Skipping breakfast may be good for you'.

An ambivalent picture emerges, then, with newspapers simultaneously appearing to both advocate but also advise eschewing 'fad' diets. This also applies more generally to any form of calorie-reducing diet designed to induce weight loss over a short period of time, sometimes involving quite explicit mentions of weight-loss products.

> BUY THE SUN THIS WEEK ... Get exclusive recipes and workouts from Joe's new book The Fat-Loss Plan
>
> (*Sun*, 30 December 2017)

> Buy The Paleo Diet Made Easy by Joy Skipper (Hamlyn) from Telegraph Books at 7.99 + 1.10 p&p.
>
> (*Telegraph*, 8 January 2014)

The tabloids tend to be most positively inclined towards two weight loss organisations which require members to take out subscriptions, *Slimming World* (1,256 occurrences) and *Weight Watchers* (1,558). It is not unusual to find contact information relating to these organisations at the end of slimming narratives.

> For your nearest Slimming World group call 0844 897 8000 or log on to slimmingworld.com
>
> (*Express*, 1 August 2013)

> For more inspiring success stories look out for the June issue of Weight Watchers magazine in shops now, only £2.75.
>
> (*Express*, 13 April 2012)

Weight Watchers produces meal replacements, and these also form part of slimming narratives, as descriptions of the food consumed by people who have lost a lot of weight.

> Fay and Lorraine's diet now...
> Breakfast
> - Porridge and a banana
> - Snack Grapes
> Lunch
> - Soup with Weight Watchers bread
> Snack
> - Weight Watchers crisps
> Dinner
> - Healthy recipes which Lorraine cooks, like chicken with vegetables and a Weight Watchers chocolate bar snack
>
> (*Mail*, 14 November 2014)

Slimming World seems to have a close relationship with the tabloids, particularly the *Mirror* (see also Chapter 3), which mentions the weight loss organisation 155.29 times PMW (the newspaper with the second most mentions is the *Express* with a much lower 56.95 occurrences PMW). Some of the weight loss narratives in the *Mirror* appear to have been taken from stories published on the Slimming World website. For example, the *Mirror* reported on a couple called Andrew and Paula who could not fasten their seatbelts on a plane, which inspired them to join Slimming World. The same story was also published on the same day, with a few changes, on Slimming World's website.[1] The article (on both websites) contains the following quote attributed to the dieting couple:

> "Now we can do all of those things without fear – and we can't wait to get started. Thanks to Slimming World the world is our oyster."
>
> (*Mirror/Slimming World website*, 18 March 2016)

The *Mirror* also advertises free supplement magazines from Slimming World.

> Don't miss our five exclusive magazines starting FREE inside the Daily Mirror and Sunday Mirror 7-DAY SLIMMING WORLD EATING PLAN
>
> (*Mirror*, 4 January 2013)

The *Mirror's* advocacy of Slimming World could be seen as urging readers to participate in a community in which they can share their stories, make friends and receive advice from others – practices that are perhaps congruent with the *Mirror's* left-leaning ideological perspective, which values participation in a co-operative community with shared goals. However, as noted in Chapter 3, readers who join Slimming World are implied to be taking responsibility for their weight, and the fact that there is a weekly membership fee indicates that the neoliberal aspects to the membership are also wrapped up with the commercial, profit-making object-ives of the organisation. The tabloids write about Slimming World and Weight Watchers in stories that feel like advertorials (Zhou 2012), a hybrid genre of advertisement and editorial or journalistic article, which also suggests a framing of slimming as falling within commercial concerns. On the *Mirror's* website, many of its weight-loss stories are filed in a section called 'Slimming World', which is itself part of a larger section called 'Lifestyle'. However, a casual reader of the newspaper, particularly the print version, would perhaps not be aware that what they are reading is not impartial journalism per se but a story that appears to have been largely reproduced from a commercial text. Although Chapter 4 noted the relatively low amount of language devoted to discussion of businesses and economic frames, it seems that references to these well-established commercial slimming organisations are exceptions to this.

Metaphors of the Body

In this section, we consider metaphorical language related to the body and body weight. Metaphors are figures of speech which refer to one thing in terms of another, e.g. 'His eyes were hot coals.' Related to metaphors are similes, which contain a more explicit linguistic marker of comparison, such as *like* or *as*, e.g. 'His eyes were like hot coals.' Metaphor use can be subtle, with something being described using language normally associated with another

---

[1] www.slimmingworld.co.uk/press/couple-flying-high-after-15st-weight-loss

concept or domain. For example, Semino et al. (2017) report how people with cancer use violence and journey metaphors when describing their illness, e.g. 'I feel such a failure that I am not winning this battle' or having cancer 'is like trying to drive a coach and horses uphill with no back wheels on the coach'. Lakoff and Johnson (1980: 3) write, '[o]ur conceptual system ... plays a central role in defining our everyday realities. If we are right in suggesting that our conceptual system is largely metaphorical, then the way we think, what we experience, and what we do every day is very much a matter of metaphor.' Considering the ways and extent to which journalists employ metaphor around the body and weight loss is thus likely to provide further insight into the ways that representations of obesity can potentially shape individuals'/readers' under-standings and experiences of obesity and weight loss.

Examining a random sample of concordance lines of *diet* did not identify many cases of metaphor. Nor did phrases such as *weight loss* or *lose weight*. Therefore, to consider metaphors around weight loss we instead decided to focus our analysis on metaphorical language used around the word *body*. In Chapter 3, we saw that this word is key in the right-leaning tabloids compared to the rest of the corpus. It is also the 25th most common content word in the whole corpus, occurring 33,563 times. Among its twenty strongest MI^3 collocates, we find *mass* and *index* (almost always used in *Body Mass Index*), *weight* (occurring in *body weight*), *clock* (*body clock*) and *image* (*body image*). Three other collocates are possessive pronouns (*your*, *my* and *her*), while the determiner *the* is also a top ten collocate. *Body clock* is a metaphor in itself, while *body image*, *body mass index* and *body weight* tend not to be used metaphorically. Examining how *body* collocates with possessive pronouns or *the* was more useful for identifying metaphors, particularly indirect ones, which tended to be expressed through a wide range of verb choices. For this reason, we decided to focus on cases where possessive pronouns or the word *the* were used with *body*. For completeness, we also considered the possessive pronouns *your*, *her*, *his*, *our*, *my* and *their*.

We examined 2,000 randomly ordered concordance lines of two phrases. The first phrase, [POSSESSIVE PRONOUN/*the*] *body* [VERB], covered cases such as *her body believes*, where the body is usually positioned as the grammatical agent of a verb process. The second phrase, [VERB] [POSSESSIVE PRONOUN/*the*] *body*, positioned the body as the grammatical patient of verb processes, e.g. *tell your body*. We noted all cases where the processes involved some form of metaphorical representation, the results of which are shown in Table 6.3.

The most common type of metaphor is one which represents the body as a sentient being. Verbs which position the body as the grammatical patient mostly construe it as being communicated with or persuaded, e.g. *teach*, *encourage*, *tell* and *train*.

Table 6.3. *Metaphors involving verbs relating to the body*

Metaphor	Body as grammatical agent, ordered alphabetically (frequency in brackets)	Total	Body as grammatical patient, ordered alphabetically (frequency in brackets)	Total
Body as sentient being	*achieve (1), activate (1), adapt (1), adjust (1), anticipate (1), ask (1), aim for (1), associate (1), become accustomed (2), believe (1), bounce back (3), cannibalise (1), choose (1), cling on to (1), complain (1), comply (1), compensate (1), cope (6), count (1), crave (7), cry out for (2), deal with (1), eat (1), encourage (1), expect (1), feel (1), find (4), get ready (1), get used to (3), get accustomed to (1), handle (5), hoard (1), hold (4), interpret (1), keep (1), know (7), let down (1), like (1), lose track (1), mask (1) notice (1), overcome (1), pile on (1), play catch-up (1), pour out (1), prepare (2), react (10), rebel (1), recognise (4), require (2), resist (1), respond (6), rid (1), say (2), send (2), store (6), struggle (1), tell (15), thank (2), think (12), thrive (1), tolerate (1), try (5), want (5)*	156	*allow (6), direct (1), embrace (2), encourage (7), instruct (1), prompt (5), signal (1), teach (1), tell (19), train (2)*	45
Body as enemy	*battle (1), defend (1), destroy (1), fight (3), give up (1), get you back (2), go into red alert (1), plunder (1), trick (1)*	12	*confuse (1), fight (1), force (2), purge (1), push (1), shock (1), trick (11)*	18
Body as a machine/vehicle	*break down (2), burn (35), close down (1), drive up (1), gear up (1), go into lockdown (1), hum (1), perform (1), run (3), switch (6), tick over (1), work (8)*	58	*drive (1), fuel (1), mend (1), overhaul (4), recalibrate (1), re-engineer (1), set on course (1), take along to the garage (1), wear down (1)*	12
Body as computer	*go into [*] mode (5), shut down (10)*	15	*program (1), reboot (1), reset (1), send into [*] mode (4)*	7
Other			*block (1), inflame (1), flood (2), flush (1), hone (1), penetrate (1), sculpt (1), trigger (2)*	10

By exercising to lower carbohydrates stored in the body and by limiting the amount of carbs you ingest, you can effectively **teach your body** to 'shift' it's [sic] fuel source from Saturday's carb-heavy pizza to the fat on your waistline.

(Telegraph, 13 January 2015)

A much larger set of verbs in this category occur when the body is the agent, although there are still communicative ones, such as *say, thank* and *tell*.

Do something simple like go to sleep half an hour earlier and **your body will thank you**.

(Mail, 26 November 2016)

However, even when our bodies are not communicating with us directly, they are still frequently represented as entities with cognition, through verbs such as *interpret, notice, recognise* and *think*.

What's interesting is that the subjects didn't make up for the reduced calories from their portion-controlled lunches at other snack and meal times, and were able to almost sneak in small caloric reductions without **the body noticing**, the researchers said.

(Independent, 1 September 2011)

A related metaphor also positions the body as a conscious social actor, although we have categorised this separately as it involves cases where the body is either an aggressor or is the victim of aggression from some other entity (usually the person dieting). In this sense, then, the body is viewed as an enemy of something and is the grammatical patient of verbs such as *trick, confuse* and *force*, and the agent of verbs such as *battle, defend* and *plunder*.

Using smaller spoons, plates and cups to **trick your body** into thinking you're getting more than you actually are is a great way to help reduce portions.

(Mirror, 19 May 2016)

Most studies show when you lose a lot of weight, then **your body fights** fiercely against it.

(Independent, 14 April 2016)

Thus, the body is most frequently metaphorically constructed as something separate from the self, a constant companion who has conscious thoughts and motivations to which the self is not privy but is able to influence. Two less frequent metaphors also conceptualise the body as a separate entity, although in both cases they do not imply any sort of conscious motivation. The first involves the body as a machine or vehicle (see also Madden and Chamberlain 2004: 250). This is a centuries-old metaphor which has been traced to the

French philosopher René Descartes (1596–1650), who is quoted by Synnott (1992: 93) as saying, "'The rules of mechanics" are "the rules of nature"'. Some journalists make this representation explicit, as in the following article from the *Mail*, which employs both metaphors and similes belonging to the domain, BODY AS A MACHINE.

> We tend to **treat our bodies like a car**: we keep it topped up with high-calorie fuel and drive it hard. If you do that it will, eventually, break down. It's only when you go for long periods without food (around 12 hours) that **your body switches to 'clean up and repair' mode**. Going on a short fast is a bit like **taking your body along to the garage**. Freed from their normal routine work, the little gene mechanics start doing urgent maintenance tasks.
>
> (*Mail*, 18 March 2017)

In the corpus we also find references to keeping a body *ticking over*, *humming* (like a car engine) or *gearing it up*. Additionally, the body can be *set on course*, *re-calibrated* or *fuelled*. In this sense, the body is the machine and the person dieting is the operator or driver. We have kept the domain BODY AS A COMPUTER separate, although this metaphor also construes the body as a type of machine, albeit one that the dieter (who is positioned as a programmer or operator) can *program*, *reboot*, *reset* and *send* into various *modes* or *shut down*.

> Researchers at the University of Southern California believe that a near-fasting regime over a few months is a way to **"reboot" the body**.
>
> (*Mirror*, 10 March 2017)

A final, smaller category (ten cases) contains verbs which position the body as the grammatical patient in different ways that could not be easily categorised into the sets just described. Two verbs draw on the BODY AS A CONTAINER metaphor (*flood*, *flush*), although an argument could be made that some sort of equivalence is being made to treating the body mechanistic-ally either as a vehicle or a utility (e.g. *flood the engine*, *flush the toilet*), while most of the others suggest that somewhat violent actions (*block*, *inflame*, *hone*, *penetrate*, *trigger*) are being carried out on the body. Another verb, *sculpt*, implies that the body is a work of art (see also Ogden 2003).

> Those who loathe competitive sports can get fit with dance classes, or work on strength and conditioning: maybe using a personal trainer to shed a few pounds, to get fit after an injury or to **sculpt the body** into something approaching an ideal shape.
>
> (*Times*, 4 July 2009)

Bordo (1993: 52) quotes a female bodybuilder as saying, 'It's up to you to do the chiselling; you become the master sculptress.' While this metaphor might be more frequent in other contexts, such as bodybuilding magazines, it was relatively rare in our corpus, where the focus of articles around obesity was simply for people to lose weight rather than to have sculpted bodies. Similarly, another rare metaphor involved the verb *hone*, which depicts the body as a blade or weapon to be sharpened.

> Because he has **honed his body** to Greek god standard ('yes, the ladies do like it'), he takes a rather dim view of anyone who hasn't.
>
> (*Mail*, 31 May 2016)

Thus, the metaphors examined largely represent the body as a distinct entity from the self, most usually a conscious entity, although sometimes not. We could ask whether such a view of the body is always helpful – particularly in the context of discourse around obesity and weight loss, where readers are presented with information and encouragement about a range of ways to alter themselves, sometimes involving language that encourages a view of the body as an enemy and which frames actions to be carried out on it as somewhat hostile or aggressive.

The range of metaphors identified here suggests that there is a lack of consensus around how we understand our relationships with our bodies. This inconsistency has the potential to send mixed messages to readers about how they should conceptualise their bodies and their relationships to food and weight loss. Is the body an enemy to be tricked into complying, a computer that needs to be rebooted, a vehicle to be driven, or a work of art to be sculpted? Is our body a conscious being that is attempting to communicate with us and, if so, how do we understand it, and which messages should we pay attention to? Or is it the case that the body is an unthinking machine that needs to be controlled? Considering the wide range of new diets about which newspapers regularly inform their readers, it might be easier to justify subjecting our bodies to various food restrictions or excesses if they are viewed as separate from our selves. The same point applies to the different forms of exercise we can also put our bodies through, which are discussed later in the chapter. Before that, we turn to a word which collocates with both *exercise* and *diet*: *healthy*.

Good, Clean and Healthy?

One aspect of language around weight loss that has been commented on, both in academic research and the press itself, is the use of terminology evoking religious or moral discourse. For example, Turner (2019) writes,

[I]t's fair to say that all of us use the language of religion when talking about diets and food. We use phrases like 'I'm converted', 'It's changed my life', 'I've been good', 'A little taste of heaven' ... Even diet books have a tendency to use the word 'bible' in the title. 'Temptation', 'sinful' (come on, Slimming World uses 'syns' to categorise foods, for God's sake), 'guilty' - all these words have religious connotations ... Moralising and theologising food and health is now the norm.

(ebook: no page number)

We also found a small number of articles in left-leaning broadsheet newspapers where the language around eating and dieting was criticised.

It fascinates me that so much religious language is purloined into the lexicography of dieting. Calories are sinful. Eating fatty food is giving in to temptation. Why do we create such a pathology of desire?

(*Guardian*, 5 January 2013)

How clean was your bank holiday weekend? Don't worry, I'm not suggesting anything sordid (this is a family newspaper) – I'm just enquiring about your food choices. Any naughty little indulgences? A cheeky glass of wine, maybe? Or a devilish dessert? The language we associate with food has always been loaded. We have cheat days, or are "being good" when on a diet. And perhaps no phrase is as loaded as one of the newest: clean eating.

(*i*, 30 May 2016)

Orbach, quoted by Jones (2018), describes a change in the language used around dieting,

Instead of saying 'this is going to make me thin,' the language takes on an almost moral quality. We talk about purity, about 'healthy,' 'natural' and 'clean' foods. We use euphemisms (like saying we're undertaking a 'transformation') to signify that we're going on a diet. But the effect, and the impact on us, is much the same."

(online article: no page number[2])

When examining newspaper discourse around obesity, we should bear in mind that journalists are not inventing new ways to present the topic, or related ones such as dieting and the body but instead draw, more or less uncritically, on existing discourses. Phrases such as *crash diet* (166 occurrences) or *junk food* (5,003) contain metaphors that are long-established (both occur in the BNC, which contains text from the early 1990s) and used in other contexts. Other

---

[2] www.bbc.co.uk/bbcthree/article/6b0548de-903f-4b15-8dd8-5c11bed79efc

metaphoric phrases, such as *clean eating* (234 cases), do not appear in the BNC and refer to more recently conceived diets, relating to the news value of recency. It is important not to conceive of the press as always being compliant with all metaphorical language around eating. For example, of references to *clean eating* in the press, 70 per cent of cases are critical and describe it, for example, as 'a hobby for the rich, bored and superior', 'really annoying' and a 'fad', while at other points it is associated with eating disorders.

Examination of a set of 'moral' words related to the previous examples (*sin (s), naughty, cheat, tempt, guilty*) found a range of cases where these words referred to eating, with the vast majority being used uncritically.

> Surprising dieting **sins**: Are these stopping you from losing weight?
>
> (*Express*, 16 June 2016)

> It is easy to fall off the wagon with diets but Paul is really good and doesn't **tempt** me with any **naughty** foods.
>
> (*Mail*, 29 July 2014)

> During the week we both eat healthily and then at weekend we can relax a bit more. We have a "**cheat**" day on a Sunday where we might have a kebab, chips or a Chinese or Indian takeaway and snuggle up on the sofa to watch The X Factor.
>
> (*Mirror*, 5 September 2009)

> I have resigned myself to my fate – lardy and **guilty**.
>
> (*Times*, 18 December 2012)

While there were 2,160 instances of these five terms in the corpus, in a random sample of 100 concordance lines, 27 cases were related to food, which would extrapolate to around 600 instances in total. However, there are numerous other words which could reference the eating-as-morality discourse, so the actual number of references to it in the corpus is likely to be much higher.

One word which we would like to place more focus on is *healthy*, which we identified as one of the shared keywords in Chapter 2. In the past, this term has been noted to be used euphemistically to refer to a person's weight, although there are different ways in which this can manifest. For example, the actress Portia de Rossi writes in her autobiography, 'My mother told me a long time ago that "healthy" was a euphemism for "fat". She'd say to me "Don't you just hate it when you see someone at the supermarket and they tell you, "You look healthy"? They are clearly trying to tell you that they think you look fat' (de Rossi 2010: 81). However, the aforementioned article quoting Susie Orbach (Jones 2018) goes on to say that '"healthy" has become just a euphemism for "thin"'. In order to examine whether *healthy* is used in our corpus to imply that someone has obesity or is thin, we initially examined concordance lines containing this term. However, it was difficult to identify any cases of *healthy* being used euphemistically through this method. Thus, we can instead examine contexts where *healthy* appears with other adjectives to gain a sense of how it is characterised. For example, if we take the word *overweight*, it can be implied to be an alternative and thus incompatible state from *healthy* in the following case,

> US researchers put 45 **healthy, overweight or obese participants** aged from 21 to 70 on three cholesterol-lowering diets for five weeks.
>
> (*Mail*, 8 January 2015)

However, in the following example, *healthy* modifies *overweight*, implying that it is possible to be both overweight and healthy.

> Researchers recruited 15 **healthy overweight and obese men** for the study.
>
> (*Mirror*, 29 March 2017)

We scanned the most frequent adjective collocates of *healthy* to identify those referring to a person's weight, finding *overweight* (172), *obese* (168), *slim* (107), *fat* (84), *lean* (46) and *thin* (25). We will take the words *fit, slim, lean* and *thin* first.

Slim tends to equate with *healthy* (in 96 per cent of cases analysed), e.g. 'In a healthy, slim person, 40 per cent of the sugar they eat is converted to fat' (*Times*, 28 May 2016). Similarly, only one of the forty-six cases of *lean* collocating with *healthy* was critical of the idea that lean and healthy were not equivalents.

> The research will provide new insights into why not all **lean** people are **healthy** and, conversely, why not all overweight people are at risk of metabolic diseases.
>
> (*Mail*, 26 June 2011)

Of the twenty-five cases of *thin* and *healthy* collocating, fifteen implied that the two qualities were linked, for example,

> Achieving a **thin, healthy** body was so lifechanging that she decided to help others.
>
> (*Mail*, 25 March 2008)

However, the other ten cases questioned the supposed relationship between the two states.

> Half of those classed as clinically obese were as **healthy** as **thin** people, the study found.
>
> (*Express*, 5 September 2012)

So, while there is a small amount of evidence that *thin* is implied to be healthy, this is not always the case, and associations of *health* with *thin* are generally infrequent. With that said, words that are similar to *thin*, such as *lean* and *slim*, tend to be used to imply good health. How about the adjectives which indicate the opposite state to thin: *overweight, obese* and *fat*?

Examination of 100 random cases of *healthy* collocating with *overweight* found five which did not imply either a link or lack of link between the two concepts (for instance, reference to an 'overweight man eating healthy food' does not tell us whether the overweight person is classed as healthy or not). The majority of cases (68) implied that being healthy was distinct to being overweight. This was frequently in the context of descriptions of the BMI, also noted in Chapter 2.

> BMI: 18–25 is **healthy**, 25–29 overweight and 30 or higher suggest obesity.
>
> (*Mirror*, 8 February 2016)

In the following example, while the volunteers are described as both 'overweight' and 'healthy', the use of *but otherwise* implies that being overweight is *not* healthy.

> He gave overweight but otherwise **healthy** volunteers two eggs a day for 12 weeks
>
> (*Mail*, 30 September 2008)

Another twenty-seven uses did suggest that *healthy* and *overweight* were not mutually exclusive, although such cases often implied that this view is not typical, with the first example that follows putting the modal verb *can* in block capitals for emphasis and the second appearing to contradict received wisdom using the phrase, 'there is such a thing as'.

> Size 26 model Tess Holliday says she CAN be **healthy** and overweight . . .
>
> (*Mail*, 20 May 2016)

> There is such a thing as being overweight and **healthy** – not everyone has to be skinny.
>
> (*Mirror*, 4 April 2016)

Considering 100 random cases of the collocation of *healthy* with *obese* produces a surprising finding. There are forty-three cases of the two states being seen as compatible and only thirty-five where they are not compatible. Twenty-two cases were unclear or did not indicate any sort of relationship. Thus, it appears that the press is more likely to equate healthiness with obesity as opposed to being overweight, despite the fact that people with obesity are defined as having higher BMIs than overweight people. However, looking closely at some of the cases where *healthy* and *obese* are linked together indicates that, although articles accept that healthy people with obesity exist, such a status is still viewed as problematic, either because it is seen as a temporary state on the way to becoming unhealthy,

> We can now see that **healthy** obese adults tend to become unhealthy obese in the long-term, with about half making this transition over 20 years in our study.
>
> *(Mail, 5 January 2015)*

Or because it is still associated with health problems,

> While there was an overall lower risk of peripheral vascular disease, **healthy** obese people who never smoked had an increased risk.
>
> *(Telegraph, 17 May 2017)*

For the eighty-four cases of *healthy* collocating with *fat*, forty-nine (58 per cent) did not show a relationship between the two states, while twenty (24 per cent) suggested that the two are incompatible and fifteen (18 per cent) indicated that they can be mutual (although again using linguistic markers of unexpectedness, such as the use of all-caps AND in the second example).

> I've never met a **healthy**, fat person
>
> *(Telegraph, 3 December 2013)*

> You can be fat AND **healthy**: Obese middle aged are at no greater risk of a heart attack ...
>
> *(Mail, 1 March 2017)*

What emerges, then, is a confusing picture. Healthiness is clearly linked with qualities such as *slim* and *lean* (less so for *thin*), while there is considerable disagreement among the press about whether it is possible to be *healthy* and *fat*, *obese* or *overweight*, though some of the articles which do accept this to be the case are still likely to warn about its long-term effects. Thus, readers concerned about their health will again receive mixed messages from the press, which could result in confusion or help to reaffirm almost any position they wish to take on the subject.

Exercise

We now turn to the final word analysed here, *exercise*. As noted earlier in the chapter, while reference to *diet* is both highly frequent and growing over time, *exercise* has always been less frequent and has remained more stable over time (see Figure 6.2). *Exercise* appears to take a secondary role in the personal responsibility discourse, regularly following *diet* in phrases such as *diet and exercise*.

However, in a very small number of cases, the word *exercise* is presented as problematic in the corpus.

> **Exercise** is a dirty word to many people, so I just advise patients to walk 15 minutes from home every day, come rain or shine.
>
> (*Express*, 9 June 2012)

> Among other forbidden words is "**exercise**". Will Cavendish, director of health and wellbeing at the department, said that this, too, conveyed an unhelpful image to parents. Being "physically active" is preferred.
>
> (*Times*, 5 August 2008)

Could it be, then, that this apparent censorship around the term *exercise* helps to explain the lack of change in its frequency over time, with alternative terms replacing it? This seems unlikely, given that, taken together, the frequency of the terms *physical activity* and *physically active* has only increased marginally over time (the trend line slope for these two phrases combined is 6.94), and there are only 4,441 instances of these terms across the corpus overall, as opposed to 21,538 of *exercise*.

Perhaps another reason for the increasing focus on *diet* as opposed to *exercise* is the view that cutting calories through reducing food intake is more effective than physical activity for losing weight. This perspective is occasionally voiced in the corpus.

> But the main cause of the burgeoning epidemic of type 2 diabetes is obesity which, as my mother used to say, is usually caused by "gluttony and sloth". Of these, over-eating is more important than a lack of **exercise**, and how much you eat is more important than what you eat.
>
> (*Telegraph*, 8 August 2016)

However, as with other debates considered in this chapter, there is also evidence that alternative positions are taken up.

> As with any weight-loss regime, **exercise** plays an important part, and the 42 year old has taken to jogging – even sporting a £99 wristband that measures his progress.
>
> (*Express*, 20 February 2014)

> Professor says there is 'no obesity crisis' and regular **exercise** is more important than weight
>
> (*Independent*, 10 July 2017)

A related reason for the lack of increase in the term *exercise* could be that exercise is perceived as more taxing and time-consuming. People do not have to exercise, whereas they do have to eat, so changing what is eaten, or eating

Table 6.4. *Collocates of* exercise

Category	Collocates
Grammatical words	*and, of, to, the, a, is, do, doing, as, for, that, in, an, or, can, you, not, with, they, little, but, I, n't, through, on, at, your, it, such, are, their, who, how, too, did, during, than, also, be, should*
Frequency	*regular, lack, regime, more, minutes, enough, less, regularly, daily, day, much, week, bursts, amount, hour, regimes, habits, routine, any, no, programme, plan*
Intensity	*moderate, vigorous, strenuous, intense, intensity, gentle, high-intensity, moderate-intensity*
Type	*aerobic, physical, classes, bike, weight-bearing, 30*
Food	*diet, eating, healthy, eat, nutrition, healthily*
Punctuation	*. , - " ' :*
Others	*take, taking, getting, sport, benefits, get, weight, people, help, form*

less, is perhaps viewed as less trouble than making time to exercise. Put simply, a diet often involves doing less of something, while exercise involves doing more, a point which is sometimes made explicit in the corpus.

> We know we need to do more **exercise**, but with busy work lives it's not always easy.
>
> (*i*, 9 September 2011)

Table 6.4 shows the 100 strongest collocates (MI^3) of *exercise*, categorised by hand. We have placed *health* and *healthily* in the category 'Food' because they tend to occur in phrases such as *healthy eating and exercise*, as opposed to *healthy exercise*.

After grammatical words, the largest category in Table 6.4 refers to the frequency of exercise, with numerous collocates suggesting that exercise is presented as occurring repeatedly: *regular, regime, daily, regimes, routine, habits, strict, programme, plan*. The word *regime* almost always collocates with *exercise* in the phrase *exercise regime*. These types of exercise regimes are most frequently described with adjectives which emphasise their exhausting nature and construe them as being difficult to maintain: *gruelling, strict, rigorous, intense, punishing, extreme, brutal, ambitious, desperate, stringent, tiring* and *tough*.

> She shed a mind-blowing 12 stone after putting herself on a strict diet and **gruelling exercise** regime for 18 months.
>
> (*Mail*, 27 October 2017)

Exercise routine tends not to be prefaced with these kinds of adjectives, instead being described in terms of how often the routine takes place (*daily, regular*), with the same pattern appearing for *exercise programme* and *exercise plan*. There are different kinds of routines, plans and programmes, though – some are *weekly* while others are *daily*. Another type of exercise routine involves exercising in *bursts*, which are usually described as *intense* or *vigorous*.

> Scientists at the universities of Nottingham, Birmingham and Bath claim a few 30-second bursts of **intense exercise** could deliver the same health benefits as slogging it out for hours in a smelly gym.
>
> (*Mirror*, 11 April 2013)

However, other collocates of *exercise*, in the Intensity category, include *moderate* and *gentle*, advising a different approach.

> Those researchers concluded that regular **gentle exercise** may be better for health than occasional heavy exercise.
>
> (*Mail*, 31 October 2008)

> Walking 'is better than the gym': Long periods of **gentle exercise** are more beneficial than a high-intensity workout
>
> (*Mail*, 14 February 2013)

> Official advice is for adults to do at least 150 minutes of **moderate** intensity **exercise**, such as brisk walking or cycling, each week in bouts of 10 minutes or more.
>
> (*Independent*, 30 November 2012)

Not all articles appear to advocate gentle exercise as a form of weight loss or maintenance, though.

> A study found those who exercised for 60 to 90 minutes a day – walking the equivalent of a marathon each week – tended to shed at least two stones and kept the weight off for six years. The data contradicts the theory that **gentle exercise** is enough to stay slim.
>
> (*Mail*, 18 February 2008)

> Swimming, gardening or golf not enough to prevent early death; Study shows that **gentle exercise** is not enough to ward off issues like heart disease and diabetes ... The results indicate that whether or not you are obese, and whether or not you have heart disease or diabetes, if you can manage some vigorous activity it could offer significant benefits for longevity.
>
> (*Telegraph*, 6 April 2015)

Newspapers thus present a wide, and at times contradictory, range of advice about exercise in terms of amount, type and intensity, mirroring the plethora of diets that we observed earlier.

As with diets, some forms of exercise can become newsworthy for relatively short periods. For example, a type of exercise called HIT (High Intensity Training), which involves short bursts of high intensity workouts, started to be discussed by the UK press in 2012, with the acronym *HIT* exhibiting fifteen mentions across articles in the *Mail*, *Star* and *Express* during that year. HIT is implicitly legitimated, again through invocations of the authority of expertise (van Leeuwen 2008), as it is described as having been designed in laboratories, with the following example referring to it in terms of 'exercise science'.

> **HIT** is a new kid on the block in the world of exercise science, but it's making a big impact. Jamie has a 65 million grant to carry out follow-up research and see if this ultra-short protocol can be made even shorter. I have a new resolution: to keep doing **HIT**. It's one that I may even keep.
>
> (*Mail*, 26 February 2012)

The author of the article is the television presenter and doctor Mike Mosley, who also presented a BBC documentary about HIT which aired during the same week in which this article was published. During the programme and in the article, Mosley volunteers to try out HIT, concluding that he will 'keep doing HIT'.

Information about the extent to which HIT can help people to lose weight is somewhat contradictory across different newspapers. For example, the *Times* notes that 'Fast Exercise' burns an 'impressive' number of calories, and that 'you keep burning calories even when you are resting after HIT'.

> A Fast Exercise session burns up to 20 calories a minute – that's an impressive 200 in a ten-minute session. You would need to jog for at least three times longer for the same return Researchers have also observed an increased level of catecholamines and growth hormone in the blood during and after **HIT** sessions. 10 Boosts metabolism Because Fast Exercise recruits large muscle groups, pushing them close to their limits, it has been shown to elicit a metabolism-boosting effect that can last for 72 hours. That means you keep burning calories even when you are resting after **HIT**.
>
> (*Times*, 7 January 2014)

However, the February 2012 *Mail* article on HIT mentioned previously warns 'Don't expect the weight to fall off', noting that 'One obvious disadvantage of short, sharp bursts of exercise is that you won't burn many calories'. Instead, for weight loss, the article advocates increasing time spent active, by walking.

In 2013 there were forty-nine mentions of *HIT*, with the *Independent* extolling this form of exercise in the following excerpt,

All you have to do is exercise three times a week for three bursts of 20 seconds, with a two-minute break in-between each 20-second burst. The only piece of exercise equipment you need is a stationary exercise bike. Or use a regular cycle or rowing machine. High impact activities, e.g. running, walking, jogging or jumping, are not recommended as they put too much stress on the muscles. "Anyone can do **HIT**: It doesn't matter if you're overweight or completely unfit," says Professor Timmons.

(*Independent*, 6 September 2013)

However, a few months earlier, another television presenter, Andrew Marr, suffered a stroke just after exercising in a way congruent with a HIT program.

Not content to idle his way through a gym session, Marr, 53, took to the rowing machine with such ferocity of effort that when he finished, he says, he saw flashes of light, and woke next morning " on the floor unable to move". Turns out he'd torn a carotid artery that triggered the stroke that might have killed him. Of course, there were underlying problems; two earlier strokes had gone unnoticed. But it is the manner in which he exercised, the limits to which he pushed himself, that will make many draw parallels.

(*Times*, 16 April 2013)

After Andrew Marr blames his stroke on overdoing it on the rowing machine at 53, how risky is high-intensity exercise for the over-fifties? Andrew Marr thinks his stroke three months ago caused by intense exercise

(*Mail*, 15 April 2013)

A commentary by Professor Timmons attached at the end of the *Mail* article just quoted presents a different perspective on HIT, with Timmons writing that the likely causes of Marr's stroke were factors such as his high-pressure job and years of hard drinking and smoking, as well as his genetic make-up.

For Andrew Marr to claim he knows that HIT caused his stroke is to claim something it is not possible to know. The problem is that he may have put people off doing HIT, which has been shown to have real health benefits; not least in reducing risk factors for type 2 diabetes.

(*Mail*, 15 April 2013)

After this point, HIT does not appear to have had much more impact in the press, with only the *Times* referring to it in 2014 (three articles), 2015 (one article), 2016 (five articles) and not at all in 2017. However, a related form of exercise, *HIIT* (High Interval Intensity Training), received ninety-eight mentions between 2014 and 2017 and does not yet appear to have attracted the same controversy as HIT.

Conclusion

Although the newspapers in our corpus seem to generally agree that food intake is one of, if not *the*, most important factors relating to obesity, our analysis found considerable disagreement in terms of how and which foods should be consumed in order to lose or maintain weight. Some of the more commercially viable diets seemed to be associated with certain newspapers, while a bewildering number of diets were referred to over the decade and across the different newspapers. While such diets were sometimes decried as fads, they could also be presented as successful or be supported by scientific research.

A likely consequence of the large number of named diets referred to by the newspapers is confusion, with readers potentially feeling overwhelmed by the range of diet options reported throughout single newspapers, let alone across the press in its entirety. This could result in readers who wish to lose weight trying out different diets, switching from one to the next as new diets come along, or trying diets that are difficult to maintain or which deprive the body of certain nutrients. The issue is exacerbated by news values. Newspapers want to attract readers by reporting on new stories, and stories reporting on new ways to lose weight have the potential to satisfy numerous criteria for newsworthiness at once, particularly if the article can also name-drop a celebrity or the diet features some sort of unexpected eating behaviour or unusual food.

Similarly, while exercise was also viewed as both conducive to weight loss and important to maintaining a 'healthy' body, there was little agreement or consistency regarding the type, intensity or frequency with which exercise should be undertaken. While some articles seemed to revel in sadistic descriptions of *gruelling*, *brutal* and *punishing* exercise regimes (likely to put off all but the most committed), a growing trend we found was the sense that exercise was an unpleasant, sweaty chore, perhaps helping to account for the lack of growth in discussion of it over time. Reading articles referring to exercise gave us the impression that if done at all, people should find ways of exercising either in as little time as possible (with programmes that take minutes such as HIT and HIIT) or in a manner that is so gentle as to be almost unnoticeable, incorporating everyday activities such as walking or housework. At the same time, there are contradictory voices, with some warning of the dangers of too strenuous exercise while others allude to the pointlessness of exercise that is too moderate.

Added to the confusion around diet and exercise were similarly contradictory representations of the body and what counts as 'healthy'. Metaphors around the body conceptualised it, variously and among other things, as a computer to be programmed, a vehicle to be controlled and an enemy to be defeated. It was frequently cast as independent from the self, rendered as a separate and sentient social actor. Earlier in this chapter we noted the presence of different metaphors around illnesses like cancer, specifically metaphors of battle and journey (Semino et al. 2017). A wide availability of metaphors relating to a particular health-related phenomenon can be viewed as beneficial, as individuals can then exercise a degree of selectivity in adopting the metaphors that feel right for them, while rejecting ones which do not (at least in their own language use). In our corpus, the different metaphors relating to the body could be interpreted as being utilised in ways which help readers to understand complex bio-medical processes, for example how metabolism works or how food is absorbed. However, body metaphors are also used to represent actions that are designed to induce weight loss or to change the body's shape. As is increasingly the case for communication around other health-related issues, these metaphors could be presented as a possible set of options for people wishing to lose weight. On the other hand, we also wondered whether more harm than good could follow from the adoption of metaphorical language which conceptualises, and thus implies and encourages a view of, the body as being separate from the self, particularly if those metaphors are used to discuss or even promote practices that involve subjecting the body to punishing diet and exercise programmes or treating it as an enemy to be tricked or battled into submission. Perhaps the view that the body is not separate from the self would be more likely to encourage people to treat themselves more kindly and carefully, including in terms of how they perceive their bodies and the things they do to them, as well as engendering a more holistic approach to health and wellbeing overall.

Similarly, the language around eating behaviours was sometimes couched in metaphors of morality: *sins*, *temptations*, *naughty*, *treats*, etc., which helped to frame weight as personal responsibility, where good = thin and bad = fat. Flint et al. (2016) have noted the incorporation of Protestant ethical values in news reporting on obesity, according to which obesity comes to be viewed as a form of deviant and immoral behaviour. We discussed the more clearly stigmatising and shaming representations around obesity in the previous chapter, and here we note the presence of more subtly judgemental language, particularly the term *healthy*, which while appearing less overtly judgemental is nevertheless linked to terms such as *fat*, *overweight* and *obese*. Yet even this link is inconsistent and contested within the press, as evidenced by the apparent disagreement over whether it is possible to be healthy and overweight, the result surely being further confusion for the already bewildered reader.

Press discourses around weight loss, dieting and exercise can thus be characterised as comprising a series of mixed messages which, even if well-intended, nevertheless present a multitude of different weight-loss choices, many of which are subsequently criticised and devalued.

Rates of obesity remained fairly stable in the United Kingdom over the time period under study, increasing by only a small amount (see Chapter 4), although the number of articles written about obesity increased much more over this period. One might naively think that faced with the parade of weight loss options, readers wanting to lose weight would eventually hit on the right one for them, even if by accident. However, evidence for this, while present in anecdotal cases (that often reflect amazing transformations that have recently happened, with no guarantee that they will be maintained), is not reflected in the statistics. Perhaps this is because solutions based on personal responsibility can only take us so far, although it could also be the inadvertent result of the large number of solutions proposed and the sense of urgency and shame that newspapers project onto readers who might consider themselves to be over-weight or obese, implicitly inspiring them to try out and switch between increasingly faddy diets or exercise programmes that cannot be maintained for long. For readers who turn to the mass media for guidance and information on losing weight or maintaining a 'healthy' body, they can find no end of advice in the press. Yet, for many readers, it seems that that advice is not enough.

7   Gendered Discourses of Obesity

Introduction

In this chapter and the next, we turn our attention to how representations of obesity intersect with social identity. This chapter compares the ways in which the press represents men and women in obesity coverage. We begin by introducing the related concepts of sex and gender, which are central to our analysis. The term *gender* has a related but not identical meaning to *sex* (Udry 1994). Where *sex* refers to the anatomy of a person's reproductive system, along with secondary characteristics such as body hair (Kimmel 2000), *gender* largely refers to differences between male and female behaviour and roles or an individual's internal identification. As Eckert and McConnell-Ginet (2003: 305) put it, 'gender is not part of one's essence, what one is, but an achievement, what one does. Gender is a set of practices through which people construct and claim identities, not simply a system for categorising people'. Thus, where sex tends to reflect biological distinctions (e.g. male and female), gender is more concerned with social or cultural understandings of sex roles (e.g. masculine and feminine). However, the two terms are very much linked together – with various gendered behaviours being associated with different sexes and, subsequently, informing perceptions about 'normal' ways of being a man or woman, boy or girl.

In this chapter, we analyse how men and women are represented with respect to obesity, linking these representations to wider discourses around gender at the societal level. In this sense, our analysis will explore how obesity interacts with notions of both sex and gender in the press. Before presenting our analysis, we will first consider how sex and gender relate to health and obesity in particular.

Sex, Gender and Obesity

Sex has long been understood to be a key indicator of health; women tend to live longer than men and both men and women are each more likely to experience certain causes and forms of ill-health. In terms of obesity, men

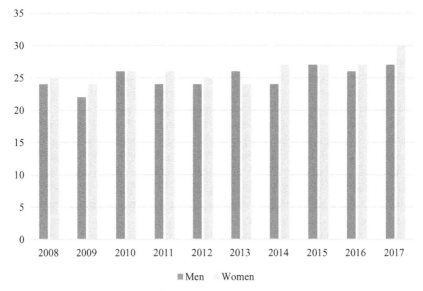

Figure 7.1 Percentage of men and women with obesity in the UK
(2008–2017)
(Source: Statista 2019)

and women are affected in roughly equal measure. As Figure 7.1 shows, over
the ten years represented by our corpus, around a quarter of men and women in
the United Kingdom were affected by obesity.

As this figure indicates, women tend to be affected by obesity slightly more
than men (except for 2013, when men were affected more, and 2010 and 2015,
when levels were equal). However, the margins of difference are very tight (at
most 3 per cent (2014 and 2017)) and if we include figures for being overweight too, we find that men are affected more than women and by a
greater margin.

A now considerable body of social scientific research has described the pro-
foundly gendered ways in which the body and its ailments are experienced and
understood. For example, Courtenay (2000: 1385) argues that 'health-related
beliefs and behaviours, like other social practices that women and men engage
in, are a means for demonstrating femininities and masculinities', while Connell
(2000: 177) asserts that '[l]ike other institutions in modern society, the health
system has a gender regime – an internal set of gender arrangements – which
marks out places for men as well as for women'.

A great deal of research has focussed on the differing representations of
'ideal' male and female body sizes and shapes, with many observing

'a gendered aesthetic of slimness for women in particular', as well as slimness being 'already strongly entrenched in the Western cultural requirements of heterosexual femininity' (Markula et al. 2008: 3–4). Indeed, scholars writing from a critical feminist perspective in particular have observed how the types of bodies represented as ideally feminine, attractive and sexually desirable across a diverse range of media have typically promoted a slender and difficult-to-achieve body shape as that to which all women should aspire (Bordo 1993).

Another area of focus in studies of gender and health is the gendered roles ascribed to women in relation to health. In many societies, including Britain (the context of our study), women are often regarded as the primary caregivers in families. Consequently, health and illness tend to be conceived of as topics that only women really know anything about, as O'Brien et al. (2005: 504) point out, 'men are often portrayed as reliant on female partners (or other female relatives) in health matters, and women are said to encourage aware-ness of health issues, to assist men in interpreting symptoms, and to play a key role in persuading men to seek help'. This role also extends to food-related activities, such as shopping, cooking and eating, which are 'conventionally presented as female-centred' (Gough 2007: 326).

While slimness is traditionally associated with femininity, we can increas-ingly observe similarly unobtainable bodily ideals in media depictions of men, with particular emphasis on toned muscularity, bulging biceps and washboard abs. Gill et al. (2000) refer to the expectations and body dissatisfaction arising from such representations as the 'tyranny of the six-pack', while Pope et al. (2000) dub it the 'Adonis complex'. In recent decades this imbalance has begun to be redressed, with slender male bodies becoming more visible and revered over time. Gill (2008: 102) puts this shift down to the 'growing visibility of gay culture and the economic significance of the pink pound/ euro/dollar; the ongoing impact of feminist critiques of masculinity, with the corresponding hunger for a "new man"; the significance of changes within the fashion industry and attempts to attract men as consumers of style; and the political economy of the magazine industry, seeking (in the mid-1980s) to produce mainstream men's magazines that would satisfy advertisers eager to sell expensive cars, hi-fis and watches to a powerful high-spending demo-graphic'. A consequence of this is that male bodies classed as obese, which are neither muscular nor slim, are frequently portrayed as 'soft, flabby, lacking the muscularity and strength of the "normal" idealized male body', being 'there-fore considered as far closer to the stereotypical feminine body in their softness, roundness and fleshiness' (Lupton 2017: 66).

Research on masculinity and health has drawn on the concept of 'hegemonic masculinity' (Connell 1995; Connell and Messerschmidt 2005) to account for the cultural predominance of particular configurations of gender practice, or ways of performing masculinity, over others. Hegemonic masculinity stabilises power structures in the gender order as a whole (i.e. positioning men above women) but also *within* genders, with certain types of masculinity positioned as more desirable and legitimate than others. The prevailing, hegemonic model of masculinity in Western cultural contexts essentialises 'real men' as being, among other things, aggressive, assertive, competitive, decisive, cavalier, independent, rational, stoical, strong and tough.

Gender performances orienting to the hegemonic ideal have been characterised as having deleterious effects on men's health, causing them to display little or no concern about their health and appearance, to perceive themselves as invulnerable, to refuse or delay seeking medical support unless in extreme circumstances, to avoid emotional disclosure (cf. Galasiński 2004) and to take risks (including 'deviant' risks such as drinking alcohol and eating red meat but also socially sanctioned ones such as extreme sports) (Courtenay 2000; O'Brien et al. 2005).

Obesity poses a threat to 'ideal' models of both femininity and masculinity, then. With all this said, there is good reason to suspect that gender is a salient category in discussions and representations of obesity in the press. While there is an impressive body of work exploring media depictions of women and women's weight issues, parallel studies focussing on men are in the minority, and studies focussing on print media representations of obesity in men or women even more so (Gough 2010). In this chapter, we examine the gendered discourses used to represent men and women in relation to obesity. For this purpose, we follow Sunderland's definition of 'gendered discourses' as those discourses which establish 'boundaries of social practice through which appropriate gendered behaviour is regulated', and which provide parameters through which people are 'represented or expected to behave *in particular gendered ways*' (Sunderland 2004: 21, original emphasis). The identification of gendered discourses can pose challenges for discourse analysts, as gender can be indexed not only directly but also indirectly, with indirect instances more difficult to spot. Our identification and subsequent analysis of gendered discourses will aim to account for cases in which gender is indexed both directly and indirectly in obesity coverage. We begin with cases where gender is indexed directly, relying on mentions of men and women, which we then examine using collocation and concordance analysis. In the second half of the chapter, we focus on instances where gender is indexed less directly, as we compare press weight loss narratives about men and women.

Collocation Analysis: WOMAN and MAN

Starting with direct indexing, our analysis begins by focussing on the use of frequent gender-marked nouns in the corpus. This approach offers the practical advantage that it allows us to quickly and reliably locate instances where gender is likely to be relevant to given representations of obesity and people with obesity. Moreover, by focussing on cases where gender is oriented to explicitly, we can probably have greater confidence that gender is indeed in some way relevant to the particular representations being analysed, in a sense narrowing the gap between our observations and interpretations.

The first step in our procedure was to search for the most common gender-marked nouns in the corpus. The most frequent terms denoting men and women were captured by the lemmas MAN (36,069 occurrences) and WOMAN (53,465). The lemma MAN includes the constituent terms *man* (13,143 occurrences in 7,084 texts) and *men* (22,926 in 8,585 texts), while WOMAN comprises the singular *woman* (12,157 in 6,771 texts) and plural *women* (41,308 in 11,966 texts). These lemmas occur together in noun phrases such as *men and women* and *man and woman* a total of 2,215 times, meaning that men and women tend to be talked about separately rather than being grouped together. From the outset, these frequency differences suggest that, despite their comparable rates of obesity prevalence throughout the period under study, women are mentioned disproportionately more often than men in the obesity coverage. This trend also runs counter to the more general under-representation of women in the media (Conboy 2005), indicating a more intense focus on women in the context of obesity.

To achieve a better understanding of the discourses surrounding uses of these gender-marked nouns, we then compared collocates for the lemmas MAN and WOMAN (MI^3, span: +/−5). There was a great deal of overlap between the collocates for each lemma. To focus more on differences, we took the top 100 collocates from each list and removed collocates that appeared in both lists. This left us with seventeen unique collocates for each lemma.

Taking the collocates of WOMAN first, these were *pregnant, breast, her, should, she, pregnancy, loose, birth, after, said, other, UK, babies, postmenopausal, black, will* and *size*. The unique collocates were not all equally useful for identifying gendered discourses. For example, we would expect the pronouns *her* and *she* to collocate more strongly with WOMAN than MAN. Likewise, the two strongest unique collocates of MAN are *he* and *his*. Beyond these pronouns, just under a third of the unique collocates of WOMAN refer more and less directly to pregnancy and motherhood (*pregnant, pregnancy, birth* and *babies*). Collectively, in the majority of cases (73 per cent) these words feature in articles reporting the health risks that expectant mothers' obesity and, by extension, their lifestyle choices, pose to their unborn babies' health, including future obesity in the child and the mother.

> Obesity in **pregnant women** can lead to all sorts of problems, including the death of the mother, or the death of the baby through stillbirth or the baby having foetal abnormalities
>
> (*Observer*, 10 January 2010)

Pregnant women who are obese risk a myriad of health issues afflicting their unborn baby including diabetes, weight problems and heart disease.

(*Mail*, 7 June 2016)

So, use of these pregnancy-related collocates tends to reinforce the types of responsibilising discourses we have encountered elsewhere, except that this responsibility is for children's welfare specifically and is particularised to women (or mothers). The affirmative modal verb *should* tends to collocate with WOMAN in such advice-giving passages (81 per cent), which again reflect the type of responsibilising messages noted earlier, except that here we see more intense focus on the actions of pregnant women and what they should do to preserve not only their own but also their babies' health and to mitigate their risk of obesity.

The myth that **women should** "eat for two" was also encouraging them to put on too much weight during pregnancy, said experts. A recent report found that half of mothers who died during pregnancy, while giving birth or shortly afterwards were overweight or obese.

(*Telegraph*, 29 September 2008)

These patterns accord with the observation made by Lupton (2017) that mothers' responsibility for their children's weight begins in pregnancy; 'If women are deemed to be too fat for a "normal" pregnant woman, they must contend with fat-shaming that seeks to position them as "bad" mothers because of the risk they are allegedly posing to the health of their foetuses' (Lupton 2017: 39–40).

The collocate *breast* tends overwhelmingly (96 per cent) to be used in relation to breast cancer. In almost three-quarters of cases (74 per cent), articles mentioning breast cancer cited it as a potential consequence of obesity. In almost all cases, these articles were reporting on research findings.

During the monitoring period, 1,090 **women** developed **breast** cancer, giving an absolute risk of just over 1%. Infertility treatment, family history of breast or ovarian cancer, and use of HRT were all significantly associated with a heightened risk of being diagnosed with the disease, while pregnancies were protective. But after taking account of other influential factors, increases in skirt size emerged as the strongest pre-dictor of breast cancer risk.

(*Telegraph*, 24 September 2014)

In 13 per cent of cases, the research being cited presented obesity as something that reduced women's chances of recovering from breast cancer and which increased their chances of dying from it.

Dr Ligibel found body mass index – the relationship between weight and height – was linked to recurrence and death rates. Overall, a woman of healthy weight had a 77% chance of surviving for 10 years, compared with a 70% chance of survival for overweight and obese **women** diagnosed with **breast** cancer.

(Mail, 23 March 2012)

This focus on breast cancer explains the collocate *postmenopausal*, as women in this age bracket are identified as being at particular risk of breast cancer both in the studies being reported and then subsequently in the newspaper articles themselves.

The best way to improve this condition – which can cause leg pain – is to lose weight, say podiatrists. Lower breast cancer risk Many studies have found a strong link between obesity and **breast** cancer, especially in **postmenopausal women**.

(Mirror, 7 January 2015)

Another group singled out for focus in this regard is *black* women. In 64 per cent of the co-occurrences of *black* with WOMAN, black women are highlighted as either being particularly at-risk of breast cancer or as being at equal risk as women from other ethnicity groups, where previously they had been less susceptible. As this example demonstrates, even where breast cancer diagnoses between black and white women levelled out, the mortality rates for black women were reportedly higher.

For decades, breast cancer has been less common in **black women** than their white peers. Yet, the disease has historically killed black women at a higher rate. A new study has now revealed one of those gaps has finally closed – the first. This is because diagnoses have grown more common in **black women**, while rates among white women have levelled off. Meanwhile, the death gap has actually increased.

(Mail, 29 October 2015)

Of these articles, a small minority (3 per cent; all from the *Guardian*) used these statistics as an opportunity to engage in more critical reportage regarding ethnicity-based health inequalities, which were given as a reason for the increasing rates of breast cancer in black women.

Although **black women** and white women are diagnosed with breast cancer at the same rate, **black women** die from the disease at a higher rate, according to the report. "The gap between **black women** and white women has gotten wider over time and that reflects who gets access to quality treatment," said Linda Goler Blount, an epidemiologist and CEO of **Black Women**'s Health Imperative, an organization that promotes women's health.

(Guardian, 7 January 2016)

As well as being depicted in relation to breast cancer, black women were also represented as being particularly at-risk of obesity (21 per cent of the sample).

In 15 per cent of cases, black women were reported on in the context of eating disorders. Although, by contrast, black women were presented as being affected less by eating disorders than women from other ethnicity groups, this was a clinical group reportedly on the rise. Like articles about breast cancer, articles about eating disorders in black women also opened up the possibility for more critical reportage relating to health inequalities (again, from the *Guardian*), this time about the health effects of black women pursuing changing and more westernised standards of beauty.

> ... notions of what is deemed attractive in different cultures may also be the reason why so many black girls' eating disorders go undetected and underreported. A black woman with an eating disorder may not be willing to talk about it for fear of being ridiculed for going against cultural norms. Similarly, if researchers believe that **black women** are less likely to suffer from eating disorders, they are probably less likely to study them.
>
> (*Guardian*, 7 April 2009)

Whichever condition or minority group is under focus, what is fairly consistent is that the articles either report on, or make reference to, research into the prevalence, causes and consequences of the conditions in question. This helps to account for other collocates such as the reporting verb *said*, which tends to be used to quote scientists and researchers, *UK*, which is used when citing prevalence figures (e.g. 'Lest we forget, 25% of adult **women** in the **UK** are now obese' (*Guardian*, 27 June 2011)), and then the future-tense modal verb *will*, which tends to be used when citing projections about the prevalence of obesity in women in the future.

> A government report last year suggested that if current eating habits and exercise trends persist, nearly 60% of men and 50% of **women will** be obese by 2050.
>
> (*Guardian*, 27 August 2008)

The collocate *other* is used overwhelmingly (95 per cent) to refer to some relationship between women. These relationships could be evaluated as positive or negative, and included stories about women who wanted to help other women to lose weight, for example by 'inspiring' them.

> In response to her Facebook post, Miss Bennett received numerous positive comments, with many telling her that she was 'courageous', looked 'great' and was an 'inspiration' to **other** obese **women** ... She added that she hopes her images – and attitude toward the bullying – will encourage **other women** to embrace their own bodies.
>
> (*Mirror*, 29 September 2015)

The collocate *size* is used in 62 per cent of cases to refer to dress size. Dress sizes are referenced in a range of contexts, including as a way of quantifying body size, for instance to describe weight loss in the types of tabloid weight loss narratives flagged up in Chapter 3 and to which we will turn in the second half of this chapter.

> A **size** 22 **woman** (UK 26) has revealed the quirky secret behind her weight loss of more than 110 lbs (eight stone) – eating 10 grapefruits a day.
>
> *(Mail*, 8 September 2017)

The final keyword, *loose*, is almost always used in the proper noun bigram *Loose Women* (98 per cent) – a daytime panel show in the United Kingdom. Mentions of this are mostly incidental, for example in TV listings appended to the end of some articles. However, a minority of uses (8 per cent) report on comments made by one of the panellists, Jamelia Davis, expressing the view that the availability and affordability of 'plus size' clothing was 'encouraging' obesity. Although this is not a gendered discourse as such, *Loose Women* is a programme targeted primarily at women and discussions around clothing come up again in the representation of obesity in women, so this story is worth bearing in mind.

We now want to move on to the lemma MAN, whose unique collocates are *his, he, fattest, sperm, testosterone, both, woman, health, 2,500, prostate, world, v, 40, three, 65, up* and *60*.

Again, like the collocates of WOMAN considered earlier, not all unique collocates of MAN are equally useful for identifying gendered discourses. This includes the pronouns *he* and *his*, which we would expect to collocate strongly with the male nouns and not the female nouns, but also *health*, which tends to be used to refer to the magazine *Men's Health*, and *v*, which refers mostly to the TV show, *Man v Food*.

The first feature of the representation of men we want to explore here is their tendency to be grouped with women. This was initially indicated by the strong association between the lemma MAN and *both*, which is mostly used (62 per cent) to group men and women together, usually to present the prevalence of and health problems associated with obesity.

> In the UK, the prevalence of obesity is over 25% in **both** women and **men**.
>
> *(Guardian*, 12 October 2016)

This trend also helps to explain the strong association between MAN and *woman*, for example with the trigrams 'man and woman' and 'woman and man' alone accounting for over a quarter of the co-occurrences of these items (107). What is telling here is that men and women are grouped to the extent that we see *both* and *woman* emerge as strong collocates for MAN but we do not see equivalent collocates for WOMAN. The closest we get to this for the collocates of WOMAN is *other*. However, as we have seen, this tends to be used to refer to two or more women between whom some relationship is established (e.g. of support). It is perhaps because of the comparatively lower frequencies of the male terms that words indicating linguistic grouping are strong collocates, whereas women are, proportionally speaking, more likely to be talked about alone (i.e. not with men) or grouped with other women.

Another of the strongest collocates of MAN is the superlative adjective *fattest*. Of the 308 pairings of these items, 267 are with the singular form *man*, in all but four cases forming the noun phrase bigram 'fattest man' (263). This is used consistently in stories about the 'fattest man' either in the world or in specific countries (mostly the United Kingdom). So, these are articles which focus on obesity in men in quite exceptional or marked cases. Analysing a random sample of 100 of these texts, we found that they reported on these men in a variety of contexts and adopted a range of perspectives, with no clear overall trend. However, the most common pattern (37 per cent) was weight loss narratives about men who were formerly the 'fattest' in their country or the world but had since lost weight.

> Former world's **fattest man** reveals he can now fit into a cinema seat 'for the first time in 30 years' after he had 50lb (4st) of excess skin cut away at a New York clinic
>
> (*Mail*, 15 June 2015)

Then, in 30 per cent of cases, stories reported on the death of the men in question, such as in this headline and lead paragraph from the *Mirror*.

> **Fattest Man** Keith Martin: Dead The doctor who treated the world's **fattest man** – Brit Keith Martin – called on the government to make fast food more expensive to curb the current obesity crisis.
>
> (*Mirror*, 5 December 2014)

Slightly less frequently, 26 per cent of the articles simply reported on the existence of the 'fattest man'. Such articles provide accounts of the men's living circumstances and the amounts of food they would typically eat in a day, with the implication that this has resulted in their obesity. This focus on extreme and exceptional cases in the men is notable, then, and can be contrasted against the representation of obesity in women, which instead focussed on larger and more general groups, such as pregnant women, black women and postmenopausal women. This isn't to say that men weren't grouped together at all though, as the numerical collocates (*2500*, *40*, *three*, *65* and *60*) indicate. Not all of these are revealing of gendered discourses, but they instead tend to be used in contexts relating to men's age, statistics about obesity projections or recommended calorie intake. One numerical collocate we want to discuss here, *40*, exhibits a wide range of uses, including referring to percentages, weight, waist size and age. Although there was no clear overall pattern in the use of this collocate, one interesting pattern we found in three uses of it as an age quantifier was to establish equivalence between men aged over forty years and women post-menopause. Specifically, each of these articles reproduced advice that small amounts of alcohol could have health benefits for people at risk of heart disease, which included men over 40 and postmenopausal women.

> Drinking alcohol has long been known to have a protective effect on the heart. However, doctors say this is a benefit only among **men** older than **40** and postmenopausal women.
>
> (*Telegraph*, 2 January 2013)

Cases like these suggest a medicalisation of women's life course that we do not see with men, whereby men's age is quantified in terms of years but women's in terms of a (medicalised) bodily process. This could be why we are seeing *40* collocate strongly with men and not women, as men and women of this age (and over) are characterised in different ways.

Another set of collocates which mirrors those for the female words are those which refer to the body, particularly relating to health (*sperm*, *testosterone*, *prostate*). Like mentions of breast cancer in women, obesity tended to be construed as contributing towards or exacerbating men's health problems, in this case sperm quality and prostate cancer.

> Overweight and obese men are more likely to find it difficult to conceive as they have a worse **sperm** quality than **men** with a healthy weight.
>
> (*Express*, 27 May 2016)

> Dr Aine McCarthy, Cancer Research UK's science information officer, told BBC: "This research in mice sheds light on why obese **men** with **prostate** cancer are more likely to have aggressive tumors."
>
> (*Mail*, 13 January 2016)

Implicit in such articles is the message that men need to fulfil the neoliberal imperative to monitor and control their body weight in order to maintain the quality of their sperm (and thus their chances of conceiving a child) and to reduce their risk of developing prostate cancer or, if they already have it, to improve their chances of recovery. However, while such implorations were *explicit* in articles about breast cancer and obesity in pregnant women, this was not the case for articles about sperm quality and prostate cancer in men, where these messages were *implicit*. Rather, such articles were more likely to advocate medical solutions to the men's health problems.

Doctors should consider **testosterone** therapy when **men** report problems with sexual function.

(Mail, 4 August 2015)

Detecting differences in molecular composition between samples of 'good' and 'poor' sperm might one day allow us to design specific therapies for **men** with poor **sperm** that might help give them a boost.

(Express, 24 May 2017)

The analysis presented in this chapter so far has uncovered a number of differences in the ways that women and men are represented with respect to obesity. However, the approach we have taken is limited in the sense that it narrows our analytical scope to just those instances where women and men are mentioned explicitly and, thus, to those cases where gender is marked or topicalised in some way. Although gender is often considered a salient social category, it can manifest in discourse in diverse and often non-obvious ways. With this in mind, we decided to take a second approach to the identification of gendered discourses around obesity, focussing specifically on weight loss narratives.

Gendered Weight Loss Narratives

By weight loss narratives, we mean articles published by newspapers, mostly tabloids, that report on the weight loss of an individual but sometimes couples. They can be about celebrities or 'ordinary' people and they tend to be multimodal, often featuring 'before-and-after' images. They can be presented either in third- or first-person, but in either case are carefully selected and crafted by the editor for the newspapers' imagined readership (Bell 1991). Thus, while they reflect the experiences of individuals, such articles can't be treated as subjective disclosures or accounts of weight loss.

To identify weight loss narratives, we read through tabloid articles, taken at random, and extracted the first 100 weight loss stories about women and the first 100 stories about men that we encountered. We then, stored these, in their entirety, as two sub-corpora. We restricted our search to just the tabloids, as our prior analysis has shown that these types of articles are particularly characteristic of the tabloids rather than the broadsheets (see Chapter 3). Random sampling located the 100 weight loss articles about women faster than the 100 about men – a trend that fits with our prior analysis which found that women are reported on in the context of obesity much more often than men and is also supported by our prior analysis where we found female pronouns (e.g. *she* and *her*) to be indicative of weight loss narratives in the tabloids (Chapter 3).

Our narrative sub-corpora are fairly evenly matched in terms of size, with the men's narratives containing 106,269 words and the women's reaching 100,187. A more comprehensive profile of each sub-corpus is given in Table 7.1.

Table 7.1. *Breakdown of the weight loss narrative sub-corpora*

Newspaper	Men's narratives		Women's narratives	
	Texts	Words	Texts	Words
Express	12	10,773	12	9,653
Mail	58	71,126	50	57,836
Mirror	25	20,895	27	23,092
Star	2	2,242	8	8,155
Sun	3	1,233	3	1,451
Total	100	106,269	100	100,187

As this table shows, each narrative corpus contains a cross-section of all the tabloids except for the *Morning Star*. Consistent with the make-up of the corpus more generally, the *Mail* accounts for the largest proportion of words and text in both sub-corpora. The corpora are also comparable in terms of the distribution of the texts from each newspaper, containing the same number of articles from both the *Express* (12) and *Sun* (3). The greatest difference in this regard is the *Mail*, and even here the difference between the two corpora is just eight texts (fifty-eight in the corpus of men's narratives vs. fifty in the corpus of women's narratives).

Our first analytical step was to compare these corpora against each other using the keywords procedure. We stipulated that keywords should have a minimum frequency of 5 and log-likelihood (LL) score of 10.83, which indicates a p value of <0.001, meaning that we can be 99.9 per cent sure that our keywords are in fact statistically salient and have not been flagged as keywords due to chance. These parameters gave us sixty-seven keywords for the women's narratives (LL $\geq$ 10.97) and sixty for the men's (LL $\geq$ 10.85). We present these keywords in Table 7.2. For comparative purposes, we have grouped the keywords thematically based on analysing their uses in the articles. Since we are dealing with smaller samples, it was possible for us to analyse all instances of many of the lower frequency keywords. However, for keywords occurring hundreds and thousands of times, we based our analysis on random samples of 100 uses, assigning the keyword in question to the thematic category which best accounted for most of its uses.

As this table indicates, there is considerable thematic overlap between the keywords for each corpus, suggesting that they are thematically comparable even if these themes can reify in lexically distinctive ways. However, some themes are present in the keywords for just one corpus and not the other. In the women's narratives we find keywords denoting and evaluating women and their bodies aesthetically (i.e. *look, amazing, figure, bikini, beautiful, stunning, snap*), with no comparable keywords for the men's narratives. Likewise,

Table 7.2. *Men's and women's weight loss narrative keywords, grouped thematically (frequencies in brackets)*

Theme	Men's keywords	Women's keywords
Aesthetic		*look* (111), *amazing* (52), *figure* (43), *bikini* (29), *beautiful* (22), *stunning* (18), *snap* (15)
Death and disease	*diabetes* (87), *risk* (73), *blood* (70), *death* (59), *cancer* (49), *type* (45), *disease* (42), *liver* (23), *insulin* (22), *metabolic* (16), *feared* (13)	
Diet and weight loss	*diet* (312), *sugar* (100), *calories* (98), *alcohol* (53), *waist* (51), *drinking* (45), *drink* (40), *carbs* (35), *low-fat* (22), *beer* (20), *experiment* (17), *reduce* (16)	*size* (265), *body* (215), *into* (163), *surgery* (146), *gastric* (106), *dress* (80), *10* (71), *fit* (70), *chocolate* (64), *tried* (58), *crisps* (57), *bypass* (38), *sizes* (37), *yoga* (36), *biscuits* (31), *fitted* (25), *kilos* (25), *10st* (22), *stay* (21), *11st* (17), *2lb* (13)
Emotions		*felt* (110), *embarrassed* (28), *desperate* (15)
Family and relatives	*wife* (48), *father* (45), *brother* (28)	*mother* (99), *children* (98), *mum* (95), *husband* (85), *baby* (56), *wedding* (47), *pregnant* (40), *kids* (39), *sister* (38), *pregnancy* (32), *boyfriend* (30), *model* (19)
Grammatical – other	*is* (701), *the* (3,139), *of* (1,764), *in* (1,274), *this* (290), *or* (253), *its* (30)	*was* (1,633), *had* (538), *'d* (194), *made* (124), *having* (100)
Names of people	*Richard* (42), *Paul* (32), *Martin* (31), *Mason* (27), *Sam* (27), *Brian* (21), *Daniel* (20), *Thompson* (17), *Jordan* (13)	*Claire* (45), *Scarlett* (44), *Emma* (26), *Cheryl* (18), *Debbie* (17), *Emily* (14)
Other	*people* (223), *man* (168), *Mr* (106), *part* (54), *NHS* (50), *flight* (42), *London* (40), *number* (37), *yes* (22), *Britain* (30), *2012* (26), *strictly* (21), *fattest* (18), *services* (13)	*"* (1,217), *woman* (116), *Ms* (45), *Miss* (33), *Christmas* (30), *trip* (17)
Pronouns	*he* (1,875), *his* (1,293), *him* (308), *himself* (85)	*I* (2,703), *my* (873), *me* (449), *myself* (121), *herself* (75)

among the women's keywords we find terms denoting emotions (i.e. *felt, embarrassed, desperate*). On the other hand, the men's keywords evince a focus on death and disease (i.e. *diabetes, risk, blood, death, cancer, type, disease, liver, insulin, feared*), which we don't see in the women's keywords.

Not all themes and their constituent keywords were equally productive for identifying gendered discourses, so we will focus specifically on the aesthetic and emotion keywords for our analysis of the representation of women, the death and disease keywords for men, and the diet and weight loss and family and relatives keywords for both the men's and women's narratives.

The first set of keywords we explore here are broadly concerned with the theme of family and relatives. This theme accounted for more keywords for the women's narratives (12) than the men's (3). In the women's narratives, this theme was indicated by keywords denoting familial roles for women, mostly as mothers (*mother, children, mum, baby, pregnant, kids, pregnancy, model*) but also as wives and girlfriends (*husband, wedding, boyfriend*) and sisters (*sister*). Starting with the most prevalent of these roles, motherhood, in 22 per cent of cases, the motherhood keywords featured in stories about women whose obesity is presented as preventing them from having children, with their desire to become mothers framed as the motivation for them to lose weight.

> MIRACLE OF THE GASTRIC BAND **BABY**; **MUM** IS FIRST TO GIVE BIRTH WITH BAND IN PLACE AFTER LOSING 15ST HEARTBROKEN Michelle Bowater was told nine years ago that she was too fat to ever have **children**. Weighing 25 stone, doctors said her obesity had caused serious fertility problems. But she refused to give up on her dream of being a **mum**.
>
> (*Mirror*, 17 June 2009)

Almost as frequently, in 21 per cent of cases, the process of having children was given as the cause of initial weight gain, with women depicted as struggling to lose the attested weight they gained during pregnancy.

> As a young teen Hannah had been slim but her battle with weight began when she had **children**.
>
> (*Sun*, 18 February 2013)

Earlier in this chapter, we observed how pregnancy-related collocates of the lemma WOMAN tended to be used to responsibilise pregnant women into managing their obesity risk for the sake of their own health and that of their unborn children. While we didn't find evidence of this discourse in our analysis of the motherhood keywords in the women's narratives, mothers were nevertheless responsibilised in other ways, namely as losing weight so that they could be good 'role models' to their children (18 per cent).

> Gemma said: "I couldn't carry on being obese and I was desperate to become a good role **model** for my **kids**. I didn't want them to pick up on my unhealthy eating habits and end up being fat themselves."
>
> (*Mail*, 22 September 2017)

In 11 per cent of cases, mothers' weight loss is framed as being motivated by their desire to prolong their lives to ensure that they can look after their children and see them grow older.

> The incredible shrinking woman; **Mother** loses 11 stone in just NINE MONTHS A YOUNG **mother** calls herself the incredible shrinking woman after losing 11 stone in just nine months. [...] Emma was spurred to act when she was told she was morbidly obese and in danger of not seeing her little boy grow up.
>
> (*Express*, 31 August 2011)

Such representations of the women in these narratives, as being or aiming to be responsible mothers, broadly provide support for Lupton's (2017: 40) observation that once children are born, 'mothers are then charged with the responsibility of ensuring that their children do not become fat and that they themselves act as good "role models" by engaging in practices of the self which are recommended to avoid becoming overweight'. While we might expect to find gender-marked words such as *mother* and *mum* as key in the women's narratives compared to the men's, the marked use of words such as *children*, *kids* and *model* (as in 'role model') is perhaps less obvious but indicates that narratives about women are more likely to frame their weight and weight loss in terms of their roles as parents, thereby placing childcare responsibilities more firmly within their domain compared to the men featuring in similar weight loss stories.

Other family keywords from the women's narratives, such as *husband*, *wedding* and *boyfriend*, indicate a focus on romantic relationships. The keyword *wedding* features consistently in stories about women losing weight in order to be slimmer for their wedding day, with over half of uses (51 per cent) focussing specifically on the desire to fit into a particular (smaller) wedding dress.

> Claire Davies ballooned to 22 stone but has managed to shed almost half her body weight after she struggled to squeeze into a size 28 **wedding** gown. Now, the assistant shop manager weighs a healthy 11 stone 8 lbs and is a slim size 8 after dropping eight dress sizes in just 12 months. And following her incredible transformation, in March this year, Claire walked down the aisle in her dream size 12 **wedding** gown. Claire, who has since been referred for surgery for the loose skin on her stomach, said: "I felt like a princess on my **wedding** day."
>
> (*Express*, 26 October 2017)

These stories tend to be presented in ways that recall what Sunderland (2004: 35) describes as a 'fantasy discourse' around weddings. For example, in the previous extract, Claire is reported as losing weight to fit into her 'dream' wedding dress and describes feeling like a 'princess' on her wedding day. The keywords *husband* and *boyfriend* could also feature in these narratives, giving context to the story by mentioning the groom's name and explaining when and how the couple met. More broadly, these male social actors are indexed in a wide range of ways in the women's narratives, with no clear overall pattern. However, in 15 per cent of cases, separation from husbands and boyfriends is cited as a reason for women losing weight. Also in 15 per cent of uses, *husband*(s) and *boyfriend*(s) are described as being supportive of women's weight loss, by helping them to lose weight and/or not putting pressure on them to do so, for example by not commenting on their weight.

The men's narratives contained just three family and relational keywords: *wife, father* and *brother*. Wives were mentioned in a wide range of ways, again with no clear pattern, but most frequently (13 per cent of cases) being construed as inspirations or partners in men's weight loss activities.

> His **wife** Erin, 36, and their daughter Brianna, 9 – who have both lost weight from swimming, morning walks and eating healthy – have been an added bonus of inspiration to his weight loss.
>
> (*Mail*, 23 March 2016)

However, wives could also be represented as being responsible for their husbands' weight gain by not preparing healthy meals for them (10 per cent), such as in this example in which a man accounts for his weight gain by lamenting how he had to 'fend for [him]self in the kitchen' because his wife did not cook for him like his mother used to.

> He described how his limited skills in the kitchen left him reliant on ready meals and takeaway food. He said: "I had gone from living with my mother to living with my **wife** and had never before had to fend for myself in the kitchen. 'I just didn't know how to cook and the weight began piling on."
>
> (*Mail*, 21 June 2016)

The theme of wives preparing healthy meals for their husbands was also evident in articles presenting stories about men who ate unhealthy food in secret behind their wives' backs, or who would secretly eat extra meals in addition to those prepared for them by their wives (8 per cent).

> When his shift had finished, he would stop at fast food restaurants on the way home, often eating four burgers and drink two milkshakes. He would then get home and enjoy a home-made dinner prepared by his **wife**, Lynn, who would have no idea that he'd already eaten.
>
> (*Mail*, 20 October 2015)

So, mentions of wives in men's weight loss narratives help to position married women within the traditional gendered role of family caregiver; they provide inspiration and support to men losing weight, prepare meals for their husbands and families, ensure that those meals are healthy and, as the arbiters of the family's health, are also the ones from whom the men in these stories have to hide their misdemeanours and unhealthy habits. These discourses thus reflect wider, dominant gendered frameworks which position women as family caregivers.

Moving onto the keyword *father*, in 36 per cent of its uses the men in the articles are identified as fathers. In most cases, their being fathers does not have much of a bearing on their weight loss story but is an aspect of their identity that is mentioned to set the scene of the story. In cases where weight loss *is* connected to fatherhood, this tends to be framed as preserving life so that their children do not have to grow up without a father.

> After being hospitalised he vowed to change his life for his child and wife Amber "I didn't want my son growing up with a tombstone for a **father**," he said
>
> (*Mail*, 7 November 2017)

Rather than providing a good role model to their children as we saw with the women's stories, then, the weight loss stories about men were more concerned with averting the threat of death. This is also evident in articles in which men's initial weight gain is attributed to the deaths of their fathers (25 per cent).

> Relatives described how Mr Mason began putting on weight in his late teens when his **father** Roy, a former military policeman, died. "Before he lost his **father** he was in the Salvation Army band and he was quite slim and trim," said his aunt, Margaret Smy, 71, also from Ipswich. "But he was very close to his dad and his death hit him hard."
>
> (*Mail*, 21 October 2009)

A focus on the consequences of male relatives' deaths is also evident in uses of the keyword *brother*, which in 25 per cent of cases is used in reference to the death of a brother acting as a catalyst to spur men on to lose weight.

> But determined Graham – who also used to smoke 80 cigarettes a day – turned his life around after his big **brother** suddenly died, spurring him to turn his life around. He shed a stone a month thanks to a rigorous gym routine, strict diet and two operations – thought to be one of Britain's biggest weight losses.
>
> (*Mirror*, 10 June 2015)

So, where the death of a father is presented as the cause of weight gain, the death of a brother is framed as motivating weight loss. This distinction could be explained by the fact that the death of a brother, so a relative in the same generation, acts as a warning to the men about their own weight and as a reminder of their own mortality. Whatever the case may be, it is notable that the sorrow caused by death is presented as a cause of weight gain and fear of death as a motivation for weight loss in the men's narratives. Even in cases where the narratives exhibit concern about the men's relatives, ultimately it is their own mortality that is presented as motivating them to lose weight. This can be contrasted with the use of family keywords in the women's narratives, which are all relational, saying as much about other people, including children and spouses, as they do about the women themselves.

The heightened focus on death in the men's narratives also helps to explain why we see an abundance of keywords denoting death and disease, with no equivalent keywords in the women's narratives. This includes *diabetes, risk, blood* (pressure), *death, cancer, type* (1/2 diabetes), *disease, liver* (disease), *insulin, metabolic* and *feared*. These words are all key in the men's stories because the men's weight loss was often triggered by health risks, particularly those identified by doctors.

> He rushed to A&E in 2008 after a high **blood** sugar reading in a check by his GP. He says: "I feel so stupid I didn't see the signs. I needed to pee more and more frequently until I needed a loo stop every 20 minute. Because of my age, I thought I might have prostate **cancer**. When I got to the hospital, medics assumed I realised it was **diabetes** but I had no idea. I was admitted because I had dangerously high **blood** sugar levels that could have left me in a coma if untreated. I was sent home after two days, put on metformin and gliclizade tablets and told I needed to change my diet."
>
> (*Sun*, 15 November 2012)

As this example demonstrates, these articles can also bear some of the hallmarks of the types of 'danger of death' narratives described by Labov (2013), and in these cases it is literally the threat of death, if not serious threat to health, that makes the men decide to lose weight. Notably, despite the descriptions of life-threatening events, these narratives are also relatively devoid of emotional disclosure compared to the women's narratives. The men are not described as being fearful, for example. Their decisions to lose weight are presented as being stimulated not by these men's emotions, or even necessarily concern about or responsibility for their families, but rather are based on logic and reason, and on advice from medical practitioners. Whatever the case, because we do not see these danger of death narratives in the articles about women, it could be that they are related to a kind of stoic, masculinity. Indeed, help-seeking has been interpreted as a behaviour that undermines masculine identities, as it involves the admission of not only illness but also of an inability on the part of men to solve their own problems. As White and Johnson (2000: 540) put it, 'it seems that man is not prepared to deal with his body when it makes the transition from being healthy to being ill. He is expected to be fit, productive and able to carry out the roles expected of him. There is a feeling of invincibility that is deep-seated and, when this is threatened, men have to rationalise their position and negotiate [...] about what to do.' We will return to this consideration towards the end of the chapter. The point here is that men's weight loss is frequently framed as being motivated by medical advice and health concerns, and as occurring in extreme circumstances, particularly when the men in question are faced with the prospect of death.

Moving onto the women's narratives, and where weight loss in men was presented in terms of preserving their health, for women, aside from their duty to their families, another reason for their weight loss was to improve their physical appearance, as indicated by the 'aesthetic' keywords (*look, amazing, figure, bikini, beautiful, stunning* and *snap*). The keyword *bikini* consistently performs in a similar way to the stories about wedding dresses we explored earlier, wherein the desire to wear a bikini acts as a motivation for women to lose weight, with the ability and confidence to wear a bikini presented, positively, as a result of a woman's weight loss.

> Taking to Instagram, Holly revealed that she had been sent the **bikini** three years ago – but only now felt confident enough to wear it.
> (*Mail*, 3 May 2015)

Other keywords in this category are used to provide positive evaluations of the women's new *look* or *figure*, which can be described using adjectives such as *amazing, beautiful* and *stunning*.

> **Stunning** Conner keeps a trim 10 stone **figure** with a balanced diet and regular exercise.
> (*Mirror*, 12 February 2016)

The final keyword in this category, *snap*, refers to photographs of the women that have been reproduced in the articles, with readers invited to view these images as evidence of the women's weight loss.

> Scarlett showed in the second **snap** however that while her body has changed drastically, her beloved witty personality has not.
> (*Mail*, 11 August 2016)

This focus on the aesthetic can function as a motivation for women to lose weight in the narratives but also to orient readers to the visual results of the weight loss, which are conceptualised in terms of the women's resulting physical appearance and attractiveness.

As well as this, women's experiences of obesity and their desire to lose weight could also be conceptualised in emotional terms, indicated by the verb keyword *felt*, as well as adjective keywords denoting emotional states (*embarrassed* and *desperate*). These heightened levels of self-disclosure also help to account for the marked frequency of first-person forms such as *I*, *my*, *me* and the reflexive *myself*, which were all key in the women's narratives.

> Children **I** taught at school would shout 'muffin top' and other hurtful names at **me** when **my** back was turned. But **I** was so **embarrassed** about **my** size, **I**'d pretend **I** hadn't heard.
>
> (*Mail*, 15 December 2011)

The verb *felt* could also convey more complex emotional states, some of which are not represented in the keywords in Table 7.2, such as feeling miserable, depressed and disgusting. In this extract from the *Mail*, for example, loneliness and depression are given as reasons for weight gain.

> "**I** dropped out of high school because **I** was there for everybody, but **I felt** like nobody was there for **me**," she said, "When **I** was really depressed, **I** left."
>
> (*Mail*, 19 November 2015)

The emotions attested in the women's narratives were not all negative, though, and *felt* could also be used to describe more positive emotional states following weight loss, as in this example.

> **My** friends couldn't believe it, they all thought **I** looked great. And **I felt** fantastic too. **I** joined a gym which **I** could have never done at 20 stone. In a year she lost 7 stone and now weighs a slimmer 13 stone 4. She has also dropped a staggering seven dress sizes – and has gone from a size 28 to a 14. She said: '**I**'m so much more confident in **my** body.
>
> (*Mail*, 13 September 2012)

In two-thirds of uses, the keyword *desperate* described women feeling desperate to lose weight, such as in this extract where a woman's desperation sets up a description of her abuse of laxatives to try to lose weight.

> Woman **desperate** to lose 6st took 20 laxatives a DAY – even though the pain was 'worse than childbirth'
>
> (*Mail*, 30 October 2014)

This description of weight loss practices brings us to our final keyword category: diet and weight loss. Beginning with the women's narratives, the keywords assigned to this category include words denoting the method by which the women lost weight, such as *surgery*, *gastric*, *tried*, *bypass* and *yoga*. The verb *tried* is interesting, as in 64 per cent of its uses it denotes multiple attempts, including failed attempts, to lose weight and thus attests to the difficulties that the women faced trying to lose weight, as this example shows.

Obese woman loses 17 STONE after splitting from fat fetishist boyfriend – and looks unrecognisable. The difference, though, was when
each time, met with failure, she **tried** again, as she told Reddit. Woman
known as Sprk97 loses incredible 11 stone after trying every diet She
explained: "I did a bunch of WeightWatchers, I did the Curves plan,
I did Keto for a bit, had issues with cholesterol, switched to Paleo for a
hot minute, did dairy free – you name it."

(*Mirror*, 25 November 2015)

As well as describing difficulties trying to lose weight, such articles also
provide further evidence of the desperation some women feel regarding their
weight loss, echoing the uses of *desperate* described earlier. This sense of
desperation also emerges in reports of women who resorted to surgical solutions to obesity, indicated by the keywords *surgery, gastric* and *bypass*. In
Chapter 3, we observed how surgical weight loss could be evaluated negatively by the tabloids, presented as dangerous and expensive, and was contrasted against the neoliberal 'gold standard' of dieting and exercise. However,
in the women's narratives, surgical solutions were presented in a relatively
neutral way. Rather than chastising the women for opting for surgery or
discussing its associated costs and dangers, these mentions seemed to function
to convey the sense of desperation that the women felt to lose weight.

Hazel Walsh, 26, was bullied for being a size 24
She tried and failed to lose weight by following diets
She opted for **gastric** band **surgery** and shed 7st

(*Mail*, 23 August 2013)

With this in mind, then, we can perhaps revise our earlier argument by adding
the caveat that the press stigma surrounding surgical methods of weight loss
can be mitigated in cases where those in question are desperate to lose weight
and have tried other, non-surgical methods of weight loss first.

Women's weight loss narratives also focussed on cases where women
employed more traditional methods of weight loss, such as diet and
exercise. The keywords *chocolate, crisps* and *biscuits* all feature overwhelmingly as types of foods that the women previously indulged in but have now
reduced or cut out altogether to lose weight. The keyword *yoga* featured in
89 per cent of cases as a method through which the women lost weight and
could index a holistic approach to health characterised by an all-round healthier lifestyle.

Too self-conscious to go to the gym, she first started working out at
home and says: "For an hour every night I ran, did **yoga** or step-
aerobics."

(*Sun*, 18 February 2013)

The keywords in this category also denoted weight loss results. In uses of the keywords *kilos*, *10st*, *11st* and *2lb*, this was quantified quite straightforwardly as the amount of weight that the women had lost, or comparisons of their 'before' and 'after' weights. Consistent with the patterns around wedding dresses and bikinis seen earlier, weight loss could also be characterised in terms of the women's dress sizes, including their ability to fit into clothes of a certain size, indicated by uses of *size*, *into*, *dress*, *10*, *fit* and *fitted*. This attention to clothing also provides further evidence of the focus on women's weight loss from an aesthetic perspective; that is, how they appear physically to others. An interesting keyword in this category for the women is the verb *stay*, which was used mostly in reference to the desire of, or even pressure on, the women to maintain their results in the long-term and *stay* at their new weight (25 per cent).

> After eating only grilled turkey for two weeks I'd lost half a stone and was granted the place. From then on, I knew I had to **stay** slim. I was basically blackmailed by my record company – they frightened me into thinking that if I put on weight our records wouldn't sell and I'd lose everything.
>
> (*Mail*, 16 January 2009)

The keyword *body* exhibits a wide range of uses, most commonly in the bigram 'body weight' (20 per cent). Yet in a minority of cases (5 per cent), this keyword also cued more politicised explanations of body dissatisfaction, such as in this extract from an article about soap actor Letitia Dean, who describes having body anxiety due to her job being 'in the public eye'.

> It was really depressing. At the back of my mind, I knew I should exercise but I just couldn't see myself as a gym bunny. Most women worry about their weight, but being in the public eye heightened my **body** anxiety. Red carpet events were a nightmare.
>
> (*Mail*, 16 January 2009)

Returning to the men's keywords, we find just one keyword that orients directly to the results of their weight loss: *waist*. The comparative plethora of keywords referring to the women's weight loss results might thus indicate a closer focus on their results compared to in the stories about men. Moreover, while the keyword *waist* occurs 51 times across the men's narratives, the keyword *size* alone occurs 265 times in the women's stories.

Instead, the men's stories appear to focus more on the methods of their weight loss than on the results. The most frequent keyword relevant here is *diet*, which in 83 per cent of cases is used to denote the diets that the men have embarked on in order to lose weight. Descriptions of diets help to explain some of the other keywords too, as these involve reducing *sugar*, *calories* and *carbs* and opting for *low-fat* alternatives. In the majority of cases (71 per cent), the diets described are marked as unusual in some way, particularly as being high protein and involving the consumption of meat.

> The low-fat, high-protein **diet** keeps his energy up for running 5k and 10k races.
>
> (*Mirror*, 23 September 2015)

> After signing up to a protein-rich **diet** plan, Gafyn found himself 'shovelling down' food nine times a day, often when he was not hungry. But, to his disbelief, the weight quickly began to drop off and – after getting a personal trainer – the father-of-one has now lost more than six stone of body fat.
>
> (*Mail*, 19 January 2016)

While it is not strictly to true to say that 'only women diet', the diets that men are reported as embarking on in the tabloids are at least marked or unusual in some way, which could contribute to their newsworthiness and thus explain why they are reported on in the first place. Yet, we also find evidence that the men's diets are presented in such a way that distances them from traditional diets, too. For example, the man featured in this extract is quoted as describing what he did to lose weight as not being a diet and then distinguishes 'a diet' from 'healthy eating'.

> It wasn't a **diet**, it was just healthy eating, and I was never hungry.
>
> (*Mail*, 31 May 2013)

This avoidance of labelling weight loss practices as 'diets' is most explicit in this extract, also from the *Mail*, which quotes a nutritionist who advises against using the word *diet*.

> He says: "The one biggest **diet** mistake is anything with the word **diet** in. Anything low calorie, anything depriving when you don't eat much for days and days. Because all that time all you're thinking of is food."
>
> (*Mail*, 22 November 2016)

Another way in which diets were discursively avoided was through the keyword *experiment*, where ten of its seventeen occurrences are used to describe the changes that men made to what they ate to lose weight.

> As experts question conventional wisdom on diets, the extraordinary results of one man's experiment. When most attempt to lose weight, they try the low-fat, high carb diet. But this formula is increasingly under attack. Sceptics now believe you should cut down on carbs and eat more fat.
>
> (*Mail*, 15 October 2013)

By describing the men's weight loss practices as experiments, these are not only distanced from dieting, which might be perceived as feminine (Lupton 2018), but are also framed as a kind of scientific quest for knowledge and are thus situated more firmly within a traditionally masculine domain. As Connell (1995: 6) points out, '[w]estern science and technology are culturally masculinised [...] The guiding metaphors of scientific research, the impersonality of its discourse, the structures of power and communication in science, the reproduction of its internal culture all stem from the social position of dominant men in a gendered world.'

Conclusion

The analysis in this chapter explored how the press utilises a range of gendered discourses in its reporting on obesity. Taken together, the gendered discourses identified in this chapter provide evidence that the press recycles and reinforces a restricted set of prominent and long-standing ideologies around femininity and masculinity. As well as being reported on much more than men, women were consistently represented in terms of relational aspects of their identity, with particular focus on their roles in, and responsibilities for, caring for others. Specifically, women were responsibilised into minimising the risk of obesity in their (unborn) children, husbands and boyfriends, and even other women.

The relational types of identities that were attributed to women in the articles also manifested in an aesthetic focus on their bodies, weight and weight loss, whereby both their desire to lose weight and the results of their weight loss were presented in terms of how they appeared to others, for instance in wedding dresses or bikinis, prompting evaluations of them in the articles as 'beautiful' or 'stunning'. This reflects what Conboy (2005: 146) describes as the 'linguistic flagging of female body shape', which, he argues, 'is one of the primary ways in which [the tabloids] act to define norms of the female body for readers'.

Representations of women also foregrounded the emotional aspects of their weight loss and embodied experience, with obesity presented as causing embarrassment and even depression; the process of weight loss characterised in terms of difficulty and desperation; and the results of weight loss leading to increased confidence and other more positive emotions. Men, by contrast, were portrayed in ways that backgrounded their emotions. Instead, their decisions to lose weight were construed as logical and life-preserving, as motivated by the threat of disease, or even death, that was posed by their obesity. These differences can be linked to what Charteris-Black and Seale (2010: 120–121) describe as an 'underlying distinction between masculinity, rationality, science and a world view that implies dominance and control of the material world and femininity, emotionality and influence over a private and domestic order'.

This sense in which men only diet in extreme or exceptional circumstances was reinforced by the way in which their weight loss practices were represented in the articles, particularly those featuring weight loss narratives. Although the word *diet* was key in these texts compared to the women's narratives, we found that the men's actions were frequently portrayed as *not* being diets, in some cases lexicalised instead as 'experiments'. The diets that men did engage in were marked or unusual, and frequently preserved the consumption of foodstuffs that have become symbolic of hegemonic masculinity, such as alcohol and red meat. In this sense, our analysis lends further evidence to what Gough (2006) describes as the persistence and durability of hegemonic formulations of masculinity, since even those men who engaged in 'feminised' endeavours such as dieting are presented as doing so in exceptional circumstances, with a kind of linguistic distancing between their activities and an activity, in dieting, that is likely to be perceived as 'woman-centred' and 'unmasculine'.

The discourses identified in this part of our analysis offer a relatively narrow range of gender roles and experiences which, we argue, are likely to fail to capture the complexity and variability of contemporary gender identities, including the ways in which these intersect with notions and experiences of health. It is not the case, for example, that women are the primary caregivers in all families. Therefore, press reporting that responsibilises women for the health and risk of obesity of their entire families (including children), all the while seeming to absolve others (including fathers) of these responsibilities, could be viewed as having a narrow applicability and even as being outdated. Likewise, men also have an array of discourses and 'masculine' identities open to them in the ways that they make sense of and communicate about themselves and their health. For instance, research has shown that men are increasingly sensitive to concerns around body image (Gill et al. 2000) and, contrary to the lack of focus on the aesthetic aspects of men's weight loss in our data, some men have been found to orient to concerns around physical appearance when describing their weight loss online (Bennett and Gough 2013). Yet, such masculine positions seem to be limited if not absent altogether in the context of press reporting on men's weight loss.

Similarly, while the dearth of emotional disclosure in men's weight loss narratives compared to women's might reflect traditional, stoical models of masculinity, research has demonstrated that men can and indeed do disclose their emotions in certain contexts (Galasiński 2004). Indeed, studies of emotions relating to obesity specifically have shown that men and women feel 'similar feelings of shame, humiliation and revulsion about their bodies and are also treated by others as inferior, deficient and lacking in self-control' (Lupton 2017: 66). However, the press does not seem to provide any therapeutic discourse within which men can situate themselves as 'feeling subjects, needing to talk to professionals [or anyone else] about their self-image in the light of their outcast obese status' (Gough 2010: 138).

Based on our analysis, then, the British press seems to be lagging behind in terms of representing contemporary gender identities, as well as both men's and women's evolving relationships with their diet and weight. Instead, the press seems to orient to more traditional models of femininity and (hegemonic) masculinity. One explanation for this might be that the newspapers are offering depictions of men and women that they think their older 'imagined' readers will be familiar with and able to identify with. Yet as well as reflecting society, it is important to bear in mind that media texts also have the potential to shape and indeed dictate social norms and, from a public health perspective, these kinds of gender norms haven't done women's or men's health much good in the past. For example, for women, intense focus on slenderness has been linked to the development of body image concerns and disordered bodily practices such as eating disorders (Stice et al. 1994). Meanwhile, although hegemonic discourses have privileged men in some respects, they can also have deleterious effects on their health (Buchbinder 2010), such as promoting the consumption of alcohol and red meat, as well as the notions that men are invulnerable, emotionally detached, and should only address their health concerns when they are at risk of serious illness. These aspects of masculine identity become all the more problematic when we consider that the feminine coding of conventional weight management and reduction activities, including dieting and attending weight loss groups, means that men with weight concerns are less likely to utilise these and instead rely more on the media for their health advice (Gough 2010).

We argue that the public would be better served by media coverage which at least incorporates a wider range of gendered subject positions, rather than relying on a narrow range of rigid and traditional assumptions about men and women. Not all men are beer-swillers and not all women are the primary caregivers in families and base their health decisions on their ability to squeeze into a wedding dress or a bikini. Reportage that reflects this reality is surely more likely to be successful in identifying with members of modern societies and encouraging them to engage in positive health behaviours. Ideally, though, the media should also endeavour to challenge gendered discourses that are likely to be harmful to everyone, and instead promote traits such as emotional expressivity and collaboration in health by detaching these from their associations with just femininity. There was some evidence in our corpus that debates around gender can open up space for the press to adopt such critical perspectives, for example in the *Guardian*'s articles about ethnicity-related health inequalities and tabloid narratives alluding to women's experiences of body anxiety. These were both minority discourses in the corpus, although more coverage of this kind could usefully improve the public's critical awareness of gender power relations and the potential of these to harm everyone's health.

8   'A Disease of the Poor'? Obesity and Social Class

Introduction

Following our analysis of gendered discourses in the previous chapter, in this chapter we maintain our focus on social identity but switch our attention to a different aspect of it; namely, social class. Social class is a complex phenomenon which has its intellectual basis in social and political economic theories advanced by nineteenth-century theorists such as Karl Marx and Max Weber (see Savage (2000) for a discussion). For the purpose of this chapter, we adopt the definition of social class put forward by sociolinguist Miriam Meyerhoff (2006), who describes it as 'a measure of status which is often based on occupation, income and wealth, but also can be measured in terms of aspirations and mobility' (295). These and other factors are commonly used to score individuals and to assign them to social class groups (see Block (2013) for a discussion of definitions of social class within and beyond linguistics), for example as working class, middle class and so forth, and so help to define the qualifying criteria for these various groups.

Despite strong interest from sociolinguists in the influence of social class on linguistic variables during the 1960s and 1970s (e.g. Trudgill 1974; Labov 2006), class has, in general, been largely neglected in more recent linguistic research. This lack of linguistic attention to social class is even starker in the case of discourse-based studies concerned with issues such as social inequality, as Rampton (2010: 1) points out, 'there is a great deal of contemporary work on discourse, culture, power and social inequality, but this generally focusses on gender, ethnicity and generation much more than class' (although for more recent exceptions, see studies by Bennett (2013); Baker and McEnery (2015); Baker and Levon (2016); Paterson (2020)). Savage (2000) argues that the initial linguistic focus on social class has been usurped by increased interest in other social variables (such as those aforementioned), while Mills (2017) attributes this waning focus to the difficulties associated with categorising individuals into particular class groups, as well as to the problems that arise from discussing class differences in terms of deficit.

Jones (2012: vii) and others have argued that although the true nature and extent of socioeconomic disparities in the United Kingdom were for a while obscured by the wide availability of cheap credit, the economic crisis of 2008 has helped to 'refocus attention on the unjust distribution of wealth and power in society'. As a result, class, or at least our awareness of and societal discourses around class, are now 'back with a vengeance' (*ibid.*: vii). Similarly, Mills (2017: 81) points out that while some argue that class is no longer relevant to British society, it is also the case that society is becoming more unequal, with lack of means and precarious employment indicated by increasing reliance on food banks and zero hours contracts.

Indeed, social class and inequality are, as Mills (2017: 81) puts it, 'inextricably linked'. Guy (2011: 159–160) argues that '[c]lass divisions are essentially based on status and power in a society', where '[s]tatus refers to whether people are respected and deferred to by others in their society (or, conversely, looked down on or ignored), and power refers to the social and material resources a person can command, the ability (and social right) to make decisions and influence events'. Our decision to study social class as a variable in the representation of obesity is thus motivated by our view of unequal class relations as a driver of obesity incidence and wider health inequalities in the United Kingdom. Indeed, as we briefly detailed in Chapter 1, incidence of obesity can also be connected to social class. As Bissell et al. (2016: 14) put it, 'obesity shows a well-established social gradient in its prevalence, with the most socio-economically disadvantaged having the highest rates'. Bissell and colleagues also note how evidence increasingly points to 'material lack and precarity which are increasingly features of daily life across many countries', with 'rising levels of material and financial hardship [. . .] clearly impact[ing] the food decisions of many' (*ibid.*; see also Ulijaszek 2014). It is in view of this social gradient of obesity that Marsh (2004: online) describes it as a 'symptom of social impoverishment'.

In this chapter, we answer calls from the likes of Rampton (2010: 1) to 'resuscitate' the issue of social class in linguistic research by examining the ways in which discourses around social class inform and shape representations of obesity. We do this by considering how different social class groups (i.e. upper class, middle class, working class and underclass) are represented in relation to obesity. According to Rampton (2006: 222–223), social class can be studied in terms of 'primary realities', which account for individuals' material conditions and everyday experiences, activities, practices and discourses, and/ or in terms of secondary or 'meta-level' representations, including the various ideologies and discourses that surround different social groups and the relations between these. Our analysis clearly orients to the latter of these perspectives, yet at the same time such 'meta-level' representations of social class can have ramifications for the 'primary realities' of people belonging to these different groups – a point which we will return to following our analysis.

Table 8.1. *Daily reach of UK national newspapers (000s)*[a]

Category	Newspaper	ABC1		C2DE	
		N (000)	%	N (000)	%
Broadsheet Left	*Guardian*	4,140	75.55	1,340	24.45
	Independent	2,035	68.33	943	31.67
Broadsheet Right	*Telegraph*	3,563	71.81	1,399	28.19
	Times	1,830	81.66	411	18.34
Tabloid Left	*Mirror*	8,093	54.96	6,631	45.04
Tabloid Right	*Express*	3,652	58.80	2,561	41.20
	Mail	7,345	63.52	4,219	36.48
	Star	874	45.95	1,028	54.05
	Sun	7,654	52.99	6,789	47.01

[a] These statistics reflect circulation through phone, tablet, desktop and print between July 2018 and June 2019. Figures for Sunday and online editions are combined. Statistics for *Morning Star* were not available. Source: https://pamco.co.uk/pamco-data/latest-results.

Before moving onto the analysis, we want to touch briefly on newspaper readership. As we discussed in the first chapter, newspaper articles are written, or 'designed', in ways that their editors think will appeal to the perceived sensibilities and worldviews of their 'imagined' readerships. With this in mind, it is possible that the articles in our corpus will be written in ways that will appeal to the social class of their perceived readerships. Table 8.1 gives the daily circulation of UK national newspapers, divided by social class using the National Readership Survey (NRS) social grading system. The column ABC1 represents readers in the categories A (upper middle class; higher managerial, administrative or professional occupation), B (middle class; intermediate managerial, administrative or professional occupation) and C1 (lower middle class; supervisory or clerical and junior managerial, administrative or professional occupation). The column headed C2DE represents readers in the categories C2 (skilled working class; skilled manual workers), D (working class; semi-skilled and unskilled manual workers) and E (non-working; state pensioners, casual and lowest grade workers, unemployed with state benefits only).

Although these social grades do not map directly onto the class groups that we consider in our analysis, they do give a rough impression of the likely target or 'imagined' readers for each section of the corpus. The first point of note is that all newspapers are read more by the higher social groups than the lower ones, except for the *Star*, which is read more by people in the lower groups. However, proportionally, the gaps between the numbers are tighter for the tabloids than for the broadsheets, which indicates that readers at the lower end of the social spectrum make up a much bigger proportion of the reader-ships of the tabloids compared to the broadsheets. Specifically, readers in the C2DE categories make up an average of 25.66 per cent of the readership of the broadsheets, but 44.76 per cent of the tabloids' readership. This is something that we will want to bear in mind when interpreting how the different levels of social class are represented in our data, as it is likely that newspapers will have their readers' social class in mind when crafting such representations.

Approach: Searching for Social Class

In order to examine how different social class groups are represented in relation to obesity, the first set of decisions we have to make relates to how we define and divide different levels of social class. Here we can draw inspir-ation from previous linguistic studies of social class representation. Meyerhoff observes how contemporary conceptions of social class in the social sciences have elaborated on Marx's initial distinction between those who produce social capital or resources and those who control that production. For example, Block (2013: 56–57) notes how social scientists studying class have tended to resolve people into upper, middle and working/lower class. Baker and Levon (2016) also look at these groups in their analysis of the intersections of social class, masculinity and race in press representations of men.

For our analysis, we also adopt this way of grouping but elaborate on it by introducing a fourth category, the *underclass*. The Oxford English Dictionary defines the underclass as the 'lowest social stratum in a country or community, consisting of the poor and the unemployed'. In other words, the term is applied to those who are perceived not to contribute to economic systems of produc-tion, including through labour or capital, but who depend on these neverthe-less. The underclass can thus be considered as distinct from the working class, and as sitting beneath it in any ranking of the social classes in terms of both means and prestige, as it is a label applied to those individuals and groups who are perceived to exist outside of the world of work and the processes of production along which lines social class groups are, as we have seen, typically defined. Johnson and Partington (2017) point out that the term *underclass* has 'highly negative evaluative connotations'. They elaborate, '[i]t is a class that should not exist in any well-ordered and equitable society. Or perhaps, better, it is a term which is usually heavily problematized; it is represented in terms of the problems it supposedly provides those who comprise it, but also sometimes in terms of the problems it or its members purportedly pose for the rest of society' (293–294).

In this chapter, we explore the ways in which four social class groups are represented in relation to obesity, (i) upper class, (ii) middle class, (iii) working class and (iv) underclass. The first challenge we are presented with here

Table 8.2. *Terms denoting social class groups in the corpus*

Social class group	Search terms, in order of frequency (in brackets)
Upper class	*upper class** (50), *upper-class** (40), *upperclass** (1) Total frequency: 91
Middle class	*middle-class** (763), *middle class** (495), *chattering class** (23), *middleclass** (19), *upper-middle class** (10), *lower-middle class** (1) Total frequency: 1,311
Working class	*working-class** (398), *working class** (253), *workingclass** (11) Total frequency: 662
Underclass	*underclass** (117), *lower class** (15), *lower-class** (5), *low class** (4), *under-class** (2), *lowerclass** (1), *under class** (1) Total frequency: 145

pertains to locating texts and passages within the corpus wherein these groups are represented, and so which are relevant to our purposes. In the first half of the previous chapter, we explored gendered portrayals of obesity by searching for mentions of the most frequent gendered nouns in the corpus. However, compared to gender, the linguistic indexing of social class can be less clear and is generally less frequent in our corpus. For this reason, we need to take a data-driven approach to finding search terms for distilling texts in which these social class groups are likely to be represented. To do this, we started with the noun *class* and its plural equivalent, *classes*, and analysed all their pre-modifying L1 collocates which had a minimum frequency of 5, noting pairings which denoted specific class groups. This gave us bigrams such as *upper* + class, *middle* + class and so forth. To expand the reach of our search terms, we also checked the frequencies of all pairings when they occurred closed (e.g. *upperclass*) or hyphenated (*upper-class*). We then assigned all the resulting search terms to one of our social class groups shown in Table 8.2 (frequencies in brackets). Note that single and plural forms are grouped together, hence the use of the wildcard (*).

Most of the terms in this table were easy to assign to one of our social class groups, as they corresponded directly to the title of the group in question. However, others required more careful consideration. An example of this is the term *chattering class**. To decide where to place this term, we consulted multiple definitions from dictionaries, academic work and even the media itself, where it was consistently defined as being part of the middle class. Another, less straightforward set of terms derived from the lemma LOW (*low class**, *lower class**, *lower-class**, *lowerclass**). It was not entirely clear as to how we should have categorised these terms. However, inspecting their use we found that they tended to be used to refer to people at the bottom of the socioeconomic ladder, i.e. mostly people without income or much income, and so we decided that these words best fit our 'Underclass' category.

Before moving onto the analysis, we should note that these search terms are, of course, not comprehensive, and will not give us complete coverage of all instances in which these different groups are talked about and represented in our corpus. Moreover, a limitation of our approach is that we have focussed on, and so our insights are restricted to, those instances where social class is indexed explicitly. We could have expanded our search terms by including words such as *rich* for the upper class and *unemployed* for the underclass. However, to have done so would have risked skewing our searches so that they produced results which foregrounded certain attributes and traits of these groups, such as their personal wealth and employment status, while backgrounding others. Moreover, to have introduced such terms would have hindered the present comparability of our search terms, which are at least comparable in the sense that they all pre-modify the term *class** and refer to their respective groups in an equally general sense.

Focussing on the frequencies of the terms in Table 8.2, immediately noticeable here is the pronounced frequency of terms denoting the middle class (1,311), which is mentioned almost twice as much as the working class (662). The underclass is mentioned even less (145), while the upper class is mentioned least of all (91). To understand these frequency differences and how these terms contribute to obesity representations, we have to consider how they are used in the contexts of the articles. Rather than analyse the corpus as a whole, which is how we obtained this frequency information, we instead explored representations across the different sections of the press (i.e. Broadsheet Left, Broadsheet Right, Tabloid Left, Tabloid Right). This gives us a greater level of granularity in our analysis and allows us to compare and contrast representations across these different parts of the press. Table 8.3 gives the frequencies for each set of social class search terms across the various sections of the corpus, along with normalised frequencies (per million words (PMW)).

The frequencies in this table suggest that, in both raw and relative terms, the right-leaning broadsheets engage in discussion of social class the most, followed by the left-leaning broadsheets and then the right- and left-leaning tabloids, respectively. Of course, we have to bear in mind that this is based on a relatively small set of search terms, and other parts of the press could use additional terms that would bump up their frequencies, so we should be cautious about drawing strong conclusions based on this frequency information alone. The same order also holds when we consider which sections of the press are most and least likely to mention specific social class groups, in all cases except for the working class, which is mentioned (relatively) most often by the left-leaning broadsheets, then the right-leaning broadsheets, then the

Table 8.3. *Breakdown of frequency of social class groups by section*

	Broadsheet Left		Broadsheet Right		Tabloid Left		Tabloid Right	
	Freq.	PMW	Freq.	PMW	Freq.	PMW	Freq.	PMW
Upper Class	29	3.40	32	3.71	3	1.32	27	1.63
Middle Class	418	48.94	524	60.67	13	5.74	356	21.43
Working Class	279	32.66	221	25.59	21	9.27	141	8.49
Underclass	47	5.97	56	6.48	1	0.44	37	2.23
Total	777	90.97	833	96.45	38	16.77	561	33.78

left-leaning tabloids, with the right-leaning tabloids last. In general, though, we can say that the broadsheets are more likely than the tabloids to talk explicitly about social class and specific social class groups.

In the forthcoming section, we use the search terms in Table 8.2 to examine the representations of these various social class groups, focussing in particular on their relation to obesity. Our analysis will consider each section of the corpus in-turn and our findings are grouped according to each social class group. This is to enable us to make clearer the similarities and differences in the ways that particular groups are depicted across the corpus. In line with our approach in previous chapters, for terms occurring over 100 times, for example the middle class terms in the right-leaning broadsheets which have a combined frequency of 524, we analysed a sample of 100 randomly selected texts representing all of the newspapers in that section (i.e. in this case, the *Telegraph* and *Times*). Where the combined frequencies totalled less than 100, we analysed all uses. We will focus mostly on majority patterns and also those which are relevant to the representation of obesity.

Upper Class

Beginning with the left-leaning press, and the broadsheets in particular, we identified a distinction between the *Guardian* and the more centrist, liberal *Independent*. In the *Guardian*, the upper class tends to be mentioned in ways that contrast it against lower classes, which are depicted as being at greater risk of obesity. Such articles focussed on differences in the means and living standards between the upper classes and people towards the bottom of the socio-economic stratum, for example in this extract which argues that food offers people from lower classes a form of pleasure, whereas people from the upper classes can afford to derive pleasure from other means.

> Sugar is highly addictive, highly rewarding and incredibly accessible, but it's not cocaine. It's one of the few pleasures left to many people, something that makes food delicious instead of bland. It activates neural pathways of pleasure that most middle- and **upper-class** people have opened up for them on a regular basis – just like smoking, or any other public health concern that has us all clucking our tongues.
>
> (*Guardian*, 1 December 2015)

The point here, then, is that the *Guardian* tends to discuss the upper classes in ways that contrast them and their means and living circumstances against those of people lower down the socio-economic ladder, in order to account for their differing obesity rates. Although we also found such representations in the *Independent*, more often (four cases) this newspaper presented obesity as something that affects the upper classes too, as in this extract, which, while acknowledging differences in the means of people across the social class groups, nevertheless describes the notion that only the lower classes experience obesity as a 'lie' and proclaims that the upper classes 'have weight problems' too.

> The biggest lie told about obesity is that only the lower classes are fat. And that this is because they can't cook. The middle and **upper classes** can afford to join gym clubs and go off to slimming "spas" to shed weight, but, trust me, they too have weight problems.
>
> (*Independent*, 30 November 2014)

Staying with the left-leaning newspapers but moving onto the tabloids, we again find evidence of a comparative element, whereby obesity is framed as a growing problem among the lower, rather than upper, classes. This accounts for two of the three mentions of 'upper class' in this portion of the corpus, with both coming from the same article.

> Obesity is now a 'disease of the poor' and experts warn it's because healthy foods is too expensive; A report said the child obesity rate is soaring for the poor but falling for the middle and **upper classes**. Obesity is now a "disease of the poor" as the well-off are getting the message on eating healthily, the world's leading experts warn.
>
> (*Mirror*, 10 October 2017)

So, although the upper classes aren't mentioned much in the left-leaning tabloids, the representations that are offered are comparable to those found in the *Guardian* in the sense that they present obesity as something that disproportionately affects people from the lower social classes, highlighting differences in the means and living circumstances between those from upper and lower social classes as a way of explaining this.

Moving onto the right-leaning data, and starting with the broadsheets we notice differences here compared to the left-leaning publications, whereby the diets and lifestyles of the upper classes are presented as things that should be followed by others, namely from lower social class groups, to avoid obesity (twelve of thirty-two mentions). This can also be framed as advice to the reader, such as in this extract which directs readers to 'Eat as the upper classes do'.

> Secrets of the 'good manners' diet; Eat as the **upper classes** do; it's the civilised way to lose weight, says historian
>
> (*Telegraph*, 24 November 2008)

A similar discourse can be found in the right-leaning tabloids, in which three mentions of the upper class occur in articles arguing in favour of hunting as a form of exercise, as well as for its universality – being something that can be done not just by the upper classes but others too.

> I now live on the commuter belt and have a massive mortgage on a small house, I earn a living on the building sites, so I'm as far away from **upper class** as you can get. The lads I hunt with are plumbers, tilers, factory workers, etc., and were certainly not politically well connected. Hunting is sport for the masses. [...] In a country with a population of young kids and teenagers that's rotten with obesity and drink and drugs we should be encouraging the young to get out into the countryside and enjoy the exercise of a day's hunting.
>
> (*Mail*, 21 February 2008)

Most frequently, though, in nine cases the right-leaning tabloids appeared to be more concerned with obscuring class-based differences in obesity prevalence, as we saw in the *Independent* earlier.

> A lot of **upper-class** children get equally bad food because their parents either can't cook or they get so much pocket money that they spend it all on sweets.
>
> (*Mail*, 13 December 2011)

The representation of the upper class appears to vary most according to the political leaning of the newspapers in our corpus, then. The left-leaning publications (both tabloid and broadsheet) tend to show the upper class in contrast to those lower down the socio-economic ladder, with the latter presented as being at higher risk of obesity due to the restrictions of their life circumstances. The right-leaning press, on the other hand, presented upper-class diet and lifestyle, including activities such as hunting, in positive ways, even as things to aspire to, by proposing these as means for people from other social class groups to lose weight. The right-leaning tabloids and the more centrist *Independent* also featured articles which, in contrast to the left-leaning data, obscured class differences in obesity prevalence by presenting the upper class as being just as at-risk of obesity as those from lower social class groups. Another recurring feature of the representation of the upper classes, as attested by some of the examples given in this section, is the grouping together of the upper class with the middle class, which we consider now.

Middle Class

Of the mentions of the middle class across the left-leaning broadsheets, the most common pattern of representation (30 per cent) was criticism of public health initiatives which held up middle class lifestyles as ideal. Specifically, these were criticised for acting as a subtle chastisement of lower classes for being 'insufficiently middle class', to quote this extract.

> What it ultimately looked like was an attempt not to improve national health but to replicate the **middle-class** diet across the entire population – to say, in other words, that the reason you are obese is that you are insufficiently **middle-class**. Likewise, the Start4Life campaign attempted to recreate the "**middle-class** habit", although only 1% of the population does it, of exclusively breastfeeding their baby for the first six months.
>
> (*Guardian*, 12 August 2010)

This position is converse to the types of glorification of upper class lifestyles we saw in the right-leaning press in the previous section. For these papers, then, obesity is a social class issue, and there is an acknowledgement that obesity is caused by social class differences. However, rather than encourage lower class people to be more 'middle class', these articles shift the focus away from individuals and towards issues such as town planning, with 10 per cent of cases attributing such class-based differences to the fact that, compared to those from the lower classes, middle class people tend to live in areas with more space for exercise.

> Architects such as Eric Lyons, who created leafy homes for **middle-class** families, always placed communal gardens and shared walkways at the heart of his work, which is why he had so many fans. Unfortunately, new towns such as Thamesmead in south-east London never captured that sense of community. Tower blocks might have offered fabulous views and high density in inner cities, but residents felt isolated. Their communal areas became dumping grounds, areas where everything from kicking a ball to riding a bike was banned.
>
> (*Independent*, 2 February 2014)

A feature of the left-leaning broadsheets' representation of the middle class, then, is a critical focus on the role of more powerful institutions, such as public health bodies, whose initiatives are perceived to encourage middle class lifestyles as solutions to obesity, all the while overlooking the role of Government and town planners who have not afforded to lower classes the kind of space and facilities to exercise that are granted to people living in middle class areas. A similar criticism of public health organisations could also be found in one mention of the middle class from the tabloid, the *Mirror*, criticising government initiatives for 'trying to make the developing world more like middle class yummy mummy suburbia' in a context of extreme hunger.

> We throw our money at bad governments and trying to make the developing world more like **middle-class** yummy mummy suburbia and don't understand the reality of that long, drawn-out, miserable cry of hunger.
>
> (*Mirror*, 20 March 2017)

Aside from this, the depiction of the middle class in the left-leaning tabloids was more varied, with no clear overall pattern. For example, the middle class was variously construed as being disproportionately affected by obesity (two cases) but at the same time as having reduced risk of obesity due to middle class mothers being more likely to breastfeed (two cases), as well as because they eat more healthily and lead healthier lifestyles (one case).

Moving onto the right-leaning press, and the depictions of the middle class found here tend to focus on how this group is at high, or higher than expected, risk of obesity. Beginning with the broadsheets, in 71 per cent of cases middle class families were represented as being unhealthy and at pronounced risk of obesity.

> Domino's Pizza gleefully reports an upsurge in custom as **middle-class** families cut back on eating in restaurants and take to dialling yucky fast food instead, and is claiming, rather boldly, that "staying in is the new going out". So, what, is obese the new healthy? Is heart disease the new cool?
>
> (*Times*, 26 July 2008)

Similarly, in the right-leaning tabloids we find articles reporting on the unhealthy lifestyles of the middle class that have left them at heightened risk of obesity, including consuming unhealthy food and drink (22 per cent).

> The findings bolster a growing body of evidence that **middle-class**, middle-aged Britons are the heaviest drinkers in the country. Doctors fear that older, more hardened drinkers are contributing to increasing rates of obesity, cancer and liver disease.
>
> (*Mail*, 24 July 2015)

A related trend in this portion of the corpus was the representation of members of the middle class as placing themselves at higher risk of obesity by not sleeping enough (7 per cent).

> Yet while **middle-class** parents fret endlessly over their children's exam results, eating habits and unsuitable boyfriends, they are blindly setting them up for a lifetime of ill-health by neglecting something just as vital to their well-being – their sleep.
>
> (*Mail*, 22 March 2013)

Like representations of the upper class, then, discourses around the middle class appear to differ according to newspapers' political leanings more than their format of publication. The left-leaning press take aim at powerful institutions, particularly public health organisations, for patronising the lower classes by imploring them to be 'more middle class', while the broadsheets in this section also contrast the living conditions of middle and lower class people, which make it harder for the latter to maintain a healthy weight. Meanwhile, like the depiction of the upper class in the previous section, the right-leaning newspapers seemed to smooth out class-based differences in risk of obesity by representing the middle class as being at equal or even more pronounced risk compared to other social class groups.

Working Class

Beginning with the left-leaning broadsheets, several mentions of the working class refer to fictional characters (8 per cent), as well as overseas (12 per cent) and historical (8 per cent) contexts. If we focus on the cases that relate to obesity in a contemporary and domestic context, then we see that there is no overall majority pattern. Rather, the mentions are spread across a number of different representations, all of which appear to be written in defence of the working class. For example, 10 per cent of cases were critical of the association between obesity and the working class, such as in this film review, which describes this association as an 'ancient stereotype' and as being part of 'the same old middle-class narratives assigned to the poor',

> Every ancient stereotype of the **working class** is endorsed – obesity, sexual deviancy, alcoholism, chain-smoking, and antisocial behaviour. The government has failed this community, and it is deeply unfair to then write off the residents and their lives using the same old middle-class narratives assigned to the poor
>
> (*Guardian*, 10 February 2013)

Rather than challenging such associations, other articles in this section of the corpus appeared to be more receptive to the idea that working class people were more susceptible to obesity and aimed to account for this, for example by citing their lack of material resources, relative to members of higher social class groups (20 per cent). Such cases are consistent with how we saw this section of the press talk about the upper class earlier in this chapter.

> If obesity does disproportionately affect the **working class**, it's likely because the better-off are more likely to have access to resources that identify compulsive eating as a problem and have it appropriately treated.
>
> (*Guardian*, 22 February 2013)

The responsibility and blame attached to the working class respecting obesity were also alleviated by articles which depicted members of this group as victims of the failure of the – in this case, Conservative-led – Government to regulate food and drink (including alcohol) industries (15 per cent),

> Take obesity, where a gap is opening up between children from poor and affluent families. Some researchers suggest **working-class** children are fatter because their families aren't getting messages about healthy eating and exercise; others point out that fast food is cheaper, less time-consuming, and more filling than a healthy middle-class diet. Overweight children tend to grow into obese adults, but Tories, as a breed, have little appetite for regulating supermarkets which discount unhealthy food and alcohol.
>
> (*Independent*, 24 April 2011)

This focus on the Government echoes the kind of critical discourse we have seen from this section of the press in the depiction of the other social class groups explored so far, as well as in other areas of obesity representation more generally. The Government was also criticised for its role in contributing to working class obesity in the left-leaning tabloids. Of the six references to the working class in the *Morning Star*, half featured in calls for more government initiatives to address obesity among working class groups and were critical of cuts to funding of playgrounds and free school meals. In this headline citing a Labour councillor, such actions are likened, metaphorically, to acts of violence against working class children, who are positioned as grammatical objects of the 'aim' of the 'Government *axe*', as well as being described as being '*hammered* by the Tories'.

> Britain – Government axe takes aim at kids
> Government plans to scrap hundreds of children's playground projects are further evidence that "**working-class** kids are getting hammered by the Tories," a Labour councillor declared yesterday.
>
> (*Morning Star*, 12 August 2010)

The presupposition driving such critiques is, of course, the understanding that members of the working class are disproportionately affected by obesity. This was also evident in the other left-leaning tabloid, the *Mirror*, such as in this extract, which refers to working class regions metaphorically as 'fat ghettos'.

> The statistics show huge regional differences in the UK – with "fat ghettos" in poor areas. In largely **working class** Stockton-on-Tees in North East England about one child in six starting primary school is obese.
>
> *(Mirror, 6 July 2009)*

On the whole, the left-leaning newspapers seem to acknowledge an association between obesity and the working class, with exceptions in a minority of cases in the *Guardian*. However, rather than use this association to blame and stigmatise members of that group, the left-leaning media instead frame this association as a symptom of wider social inequalities, including taking aim at the Government for policies which are viewed as upholding such inequalities.

Moving on to the right-leaning press and starting with the broadsheets, the first thing to note is that we see a departure from the left-leaning newspapers' focus on the Government, with the roles and responsibilities of working class individuals instead the focus of what causes obesity among this group. This neoliberal perspective was evident in almost a quarter (24 per cent) of the mentions of the working class in this section of the corpus, where members of this social group were represented as eating unhealthily.

A curious feature of this discourse is the intersection of social class with race. The word 'white' collocates (span: +/- 5) with the working class search terms thirty times in the right-leaning broadsheets; that is, approximately once in every seven mentions of the working class search words, compared to once in every fourteen uses in the left-leaning broadsheets, once in every twenty-four uses in the right-leaning tabloids, and not collocating at all in the left-leaning tabloids. So, there is something about the intersection of social class with race, and whiteness in particular, that is characteristic of the representation of the working class in the right-leaning broadsheets compared to other sections of the press. In these cases, obesity is presented as being a white working class issue, feeding into a wider ethno-nationalistic narrative, observed elsewhere in the right-leaning British press (Wright and Brookes 2019), wherein the privileged status of white British people is presented as being under threat from immigration and multiculturalism. In this case, this threat to privileged status manifests in purported health inequalities being experienced by white people living in the country. For example, in this extract from the *Telegraph*, 'white working class' children are contrasted with children from 'ethnically-diverse areas', where the former are depicted as eating more 'junk food',

WHITE **working-class** children eat more junk food than any other group of young people, a minister has claimed. Kevin Brennan, the Children's Minister, claimed that poor white families live on "pizza, chips and takeaways", putting them at the greatest risk of becoming overweight and suffering poor health. By contrast, he said, pupils in ethnically-diverse areas eat an "incredibly rich array" of foods, including exotic fruits. His comments were made after a series of reports claimed that white working-class children are becoming a new underclass in England. A study for the Office for National Statistics found that white **working-class** boys are the most "persistent low achievers" in schools.

(Telegraph, 23 September 2008)

It is interesting, then, that health status is being co-ordinated with school achievement as part of presenting the wider argument that white people, and working-class people in particular, are losing their advantage in society. Yet we should also not lose sight of the fact that underpinning this ethno-nationalistic rhetoric is again an at least partly responsibilising discourse which focusses on what individuals eat as the cause of obesity.

Almost as many mentions of the working class in this section were in reference to historical contexts (22 per cent). Yet even here, we find some evidence of a contrast between the working class of the past with that of the present, where members of the latter are shown to be leading comparatively sedentary lifestyles.

The fried English breakfast was conceived during the Industrial Revolution (probably) as a form of fast fuel for a **working class** that actually worked. They ate 3,000 calories in the morning, then they burnt 3,000 calories by lunchtime. Or died when the mine collapsed. But you don't burn 3,000 calories driving a forklift truck, or answering the phone at Argos, or fiddling your disability benefit. The work dies, but the breakfast lives on. Result: obesity crisis.

(Times, 17 April 2008)

In such cases, the modern working class is represented as inactive or work-shy, resulting in them burning fewer calories than their historical predecessors. In the example just shown, the modern working class is set apart from a historical one which 'actually worked'. Moreover, the contemporary 'obesity crisis' is attributed to members of the working class performing sedentary jobs but also 'fiddling' disability benefit.

The focus of the right-leaning broadsheets tends, then, to be on the lifestyles and life choices of members of the working class and how these contribute to the reportedly rising obesity rates among this group. Yet at the same time, they are also framed in a discourse of victimhood, whereby they are victims of a multicultural society, as well as of post-industrial workplaces which result in sedentary working conditions. In the case of the latter, the right-leaning broadsheets could be compared to the left-leaning press in their siding with the working class, with a difference being that their ire is directed at changes to modern society, particularly immigrants multiculturalism and working conditions, rather than towards the Government and food and drink industries.

Turning now to the tabloids and, similarly to the broadsheets, of the mentions of the working class relevant to obesity, 30 per cent originated in articles which presented the working class as having been healthier in the past compared to today, and for similar reasons. Note again how the reader (along with the author) is indexed as working class through reference to '*our* quality of life and health' diminishing.

> 'Once they survived the age of five,' says Rowbotham, 'adult life expectancy was 75 for men and 73 for women; and they generally remained in good health until their last few weeks of life ... 'For today's **working classes**, the average lifespan is around 72 for men and 76 for women. Our quality of life and health has actually diminished.
>
> (*Mail*, 26 August 2008)

We also found examples, again, of an intersection of class and race, as working class white children were once more construed as eating more unhealthily than children from other ethnic backgrounds and so as being at heightened risk of obesity (in five of the six collocations of the working class terms with *white*).

> DO WHITE KIDS EAT MORE JUNK?
> WHITE **working-class** children are more likely to eat junk food than any other group, a minister has claimed.
>
> (*Mail*, 23 September 2008)

Other than this, the depiction of the working class in the right-leaning tabloids tends to be geared more towards representations that are explicitly supportive of a neoliberal agenda. Perhaps mindful that members of this group are likely to make up much of their respective readerships, these newspapers do not use such neoliberal rhetoric to blame and stigmatise these groups (else they risk alienating them). Instead, they promote a neoliberal agenda in an arguably more positive way, for instance by foregrounding the concept of individual choice. In 24 per cent of the sample, articles critiqued institutions (in the next example, 'Big Government', 'Big Business' and 'Big Charity') for imposing measures which restrict individuals' ability to choose what they eat and drink. Note how this article also makes the point that those in 'despair' over such measures are described not only as British and working class but also as 'healthy', implying that they are able to maintain their health without such state supervision.

This conference was concerned with choice, the right to control your own body and why it is dangerous to give that essential freedom to the State. I expected tobacco executives and coughing and spluttering delegates but I found a healthy group of British **workingclass** people in despair. They believe Big Government, aided by Big Business and Big Charity, is taking control of their lives and making them miserable.

(*Express*, 1 February 2009)

This neoliberal rationality was also advocated through anti-food tax discourse. Previously, we reported on the right-leaning press's opposition to a so-called 'sugar tax'. In 4 per cent of this sample, we found evidence of this discourse being reproduced but focussed more specifically on the (negative) effect that such a tax would have on the pockets of working class people. This example from the *Sun* is notable, once more, for its use of the inclusive pronoun 'us' to refer to working class people, compared to the distancing 'they' to refer to the Government. Also note the use of parentheses to not only quote but, we would argue, discredit both the expertise of the relevant government officials (i.e. "experts") and the purported health benefits that such a tax would bring (i.e. "to make us fitter").

Just as the **working classes**, elderly and disabled are struggling to cope with job losses, paltry pensions and obscene rises in fuel and public transport bills, Government "experts" want to introduce food taxes "to make us fitter". Are they trying to cause a revolution?

(*Sun*, 30 August 2011)

This neoliberal, autonomist perspective was also evident in articles taking aim at particular public figures for what they perceive to be attempts to lecture working class people on what to eat and how to lead their lives (10 per cent). The extracts that follow, for example, criticise celebrity chef Jamie Oliver and Labour MP Emily Thornberry.

ADVICE IS A FAT LOT OF GOOD, EM
LABOUR'S Emily Thornberry, famous for sneering at a white van and the flag of St George, is possibly not the best choice to lecture the **working class** about the perils of obesity. "If you are looking at poor children now, they are not thin, they are overweight," said Thornberry, above, before waxing lyrical about the joys of growing your own carrots.

(*Sun*, 16 April 2017)

Jamie's a bossy 'tosser'
JAMIE Oliver was branded a "tosser" by an Australian MP for slamming the country's school dinners. Peter Phelps said he is sick of "middle class" meddlers telling "**working class** parents how to raise their children".

(*Star*, 13 May 2017)

These examples usefully illustrate some of the features observed in other articles criticising public figures for advising (working class) people on how to maintain a healthy weight. For example, they are established as middle class; Jamie Oliver is described as 'middle class', while Thornberry is constructed in opposition to symbols of working class Britain (i.e. as 'sneering at a white van man and the flag of St George'), and is associated with a marker of the middle class – growing vegetables (i.e. as 'waxing lyrical about the joys of growing your own carrots'). Meanwhile, other lexical choices frame them both as giving advice that is unwarranted or unsolicited, and as doing so from positions of assumed authority; Thornberry is construed as *'lecturing'*, while Oliver is branded a 'middle class *meddler*' and described as *'telling* "working class parents how to raise their children"'. Such cases can be viewed as evidence of a wider tendency for the tabloids to align themselves with their assumed working class readerships but also to challenge figures who represent authority and perhaps expertise. Interestingly then, where the working class is concerned, both the left- and right-leaning newspapers criticise powerful groups and institutions – mainly the Government and politicians. However, where the left-leaning articles are critical of what they perceive to be a lack of action to address class-based health inequalities, the right-leaning publications are critical of such powerful groups and individuals for doing too much, for imposing a so-called nanny state by restricting the choices of the working class and by telling them what to do. 'Nanny state' is a term that is often used in debates about government paternalism and the extent to which the state and other powerful institutions should intervene in people's lives and life choices. The term tends to be used pejoratively to express the irritation and resentment that is created by what is perceived to be excessive intervention by the state in individuals' lives (Le Grand and New 2015: 181). The discourses just outlined, which echo the sentiment of the nanny state, are operationalised here in defence of a neoliberal rationality which emphasises the responsibility and self-determination of people to make their own choices and to take responsibility for their lives. We will return to consider the implications of these representations, and how they compare with those of the other groups, at the end of this chapter. Now, we turn to the final social class group explored in this analysis, the underclass.

Underclass

Beginning with the left-leaning broadsheets, the underclass is mentioned most commonly in fictional contexts (fourteen cases), for example in reviews of books and films. Aside from this, the underclass tends to be construed as a social group that is especially prone to, even characterisable by, numerous social and health problems including, among other things, obesity (twelve cases).

We have had to face up to some harsh truths: generations of families
dependent on benefits; spiralling problems with obesity and alcohol
misuse, and above all the creation of a super **underclass**; an invisible
army of people disconnected and cut off from the opportunities being
created on their own doorsteps.

(*Guardian*, 18 September 2008)

From this view, obesity is a feature or even a symptom of the underclass. From
the newspapers in this section, we also find evidence of a characteristically
critical perspective on who 'creat[ed]', to borrow from the previous extract, the
underclass and the (health) inequalities that are associated with them, with
various governments covering the time-span of our data blamed (ten cases).
For example, this extract from the *Guardian* takes particular aim at successive
Labour and Conservative-led Governments for the failure of the London
2012 Olympic games to actually improve the health and living circumstances
of members of the underclass (a point that echoes some of the criticisms we
have seen of those games in other chapters).

London has been exposed to the world as a city in which a greedy and
corrupt political and economic elite consign an **underclass** to urban
dumping grounds and dismantle the welfare state built from the ruins
of war when the Olympics last came to town, in 1948. [...] No longer
can the London Games present themselves as an advert for all the
Blairite corporate gobbledegook that has littered the public sphere. If
Blairite Britain conceived the Olympic bid as a billboard for British
modernity then the former prime minister's heir, David Cameron, is left
to reassure Japanese or Californian visitors they will not have to brave a
war zone next summer. By then, draconian prison sentences will have
been imposed on many youngsters who made stupid first-time errors of
judgment (and many who deserve a long spell inside) while unemployment and inequality continue their upward trajectories. A paramilitary
police force will have it all cleaned up by then, and the so-called
underclass who the Games were meant to inspire will be demonised
or incarcerated.

(*Observer*, 14 August 2011)

The two extracts above also hint at a further theme in the depiction of the
underclass – their invisibility. In the 2008 example, the underclass are
described straightforwardly as 'invisible', while the 2011 extract makes the
same point but does so by constructing them as the objects of the processes by
which they become invisible, i.e. they will have been 'cleaned up' and 'incarcerated' by a 'parliamentary police force'. This notion of invisibility is evident
in a further four uses of the underclass search terms, so just over 10 per cent of

all cases. Yet despite their invisibility, there is an accompanying sense in which both the underclass itself and the social inequalities that have led to the formation of this social group are growing, being described in the previous extracts, for example, as an 'army' while 'unemployment and inequality continue their upward trajectories'.

Aside from health inequalities specifically, these newspapers also adopted a critical stance on the demonization of the underclass, hinted at in the previous example. Such cases are complex, as they attribute obesity to this group but do so seemingly as a means of illuminating particular stereotypes around them (six cases).

> Meanwhile, the world of the unprivileged has become a regular staple of entertainment – sometimes a source of guilty humour – for those more fortunate. On any night of the week, you will find a programme exploring, in the usual tone of concern, some horror story from the **underclass**. It might be obesity, or youth crime, or drunkenness, or teenage pregnancy.
>
> (*Independent*, 11 November 2013)

> But we are now crossing the line from austerity-lite to deep austerity. One of the chief indicators is that the kind of protests we are seeing are not coming from the much demonised "**underclass**" – who are presumably too busy breeding, smoking and eating saturated fats – but from those who are " nice " and recognised as "respectable".'
>
> (*Guardian*, 19 October 2015)

Interpreting these cases can be tricky since, as this second example demonstrates, assertions about this group being obese can be made ironically, in this particular case to make the point that it is not just members of the underclass but also 'nice' and 'respectable' members of society, to quote the extract, who are affected by the austerity policies of the British Government. Similarly, elsewhere in this section of the corpus the underclass search terms are directly preceded by adjectives including 'feral' (4), 'fecund' (1), 'lazy' (1) and 'ignorant' (1), yet all cases signal similar deployment of stereotypes either straightforwardly to challenge them or ironically, as in the examples just shown.

So, the representation of the underclass we saw in the left-leaning broadsheets tended to be sympathetic towards this group and, like the depictions of the working class analysed in the previous section, portrayed them as victims of social inequalities created and upheld by more powerful institutions, as well as being victims of demonization, not least within the media itself. Somewhat surprisingly, we found evidence of similar discourses in the right-leaning broadsheets too, where the most common pattern, accounting for just over a third of mentions (nineteen out of fifty-six), was criticism of the demonization and stigmatisation of the underclass. An interesting distinction between these newspapers and the left-leaning broadsheets, though, is that their defence of the underclass appears to be part of a rhetorical strategy in which this group is opposed to the middle and upper classes, who are criticised. For instance, this extract from the *Telegraph* points out what it perceives to be the hypocrisy of middle class associations of 'fat' with the underclass.

> But then middle-class fat is, for them, texturally different from under-class fat. Good things have poured into middle-class fat, you see: steak, Roquefort, red wine and a heartily robust enjoyment of life. **Underclass** fat, however, being composed entirely of chicken nuggets, chips and wilful idleness, is a mark of moral degeneracy. The people who are quickest to sneer at "chavs" and the perceived physical shortcomings of the "**underclass**" often seem to be those most obsessed with flaunting their own "bling" and extending their unprovoked rudeness to those with far less social and financial clout.
>
> (*Telegraph*, 17 August 2008)

Once more, this article employs irony in its references to the distinction between 'middle-class fat' and 'underclass fat', as well as in its attributing to the latter qualities such as 'wilful idleness' and 'moral degeneracy'. Likewise, consider this extract which attributes negative traits and stereotypes to the underclass (e.g. 'jobless', 'toothless', eating 'twizzlers' and smoking 'fags'), all ironically and in order to negatively portray a member of the British royal family, Sarah Ferguson ('Fergie'), for comments she made about poverty and obesity. Note also how Jamie Oliver again emerges as a target of this ire.

> Really she wants poor people to be thin because, my God, haven't they got so fat? The Twizzlers, the fags, the limited means to procure the best low-fat fresh produce. But mostly – and here's where she hopes to best Jamie Oliver and his 'ellfy school dinners – because, as she sees it, the real problem with the jobless, toothless **underclass**'s search for healthy living is that it has such low self-esteem. If there's one thing that "fat frumpy Fergie" (her words, not mine) can empathise with it's feeling bad about yourself.
>
> (*Times*, 18 May 2008)

So, much of this discourse is similar to that which we saw in the right-leaning press's treatment of the working class, whereby figures perceived to be higher up the social ladder are portrayed negatively, for example for being 'snobs' or for giving unwanted advice to members of the lower classes in relation to their weight. However, while these newspapers indexed both their readers and own authorial voices as belonging to the working class, for example through use of first-person collective pronouns and second-person direct address, we did not find much evidence of this in the depiction of the underclass. This could be a product of audience design (Bell 1991); where the label *working class* can carry positive connotations such as being honest and hard-working, *underclass* is a comparatively stigmatising label loaded with negative stereotypes (Johnson and Partington 2017), with which readers are arguably much less likely to self-identify.

The right-leaning tabloids adopted a less sympathetic tone towards the underclass and, while there was a range of representations with no dominant pattern overall, in general the depictions of them seemed to contribute, in various ways, to the very demonising and stigmatising depictions that the left- (and to a lesser extent, right-)leaning broadsheets seem to be challenging. For example, in six of the thirty-seven mentions, the underclass labels were applied in concert with terms relating to obesity in order to negatively evaluate public figures such as celebrities and reality TV stars.

> All of a sudden, Kirsty, a slightly obese, uncouth 21-year-old old female member of the **underclass**, storms into the office, shouting: "This place is a f**king joke."
>
> (*Mail*, 15 April 2010)

In the broadsheets (both left- and right-leaning), we saw how stigmatising labels were applied to members of the underclass ironically to criticise members of the middle and upper class and to illuminate and problematise assumptions and stereotypes relating to social class. Similar types of descriptors were applied to the underclass in the tabloids. However, we did not find evidence of such ironic usage here, where instead such labels formed part of a broader construction of the health problems of the underclass, including pronounced risk of obesity, as constituting a financial burden on the country and taxpayers (eight cases).

> Cost of the underclass FOR decades, governments decided it was easier to hurl money at Britain's burgeoning **underclass**, rather than try to break the cycle of welfare dependency. The results, according to a government adviser, are 500,000 problem families who cost the taxpayer about 30billion a year in benefits and use of State services. Truancy, crime and ill-health are rife. One family triggered 90 police callouts in just six months, while a single morbidly obese mother visited her GP 226 times in just seven years.
>
> (*Express*, 18 August 2014)

In three such cases, this discourse of economic burden fed into a more general, and by now familiar, attack on state intervention, framed here as 'mollycoddling advice'. Note also the use of the inclusive 'we' to refer to – and index readers as – taxpayers, compared to the distancing 'them' and 'their', which construe the underclass as an 'othered' out-group.

> The latest colossal waste of public cash – in the middle of an economic crisis don't forget – is the plan in Glasgow to take on a dozen Childhood Obesity Coaches. Not only is this a ludicrous idea, it could also have the opposite effect. We are already creating an **underclass** who rely on the state for everything, now we are offering them mollycoddling advice on how to remain slim. How on earth will they ever learn to stand on their own two feet?
>
> (*Star*, 6 February 2009)

Another telling feature of this example is the construction of taxpayers as the 'we' who are 'creating' an underclass through too much state intervention creating dependency, as opposed to the representation of the Government as the creators of the underclass that we saw earlier in the left-leaning broadsheets.

Finally, the stigmatisation of the underclass and criticism of state support is enabled, and even legitimised, by the perception that members of this group have brought obesity on themselves. We have found evidence of such responsibilising discourse throughout our corpus and in relation to numerous groups, and we also find such blame-loading rhetoric in relation to the underclass in this portion of the corpus, where in five cases the underclass are represented as consuming unhealthy food and drink. This first example illustrates how such constructions can facilitate a logic whereby responsibility for obesity serves to preclude 'sympathy and understanding' (described as 'rot'), which is instead replaced by 'condemnation'.

> Who can forget those tubby mums passing bags of chips through the school gates? Those of a liberal persuasion will doubtless claim the impoverished **underclass** deserve sympathy and understanding instead of condemnation. What rot.
>
> (*Mail*, 11 July 2009)

Hamilton (2012: 86) contends that the underclass is frequently portrayed negatively as a 'moral category' that can be defined by its 'deviant behavioural norms'. In the right-leaning press, and particularly the tabloids, members of the underclass are represented as deviant not only in terms of their (lacking) economic and labour contributions but also in terms of their purported failure to maintain a healthy lifestyle and successfully mitigate against the risks of obesity – at financial cost to the taxpayer and assumed readers.

Conclusion

In this chapter, we have identified a range of ways in which representations of social class intersect with and contribute towards the representation of obesity.

These representations are complex, with few straightforward patterns. However, we have also noted points of similarity and difference across the different sections of the press that are worth reflecting on further, specifically relating to newspapers' political leanings.

The left-leaning press, including the tabloids but mainly the broadsheets, foregrounded the role of class inequalities in contributing to disproportionate rates of obesity. This included depicting the upper and middle classes as possessing the necessary material means to eat healthily and as living in environments conducive to exercise and physical fitness. On the other hand, both the working class and underclass were constructed as the victims of government actions and policies perceived to support such health disparities, including, among other things, making cuts to public services for poorer families and failing to regulate food and drinks industries. In representations of the underclass, we also found evidence of discourses seeking to counter what are perceived to be stigmatising and demonising (media) depictions of this group, including through the use of irony. The left-leaning newspapers could therefore be viewed as siding with groups on the poorer end of the social class spectrum; for them, obesity is a class-based issue and it is the fault of the Government and other powerful institutions that this is the case. However, the political distinctions between the newspapers also brought to light some more subtle distinctions between the publications assigned to the 'left-leaning' category. For example, although both left-leaning broadsheets, the *Guardian* and the *Independent*, drew attention to the differences between the means and living circumstances of the upper and lower classes, the more centrist *Independent* also contained representations of the upper class as being equally affected by obesity, thereby flattening out social class-based differences in obesity prevalence in a way that we saw the right-leaning newspapers do. This distinction aside, much of what we found in these newspapers can nevertheless be viewed as echoing findings from previous chapters, in which we reported on the tendency for the aforementioned institutions to be evaluated negatively and assigned blame for rising rates of obesity in the left-leaning press. Here, we see that discourse extended to obesity in poorer sections of society in particular.

From the right-leaning press, a more complex picture emerges. On one hand, obesity can be constructed as an issue that exists above and independent of social class. We found evidence of representations designed to smoothen out the disparities between social class groups, for example the reporting of the upper and middle classes as being affected just as much by obesity as people from poorer groups. At other points, we found what seemed to be more of an acknowledgement of class-based differences respecting obesity rates, specifically in stories about obesity among the underclass. However, rather than frame this as a symptom of social inequality, as the left-leaning press did, such associations formed the basis of negative portrayals of the underclass as constituting a financial burden on reader-taxpayers. Inconsistent though it is, we would argue that the right-leaning press's treatment of social class and obesity is always manipulated in a way that upholds and does as little harm as possible to the neoliberal agenda that it seeks to support. Key, here, is the discursive down-playing of social class as a determining factor in the development of obesity. This is perhaps because, to attribute obesity to social class, as the left-leaning press does, is arguably to illuminate the particular social and political systems that create and maintain health inequalities through the unequal distribution of resources (Ulijaszek 2014). This, in turn, shines the spotlight on those powerful institutions, including the Government but also the producers of mass media (Jones 2012: 248), which uphold such systems and benefit from them. By backgrounding social class as a factor in obesity, then, the right-leaning press keeps the spotlight from these institutions and maintains its focus on individuals, with positive or poor life choices given as the cause of not only obesity but other forms of inequality too (Bennett 2013: 160). Therefore, when these articles associate the underclass with obesity, this is framed as a form of deviance, as this group is portrayed as actively disregarding health advice by engaging in activities such as eating high-fat and sugary foods, drinking alcohol excessively and smoking. The topos that arises from, or is implied by, such associations is that members of this social group experience obesity because of their poor lifestyle choices, rather than their lack of material means and the limitations of their living circumstances.

Another way in which the right-leaning press seeks to defend the neoliberal mindset is through its resistance to what it perceives as nanny-stateism. This manifested in numerous representations, including the negative evaluation of politicians and middle class public figures for what was perceived to be them intruding into and controlling the lives of working class people – indexed frequently as the reader. Such perceived attempts by the state to control the public also emerged in the representation of the underclass, whose very existence was constructed by some of the right-leaning articles as a consequence of over-dependency created by state intervention. Reduced intervention in people's lives is a core characteristic and indeed driver of neoliberal political systems (Brown and Baker 2012). Therefore, in contrast to the left-leaning newspapers which criticised the state for its lack of intervention and lack of social provision for society's poorest, the challenging of state intervention by the newspapers on the political right can be interpreted as contributing to their wider neoliberal agenda.

We might regard the centrality of the neoliberal approach to the right-leaning press's discourse, and that of the tabloids' in particular, to be problematic when we consider that people lower down the social class spectrum tend to read these types of newspapers more than others (see Table 8.1), given that health policies emphasising personal behaviour and responsibility usually have limited success with people from poorer socio-economic backgrounds. As Atanasova and Koteyko (2017: 652) point out, this is 'largely due to their disregard for the social determinants of health or the understanding that individual behaviour is influenced by environmental and socioeconomic settings', which means that 'policies emphasising personal behaviour fail to grasp the following: when individuals behave in ways that may be damaging to their health, this may not necessarily be due to their lack of awareness about adverse health effects; rather the constraints of their life experiences and environments may mean that they are simply unable to change their behaviours' (see also Baum and Fisher 2014).

Readers from all social class groups would probably benefit from a more balanced style of reporting, perhaps which incorporates elements of both perspectives. Unlikely though it seems, such an approach would at least (arguably) allow readers to develop more informed views on the relationship between obesity and social class. We will return to these debates surrounding neoliberalism and approaches to obesity in the final chapter of this book. However, we want to conclude this chapter with a brief reflection on the social impacts of the types of oppositional, potentially stigmatising representations found at points in this chapter. Many of the discourses described over the foregoing pages represent class-based identities in a relational way. To an extent, this is understandable, given that the class labels we have analysed only really make sense in relation to each other. However, at times, this discourse was also oppositional; the upper and middle classes could be demonised for having more material means than working class people, as well as for being perceived as lecturing working class people on how to live their lives. Meanwhile, the underclass – already the most demonised class-based group in society – were placed in opposition with everyone, depicted in the most stigmatising terms as a burden on the whole of society. Whatever our views on obesity and its causes are, the blaming of entire groups of people within society, based on the social class label that we or newspapers assign to them, is to risk projecting all of the concern and negative feeling about obesity onto those groups. In an already divided society, it is our view that addressing obesity should be an issue that unites us, rather than being one that divides us further.

9   Going 'Below-the-Line'

Reader Responses

Introduction

The analysis to this point has focussed on different aspects of press representation of obesity, examined from various thematic and methodological perspectives. While we have endeavoured to consider the possible interaction between the obesity discourses identified and the wider contexts in which the articles in our corpus were produced, including, for example, sociopolitical backdrop, editorial practices and (target) readerships, one level of context we have not taken into account is reception. We address this here by examining reader comments accompanying a sample of online articles about obesity. The affordances of Web 2.0 have had a profound influence on the ways in which news content is both created and consumed. In addition to news being more instantly and freely available, one of the most marked differences between online news and its print counterpart is the facility for readers to comment on stories. Such comments are often described as 'below-the-line', as the commenting facility and the comments themselves both tend to appear beneath the stories on-screen. Reader comments constitute a different genre and register to news articles; they appear exclusively online, are user-generated and constitute first-person perspectives; they offer views and opinions (in contrast to the (typically) fact-based reporting of 'hard news'); and they are multi-party and interactive, with commenters directing their contributions not only to the given news outlet but also to other commenters and website users.

Given these differences, reader comments pose numerous methodological challenges to (corpus) linguists, such as how to assess and ensure data representativeness and how to render non-standard orthography. We begin this chapter with a detailed introduction to below-the-line comments, including outlining prior corpus-based discourse studies of them, before describing how we selected, collected and analysed comments about obesity.

Background: Reader Comments

Jewell (2014: online) describes reader comments as a form of 'participatory journalism' and argues that they have 'transformed the relationship between reader and journalist'. While journalists previously enjoyed something of a comfortable distance from which to comment on – and shape public opinion around – society, forms of participatory journalism such as reader comments have reduced this distance, with audiences now able to challenge news content in more public and direct ways than ever before. As Jewell puts it, 'the reader's role is no longer necessarily passive' (*ibid.*).

Some impacts of the public's increased participation in news creation are clearly positive, such as helping to ensure that news outlets are held to account for the content they produce (Kovach and Rosenstiel 2007) and stimulating constructive intellectual debate (Jewell 2014). Yet other consequences are clearly more negative. The relatively anonymous nature of reader comments sections can provide fertile ground for forms of online aggression, such as trolling. Asynchronous and anonymous online platforms can produce what Suler (2004: 321) terms the 'online disinhibition effect'; that is, the phenomenon whereby individuals tend to 'loosen up, feel less restrained, and express themselves more openly' when communicating anonymously online. Studies have found the anonymity of online reader comments to be conducive to uncivil discourse, including towards journalists (Neurauter-Kessels 2011). Most news websites actively discourage such contributions in their terms and conditions and operate moderating processes to filter out comments which breach their rules, while some have disabled the comments function on stories deemed to be particularly liable to attract aggressive and offensive comments and others have removed the comments facility altogether. In view of both their positive and negative consequences, Reagle (2015: 185) argues that comments can 'inform, improve and shape people for the better or [...] alienate, manipulate and shape people for the worse'.

Other effects of online commenting facilities are less easily evaluated as either positive or negative. For example, it seems likely that journalistic practices have been shaped to an extent by news outlets' desire for users to not only read but interact with and return to their websites. Increasing the number of visits to a website can place a higher premium on advertising space and thus help news outlets to increase their revenue. As well as motivating 'click-bait' headlines, such commercial motivations could also be served by articles which encourage – provoke, even – readers to post comments. Another feature of reader comments that is less easily evaluated as positive or negative is their potential to shape other readers' opinions. Lee's (2012) study of the effects of reader comments on the reception of news articles found that, '[u]nknown readers' comments serve readers as a proxy for public opinion; user-generated comments accompanying news stories significantly altered the participants' beliefs about what other members of the society think' (41). Whatever their impacts are, it is clear that readers' comments now constitute an integral part of the online news context and should, where present, be viewed as contributing to the overall communicative import of the articles themselves.

In recent years, readers' comments have received increased attention in linguistic research, including corpus research. Such studies have tended to view comments as providing access to the ways in which audiences receive and respond to news representations, while also providing indirect evidence of public discourses around certain topics. Examples of recent corpus-based studies include Collins and Nerlich's (2015) analysis of *Guardian* reader comments on climate change, Collins's (2019) examination of comments about Antimicrobial Resistance on the websites of the *Guardian* and *Mail*, Baker and McGlashan's (2020) research into reader comments about Romanians on the website of the *Express*, and Paterson's (2020) study of comments about poverty on the website of the *Mail*.

A couple of studies have examined representations of obesity or obesity-related issues in reader comments. Focussing on the website of the Canadian Broadcasting Corporation, Glenn et al. (2012) used Content Analysis to examine the dominant obesity-related messages conveyed by both news texts and reader comments. They found that articles were 'predominantly "positive/supportive" (63%) in tone and frequently presented the voices and opinions of "experts" conveying a biomedical perspective', while comments were 'overwhelmingly "negative" (56%) and often derogatory including such language as "piggy" and "fatty"' (2012: 125). They also noted that comments were frequently directed at other commenters and people with obesity. More recently, Thomas-Meyer et al. (2017) carried out a qualitative thematic analysis of reader comments on online UK news articles reporting on proposals for the taxation of sugar-sweetened drinks. They collected and analysed 1,645 comments relating to four articles, identifying that both support and opposition to the tax could be underpinned by the following themes, 'the balance between personal responsibility and autonomy, and population need; mistrust of the intention of the proposed tax and those promoting it; and variations in the perceived complexity of unhealthy diets and obesity associated with variations in what are considered appropriate interventions' (2017: online). While these studies provide a useful, though restricted, literature on which we can draw and against which we can compare our own findings, ours is the first analysis, to our knowledge, to take a linguistic or discourse-based perspective on this context of obesity representation.

The Obesity Comments Corpus

For this analysis, we took all available comments from a sample of obesity articles published on the website of the *Mail* – *Mail Online*. Our rationale for selecting the *Mail* is two-fold; not only is it the newspaper which contributed the most articles and words to our corpus but its website is also the most-visited online news website in the United Kingdom (Paterson 2020). To ensure the data we analysed was as contemporaneous as possible but still fell within the scope of our corpus, we collected comments from a month's worth of articles in the most recent year in our data – 2017. We began at the end of the year, with December, but this month did not have many articles where comments were still viewable, so we then looked at articles in November, which was more productive, giving thirteen articles with viewable comments. Table 9.1 gives a breakdown of these articles, including their headlines, dates of publication and total number of comments.

The *Mail* website sets out a series of so-called 'House Rules' for website users,[1] which include 'dos and don'ts'. 'Dos' include giving your opinion, making comments clear and understandable, keeping contributions relevant and reporting abuse. 'Don'ts' range from rules regarding basic 'netiquette' (i.e. be kind, no swearing, no abuse) to reminders of laws regarding copyright and libel. As far as we can tell, these rules were the same in 2017 as they are now.

Being user-generated and published without rigorous spelling/grammar/punctuation checks, reader comments, like other forms of computer-mediated communication, are particularly susceptible to non-standard orthographic representation. Manually reading a sample of comments gave a glimpse into some of the creative ways in which commenters worked bad language into their comments, for example by substituting characters (e.g. *cr#p* for *crap*) and putting spaces between words which might trigger a content review, e.g. *burkhas* (*b u rk h a s*) and *white* (*w h i t e*). With this in mind, we partially cleaned our corpus by checking for cases of what we perceived to be deliberate misspellings (such as those described). For this task, we used VARD (version 2; Baron 2011), a tool which allows users to search for and replace non-standard spellings in corpora. This allowed us to standardise many but not all deliberately misspelt words. Following this process, our completed corpus amounted to 49,674 words, from 1,777 comments.

As discussed in Chapter 1, representativeness is a key consideration in corpus design, as it has a strong bearing on what the researcher can and cannot claim on the basis of their analysis. Evaluating the representativeness of a corpus such as this is difficult, though, as its anonymised nature means we cannot reliably ascertain the demographic makeup of the commenters. We should bear in mind, above all else, that these comments are likely to represent the views of a self-selecting sample of *Mail* readers. They are self-selecting in that they have elected to go online not only to access news but also to comment

---

[1] www.dailymail.co.uk/home/article-1388145/House-Rules.html.

Table 9.1. *Articles in the obesity comments corpus*

#	Headline	Date	Comments
1	Fighting fit! Obese woman sheds a remarkable SIX STONE to realise her childhood dream of moving to China to learn Kung Fu with Shaolin monks	12.11.17	5
2	Nearly a THIRD of births are now caesareans due to fears of childbirth, obesity and growing numbers of older mothers, NHS figures show	12.11.17	27
3	UK has the HIGHEST obesity rate in Western Europe after it doubled since the 1990s	13.11.17	305
4	Just one traumatic event increases a woman's risk of obesity by more than 10%, a study reveals	14.11.17	220
5	Fitbit-style wristbands on the NHS for the obese: Thousands of patients will be given the devices as part of drive to prevent diabetes	14.11.17	51
6	The children who are so fat they need hip replacements: Five under-19s had the operation last year with obesity the main cause	20.11.17	135
7	More than half of fat men don't think they are overweight: Warning chaps may now see obesity as acceptable	21.11.17	160
8	Autism risk increases 36% for children born to obese pregnant women	24.11.17	43
9	Children should be BANNED from getting treats to fight obesity, insists Bake Off's Prue Leith	25.11.17	221
10	Obesity and diabetes cause around 800,000 cancers a year, with women being nearly twice as likely to suffer as men, according to the first study of its kind	28.11.17	52
11	UK's obesity shame: Britain has highest numbers of overweight people in the EU (and we're also lazy and drink too much)	28.11.17	495
12	Obese woman whose condition left her with one breast four cup sizes larger than the other drops FIVE STONE after being told she was too big for surgery	30.11.17	9
13	Liver disease set to be the top cause of early deaths by 2020: Alcohol and obesity blamed for the increase	30.11.17	54

on these articles specifically. This also means these commenters will necessarily have Internet access, and research suggests that younger people are more likely than older people to access news online.[2] Commenters tend to be educated, affluent, employed, white and male (Baek et al. 2012). Certain types of stories are more likely to elicit comments, including those which deal with

[2] www.pewresearch.org/fact-tank/2016/10/06/younger-adults-more-likely-than-their-elders-to-prefer-reading-news/

negative and controversial topics (Weber 2014). So, neither the commenters nor the stories in our comments corpus are necessarily representative of the wider readership or content of the *Mail*, let alone of the general population. These issues should be borne in mind when making claims about what the commenters' discourse represents. However, these issues should not diminish the value of comments to the discourse analyst, given their potential to influence the views of other readers.

Keywords in the Comments

The analysis in this chapter utilises an approach based on the keywords technique that we have employed in previous chapters. Specifically, we compare both our comments and their corresponding articles to a general language corpus. As Chapter 3 demonstrated, comparing two corpora to the same reference corpus can highlight areas of similarity and difference between them, with overlapping keywords showing similarities and unique keywords indicating differences (though these are not necessarily statistically significant, as we will discuss later). Existing studies of reader comments have generated keywords for them using reference corpora of written texts (e.g. Baker and McGlashan 2020), computer-mediated texts (e.g. Collins 2019) and a combination of spoken and written language (e.g. Paterson 2020). What we required of our reference corpus was one that contained texts that were close to our comments in terms of both their interactivity and recency and which contained British English language. We therefore decided to use the spoken component of the new British National Corpus, referred to henceforth as the Spoken BNC 2014 (Love et al. 2017).

The Spoken BNC 2014 is a corpus of approximately 11 million words of conversational British English sampled between 2012 and 2016, with a median sampling point of 2014. This corpus has already provided a useful reference corpus in recent research of interactive e-language contexts (Hunt and Brookes 2020), while, as the forthcoming analysis will show, its close cultural and temporal proximity to our comments corpus can help to guard against words emerging as key simply due to their absence in reference corpora that are older or sourced from other contexts (e.g. *NHS*, *Brexit*). Admittedly, this corpus does not provide a neat comparison for the articles, which do not exhibit the same interactive elements as the comments. However, our main focus is the comments, rather than the articles. Nevertheless, this reference corpus proved productive for obtaining keywords from both the comments and articles in this analysis.

We stipulated that keywords should have a minimum log-likelihood score of 15.13 (0.01 per cent level; $p < 0.0001$). For the articles, we imposed a minimum frequency threshold of 5 but raised this slightly to 10 for the comments on account of the larger size of this corpus (the comments amount to 49,674 words, compared to 10,082 for the articles). To filter out words that

Articles   **Shared**   **Comments**

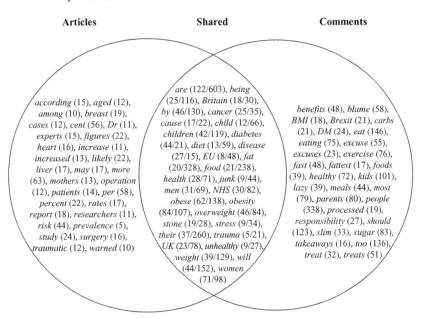

according (15), *aged* (12), *among* (10), *breast* (19), *cases* (12), *cent* (56), *Dr* (11), *experts* (15), *figures* (22), *heart* (16), *increase* (11), *increased* (13), *likely* (22), *liver* (17), *may* (17), *more* (63), *mothers* (13), *operation* (12), *patients* (14), *per* (58), *percent* (22), *rates* (17), *report* (18), *researchers* (11), *risk* (44), *prevalence* (5), *study* (24), *surgery* (16), *traumatic* (12), *warned* (10)

are (122/603), *being* (25/116), *Britain* (18/30), *by* (46/130), *cancer* (25/35), *cause* (17/22), *child* (12/66), *children* (42/119), *diabetes* (44/21), *diet* (13/59), *disease* (27/15), *EU* (8/48), *fat* (20/328), *food* (21/238), *health* (28/71), *junk* (9/44), *men* (31/69), *NHS* (30/82), *obese* (62/138), *obesity* (84/107), *overweight* (46/84), *stone* (19/28), *stress* (9/34), *their* (37/260), *trauma* (5/21), *UK* (23/78), *unhealthy* (9/27), *weight* (39/129), *will* (44/152), *women* (71/98)

benefits (48), *blame* (58), *BMI* (18), *Brexit* (21), *carbs* (21), *DM* (24), *eat* (146), *eating* (75), *excuse* (55), *excuses* (23), *exercise* (76), *fast* (48), *fattest* (17), *foods* (39), *healthy* (72), *kids* (101), *lazy* (39), *meals* (44), *most* (79), *parents* (80), *people* (338), *processed* (19), *responsibility* (27), *should* (123), *slim* (33), *sugar* (83), *takeaways* (16), *too* (136), *treat* (32), *treats* (51)

Figure 9.1 Top thirty unique and shared keywords between the articles and comments compared to the Spoken BNC 2014 (frequencies in brackets; note, for shared keywords, the first figure reflects their frequency in the articles and the second figure indicates their frequency in the comments)

were key because they were used a lot in relation to one story, and which were thus not as representative of obesity discourses generally, we also stipulated that keywords for the articles needed to occur in at least two articles, and keywords for the comments had to occur in at least two of the thirteen sets of comments. This helped to filter out keywords that were specific to one story, such as *Prue*, which refers to the TV chef Prue Leith, who is quoted extensively in one of the articles and so also appears in the corresponding set of comments but is otherwise absent. This gave a total of 134 keywords for the articles and 206 keywords for the comments. Of these keywords, fifty-one were overlapping and appeared in both lists. Considering their disparate sizes, to carry out a more balanced analysis we focussed on the top thirty keywords, ranked by log-likelihood, for the articles and comments. For the shared list, we took the overlapping keywords that had the thirty highest log-likelihood scores on average between the two lists. These three lists of keywords – (i) unique to the articles, (ii) unique to the comments, (iii) shared between both lists – are visualised in the Venn diagram in Figure 9.1.

These keywords indicate a range of themes, many of which span both the articles and comments, while some are more prominent in, or even unique to, one or the other. We do not have space to explore every keyword in detail so concentrate on the most substantial themes, in terms of both the number and frequency of their constituent keywords, as well as keywords whose uses reveal interesting similarities and differences within and across the articles and comments. We begin, though, by considering the words that the articles and comments used to refer to obesity itself. Both articles and comments included the keywords *obese*, *obesity* and *overweight*. These are not particularly surprising. However, another keyword, *fat*, is a more interesting and complex case. In Chapter 2, we saw how *fat* exhibited different preferred meanings depending on which section of the press we were looking at. While this term was key in both our sample of articles and their corresponding comments, analysis of its use in context revealed differences in its preferred meanings between these contexts. Of its twenty uses across the articles, *fat* was used in reference to bodily tissue (twelve; 60 per cent), to describe a person (six; 30 per cent) and to refer to a property of food just twice (10 per cent). By contrast, of its 328 occurrences in the comments, *fat* was used overwhelmingly as an adjective to refer to a person (70 per cent), in reference to body fat in 18 per cent of cases, and then to refer to a property of food 9 per cent of the time (with the remaining 4 per cent made up of other uses). So, in the comments, *fat* is most likely to function as an adjective used about people and in this sense is comparable to *obese* and *overweight*. This helps to explain why the superlative adjective *fattest* is key in the comments but not the articles. Despite being the term of choice for many fat activists, we saw in Chapter 5 that in the context of the British press the word *fat* tends to invoke negative connotations and can be used to shame and stigmatise people with obesity. It is notable, then, that use of *fat* as an adjective, along with *fattest*, is more characteristic of the comments than the articles and could indicate the presence of more explicitly shaming and stigmatising discourses in the comments. To explore this further, it is useful to broaden our enquiry and consider other keywords in Figure 9.1.

Turning to the words in the left-hand list, which were unique to the articles' keywords, the first point of note is the plethora of keywords relating to science and research. This includes words denoting studies (*report*, *study*), those who carry them out (*Dr*, *experts*, *researchers*), and words used to attribute findings and quotes (*according*, *warned*). A related set of keywords denotes numbers, statistics and more general quantification (*cases*, *cent*, *figures*, *increase*, *increased*, *more*, *per*, *percent*, *rates*, *prevalence*). Things that are quantified tend to be rates of obesity and risk both of obesity and diseases attributed to it, which is why *risk* is key in the articles. These figures tend to be reported as the product of research, as the following example shows (note, bracketed information accompanying each extract indicates whether it is taken from an article or comment, while the number denotes which article (or corresponding set of comments) it was taken from (with reference to the numbers given in the first column of Table 9.1)).

> Living through just one traumatic life event increased the **risk** of obesity by 11 **percent**, over that of women who reported no traumatic events. Those that had experienced four or more "negative life events" were at a 36 **percent** greater **risk** of obesity. **Dr** Albert says that the **study**'s findings suggest that "we should consider including assessment and treatment of psychosocial stress in approaches to weight management."
>
> (Article, 4)

As we have noted previously, such uses might be interpreted as invoking 'expert authority' (van Leeuwen 2008) to substantiate a claim; in this case, that traumatic events increase the likelihood of obesity. Such claims can then be further bolstered through quantification rhetoric, in this case using statistics, which can serve an evidential function to legitimate the claim (*ibid.*). Notably, there is a general absence of such scientific and quantificational lexis in the comments keywords, which suggests that readers do not engage with these aspects of the articles as much as they do with others and also that they are likely to draw on other discursive strategies to construct their arguments and persuade others. The only quantifying keyword in the comments is the vague *most*, which is used to make generalisations in support of arguments, typically that people with obesity are not exceptional in their life circumstances, and that *most* people face adversity but manage to avoid obesity, thereby locating the causes and solutions for obesity within the individual.

> Alcohol and diet both issues that **most** people can combat by living a healthy lifestyle. Diabetes now costs the NHS in excess of £10 billion each year. This is just another symptom of our lifestyle, **Most** people with diabetes 2 can resolve this problem with fitness and diet.
>
> (Comment, 13)

Other keywords emerging from the articles but not the comments denote medical procedures; specifically, *operation*, *surgery* and then *patients*, which is frequently used to refer to the people undergoing those procedures. These terms tend to refer to procedures that are either required because of obesity, such as hip replacements, or which are designed to reverse it, such as having a gastric band fitted.

Many of the keywords in Figure 9.1 refer to diseases that are framed as outcomes of obesity or whose risk is heightened by it. From the articles, this includes *breast*, *heart* and *liver*, while *cancer*, *diabetes* and *disease* were key in both corpora. In the articles, these diseases were reported as increasing in prevalence and/or as being related to increasing rates of obesity (again, helping to explain why *risk* is key for the articles). For the keywords *diabetes* and *disease*, readers' comments indicated a general acceptance of this connection between elevated risk and obesity and instead the focus turned to the financial cost of these conditions, and by extension of obesity, to the NHS and taxpayers.

> Morbidly obese people run up much higher medical expenses, the rest of us end up paying for their treatment. **Diabetes**, heart **disease**, joint replacement, high blood pressure, lost work days, you name it.
>
> (Comment, 7)

This also helps to explain why *NHS* is key in the comments, where people with obesity are also frequently constructed as financial burdens on health services.

> An act of desperation, and will not work, Diabetes 2 and obesity can easily be defeated by diet and exercise, a healthy diet is cheaper than junk food, and most exercise is free. Diabetes costs the **NHS** £10 billion each year.
>
> (Comment, 5)

NHS was also key in the articles, where it could similarly be depicted as incurring financial strain due to rising obesity rates. We might interpret this as congruence between the articles and comments, with general agreement between both that obesity and associated diseases (mainly diabetes) place the health service under financial strain. Similarly, the proposed 'solutions' to these health issues discussed in the articles, such as operations and giving children 'fitbit' devices, are also construed as placing the NHS under financial pressure.

The remaining disease keyword that was shared by the articles and comments, *cancer*, exhibited more complex patterns of use. In the articles, cancer is constructed as being caused by obesity, but also diabetes. Of its twenty-five uses in this corpus, eighteen come from article 10, titled 'Obesity and diabetes cause around 800,000 cancers a year'. In this article, the lead researcher on the study on which the article is based is quoted as saying 'Our study shows that diabetes, either on its own or combined with being overweight, is responsible for hundreds of thousands of cancer cases each year across the world.' However, analysing the comments (corresponding to all articles) we find that nineteen of the thirty-five uses of *cancer* provide counter discourses which challenge this association, for example by pointing to cases where cancer occurs in people who commenters perceive not to be overweight.

> Actually, virtually everyone I've personally known who has had **cancer** has been thin ... not even average, but thin.
>
> (Comment, 10)

We have evidence, then, that readers can challenge representations offered in the articles. However, it is notable that this counter discourse emerged around cancer and not, say, diabetes. This perhaps reveals a tension for commenters between treating something such as cancer, which in most cases is not 'blamed' on the individuals who have it, and conditions such as obesity and diabetes, which are regularly subjected to such responsibilising conceptions.

Another set of keywords that exhibit conflicting discourses between the articles and comments, and indeed within the comments, are those relating to stress and trauma. While *stress* and *trauma* were key in both the articles and comments, the word *traumatic* was key just for the articles. In the articles, the vast majority of the uses of these terms occurs in article 4, titled 'Just one traumatic event increases a woman's risk of obesity by more than 10%, a study reveals'. The article offers no explicit agreement or disagreement with these findings. However, many readers *did* make their stances on this explicit and, of these, the majority (around 66 per cent) signalled disagreement that stress and trauma cause obesity, for example by citing their own traumatic experiences as not causing obesity and by emphasising the importance of personal responsibility and self-care.

> I am fat, why am I fat **trauma**, depression, **stress**? NO the answer is simple, I have an over active fork and I don't excercise. It's that simple.
> (Comment, 4)

However, in the remaining uses of these terms (approximately 33 per cent), readers signalled agreement with the study and reinforced the link between stress and obesity.

> Nothing hurts you more than **stress**. **Stress** is the origin and cause of many other illness. Certainly what this article says is true. In most cases if you have a peaceful and happy life you are not overweight
> (Comment, 4)

Comments that were disparaging about the connection between stress and obesity, including the examples above, touch on a significant theme in the comments that we have observed in previous chapters – personal responsibility. Though discourses of personal responsibility are, as we have seen throughout this book, characteristic of the press as a whole, it is notable that words denoting an explicit focus on blame and responsibility, including *blame*, *excuse*, *excuses* and *responsibility*, emerge as key in the comments but not the articles in our sample. In most cases (72 per cent), *blame* is used in ways which imply a discourse of personal responsibility. This could be straightforwardly construing obesity as being caused by individuals (including sometimes commenters themselves) being to *blame* for not taking responsibility for what they eat and how much they exercise.

> I don't **blame** anyone but myself if I overeat and gain 5 pounds. If I see the scale go up, I put the reign on my eating and hit the treadmill.
>
> (Comment, 3)

But this discourse could also manifest less explicitly, being directed at people and groups who are perceived as enabling others not to take responsibility for their obesity risk, for example *parents* (also key in the comments) and fat acceptance advocates.

> **Blame** the fat apologists who preach "fat can be healthy"; **blame** inept parents who haven't the time to care for their children properly because of their social-media habits; **blame** the fast-food culture of the last two generations who couldn't be bothered to learn how to cook.
>
> (Comment, 3)

There is also evidence of a minority discourse in which commenters highlight the role of institutions such as the Government and food marketers and manufacturers in contributing to rising obesity rates.

> If only it were simply 'treats' that were the problem. I'm sorry but most of the processed food in the supermarkets is to **blame** for the obesity crisis. This rubbish is spoon fed to babies, children and their parents through highly suggestive tv adverts and a highly addictive combination of ingredients. Treats? Give me a break.
>
> (Comment, 9)

However, this accounted for a small portion of the comments (just 14 per cent) and we were more likely to find *blame* being used in ways that undermined such positions.

> I love how US TV is to **blame** rather than their own inability to control their eating habits.
>
> (Comment, 3)

A similarly responsibilising discourse could be found in 78 per cent of uses of *excuse* and *excuses*, both of which were key in the comments but not the articles. Within this sample, we noted that *excuse(s)* was used in one of two ways. First, it could be used in comments declaring that there is 'no excuse' for people having obesity.

> There's no **excuse** for obesity. It's caused by laziness and gluttony.
>
> (Comment, 11)

Rather than being accepted as a contributory factor in the development of obesity, the environment in which people live (specifically in the United

Kingdom) is given as a reason why people have 'no excuse' to be obese. In other cases, commenters similarly cite the UK education system, BBC and free public health system all as reasons why people have 'no excuse' for developing obesity. In the second type of use of *excuse(s)*, commenters dismissed factors other than lack of personal responsibility as simply being excuses.

> I'd say eating was the main factor. Followed by lots of **excuses** and blaming everything else.
>
> (Comment, 4)

This extract also provides a useful demonstration of the propensity for *excuse (s)* to take on a negative evaluative prosody, operating as a negatively valanced alternative to the more neutral 'reason(s)'.

The final keyword in this group, *responsibility*, exhibited similar patterns of use across the comments. In fifteen of its twenty-eight occurrences, *responsibility* appeared in statements and general implorations that people should 'take responsibility' for their health, including their risk of obesity, mostly in terms of what and how much they eat.

> People need to take **responsibility** for what they eat.
>
> (Comment, 3)

In a further seven cases, commenters focussed specifically on *parents* (which, as we have noted, was key in this corpus), who were construed as being responsible for their children's health and risk of developing obesity.

> Parents do need to step up and take **responsibility** for their children. A fat tax is not fair as responsible people are effected for something theyre not part of.
>
> (Comment, 9)

Relatedly, just as taking responsibility was proffered as the means of avoiding or reversing obesity, a perceived lack of responsibility was cited as the cause of obesity in four uses.

> They can do what they want . . . just so long as I don't have to pay via the NHS for their laziness and lack of **responsibility**. Same applies to smoking, drinking and drugs.
>
> (Comment, 11)

There was some evidence of a counter discourse which focussed on the roles and responsibilities of more powerful institutions, such as in the following extract, which places responsibility with both the Government and food industries, but such cases represented a minority discourse which accounted for just two of the twenty-eight uses of *responsibility* in the comments.

our government still allows the food industry to stick as much sugar & salt into processed foods as they like, but have got around the **responsibility** by giving the industry a voluntary code of conduct!

(Comment, 3)

As some of the extracts attest, the responsibility discourses in the comments tend to focus on what and how much people eat. This is also reflected in the plethora of keywords denoting food and eating. Both the articles and the comments contained the keywords *food, junk, unhealthy* and *diet*, while the comments also contained keywords denoting specific types of food, with other keywords for this corpus including *carbs, fast, foods, healthy, meals, processed, sugar, takeaways, treat* and *treats*, as well as verbs denoting eating (*eat, eating*) and the intensifier *too*, which could be used to refer to people eating 'too much' or too much of a particular food. The wider range of keywords denoting food and eating could indicate a more intense treatment of this topic in the comments. Yet there are also differences between the articles and the comments in the ways that the shared keywords around food and eating are used. For example, examining the shared keyword *food*, we note that a significant portion of its uses in the articles in our sample (nine out of twenty-one) are concerned with the role of food manufacturers and marketers in the production and advertising of unhealthy and 'junk' foods. However, interestingly, this does not seem to translate into the accompanying comments, where just 5 per cent of the 238 uses of *food* are related to these more powerful institutions. Rather, and as the extracts containing the responsibility-related keywords demonstrate, the comments tended overwhelmingly to talk about (unhealthy) food as something that causes obesity, in the context of a wider responsibilising discourse. This difference also helps to explain why we see *eat* and *eating* as keywords in the comments but not the articles, as well as the intensifier *too*.

I think it may have more to do with being greedy and **eating too** much – or is that not pc enough – am I now to be trolled so that I too become traumatised and obese.

(Comment, 4)

So, the responsibilising discourses around food and eating are more pervasive in the comments than in the articles, where the latter do at least consider the role of institutions that are more powerful than the individual. Such representations were present in the comments but accounted for a very small minority of these texts.

The commenters' focus on personal responsibility in the development of and responses to obesity also extends to more general lifestyle factors beyond diet. For example, both *exercise* and *lazy*, which were key in the comments but not the articles, were used to construe people with obesity as lazy and to attribute their obesity to lack of exercise.

> Fat people are **lazy**! I can say that because I was fat and I've just lost a load of weight. Do some walking and **exercise**, eat sensibly, it's not easy to keep from being overweight but it's worth it.
>
> (Comment, 3)

As well as being used to refer specifically to sedentary lifestyles, *lazy* also carried a negative evaluative prosody and could be used to represent people with obesity in a derisory way.

> That's what liberal attitudes, no blame culture and benefits for anything does to people. PC dictates that being a fat **lazy** waste of space must be down to some external force rather than the simple truth that they are just fat and **lazy**.
>
> (Comment, 11)

Another keyword in the comments that is related to the attribution of obesity to lifestyle is *benefits*. This word is consistently used to refer to welfare benefit and is raised in the comments in relation to obesity in a variety of ways, including constructing welfare dependency as contributing to laziness, suggesting that benefits should be 'cut' to overcome obesity and motivate people into work. Yet there is also a minority discourse which argues against these positions on the grounds that benefit payments are not very high and that people are not dependent on welfare benefit through choice. However, the single most common use of *benefits*, evident in 40 per cent of cases, was the construal of welfare benefit dependency as contributing towards, 'rewarding' and/or 'encouraging' obesity.

> Well people get state **benefits** for being Obese, so the government is encouraging this by paying them incapacity **benefits**, my two friends are claiming this as they are both Obese and they laugh about it.
>
> (Comment, 13)

The word *benefit* is not a keyword in the articles, where it occurs only four times and is used in the general sense of 'the good of'. Thus, the discussion of benefits in relation to obesity in the comments is – at least linguistically – unprompted by the articles. Rather, these readers are bringing to bear wider assumptions, both about people with obesity and people who are dependent on welfare benefit, in the ways in which they engage with the content of the articles and when formulating their views and writing comments.

The next set of keywords refer to places, specifically *Britain, EU (European Union)* and *UK (United Kingdom)*. These words were key in both the articles and comments. *Britain* and *UK* were used almost interchangeably in both the articles and comments and exhibited almost identical patterns in terms of the discourses that were connected to their use, so we will report the analysis of both terms together. In the articles, *Britain* (19) and *UK* (25) had a combined frequency of 44. Of these, twenty-six uses (59 per cent) feature in passages giving prevalence figures for obesity in the United Kingdom, including relative to the *EU*, with such uses accounting for all eight mentions of *EU* in this corpus. The figures usually presented UK obesity rates as high (at least relative to other countries in the EU) and/or as growing, and could be formulated in linguistically creative ways, including through use of metaphor, and in ways that provided an overtly negative evaluation of the situation, for example through the language of 'shame'.

> **UK**'s obesity shame: **Britain** has highest numbers of overweight people in the **EU** (and we're also lazy and drink too much)
>
> (Article, 11)

In nine mentions of *Britain/UK* (20 per cent), the articles offered causes for the obesity 'problems' described. These included UK residents consuming too much 'junk' food, watching too much television and binge drinking. In four cases, the articles suggest that the problem is that the United Kingdom is emulating the United States or is in some way following its lead in terms of obesity rates, including in quotes from experts.

> Mark Pearson, deputy director of employment, labour and social affairs at the OECD, said: In the **UK** we follow the lead from across the Atlantic. We are more influenced by the US than people living in Italy or other parts of Europe.
>
> (Article, 3)

While in two cases, the articles attribute rising obesity rates to the 'normalisation' of obesity in the UK.

> **Britain** has the highest obesity rates in the **EU** – with experts warning that so many people were overweight that it was now considered the 'new normal'.
>
> (Article, 11)

Moving onto the comments, and *Britain* (33) and *UK* (78) had a combined frequency of 111. In around two-thirds of these uses (seventy-four; 66 per cent), readers offered their own interpretations of the causes of the obesity statistics given in the articles. Many of the discourses across the comments identified earlier in this chapter could be viewed as performing this diagnostic function, for example those which framed obesity as an outcome of the failure of individuals to take personal responsibility, failure of parental responsibility and dependence on welfare benefit. Some of the reasons that involved mentions of *Britain/UK* reflected those given in the articles, such as British people eating too many takeaways and too much 'junk' food (14 per cent), the United Kingdom following the lead of the United States (11 per cent), and the perceived 'normalisation' of obesity in the United Kingdom (9 per cent).

> From 1939 until the mid 1950s, you rarely saw a fat person in **Britain** – so it is not rocket science to see why that has changed. A lot of people that we would have called fat in those days, would now be considered to be ok.
>
> (Comment, 3)

Of the mentions of *Britain/UK* in the comments, 11 per cent are difficult to quantify because they offer a mixture of reasons, which in some respects echoed the articles but in others seemed to add something new, such as this comment which again cites the plethora of takeaway shops but also notes the role of 'bad parenting' and there not being 'enough daily PE in schools' as reasons for rising obesity rates in 'broken Britain'.

> Bad parenting, not enough daily PE in schools and too many calorie and fat laden Kebab and Pizza Shops in broken **Britain**
>
> (Comment, 6)

Other reasons for high and rising obesity rates given in the comments include people in the United Kingdom working too much (8 per cent) and the roles of the current Conservative (7 per cent) and previous Labour (3 per cent) Governments, as well as 'politicians' generally (2 per cent).

> Its all down to Labour's entitlement **Britain**. Giving the masses so much expendable income that they can waste it on bad takeaways and not home cooking goodness.
>
> (Comment, 11)

> Fat **Britain** = Tory **Britain**
>
> (Comment, 11)

> And why not with the mediocre politicians we have in **Britain** today.
>
> (Comment, 13)

As these examples demonstrate, attributions of current obesity rates to the Conservative party were less detailed than those relating to the Labour party, which is perhaps because, as they were the party of government at the time the articles were published and the comments written, the role of the Conservative party in overseeing the current obesity rates was more self-evident than that of the Labour party, who had not been in power since 2010. As the first of the three examples demonstrates, comments blaming the Labour party did so on the basis of its welfare policies, which are perceived to have created a generation of people who do not work or cook for themselves but instead spend unemployment benefit on nutritionally poor food, so can be linked through to the food- and benefit-related keywords examined earlier. Such a discourse is evident not just in comments mentioning the Labour party directly but in other mentions of *Britain/UK*, where this is presented as a broader cultural problem in the United Kingdom (6 per cent).

> As the welfare state has expanded so has **britain**'s waistlines
>
> (Comment, 3)

> Look at this logicly, this is because people in **UK** are paid far too much in benefits. To become obese you need massive amounts of food. To get massive amounts of food you need too much money Benefits give you that The **Uk** is the only country in the world wher over 1,000 benefit seekers are getting more than the Prime Mnister
>
> (Comment, 3)

Mentions of *Britain/UK* in the comments thus exhibit both similarities and differences relative to the articles. However, the area of biggest difference was in mentions of the shared keyword *EU*. Where all uses of *EU* in the articles were to put UK obesity rates in context, seventeen of the thirty-six mentions in the comments (47 per cent) blamed UK obesity levels on the EU and the country's membership of it. Some of these cases were vague and implied causality, for example by congratulating the EU on the United Kingdom's obesity rates reported in the article.

> Well done **EU**. Oh don't tell me remoaners if we had not been in the **EU** for decades we would have been even bigger debt and all debt would be double what it is.
>
> (Comment, 3)

Some readers suggested that the United Kingdom's obesity statistics had been inflated by EU migrants with obesity moving to the country.

> Most of the **EU** underclass live here so it's not surprising.
>
> (Comment, 11)

While others attributed UK obesity rates to inferior living standards in the country relative to the rest of the EU, where it is either implied or overtly suggested that the UK's financial contributions to the EU have caused poor living conditions in Britain while enabling better living conditions elsewhere in Europe.

> We have a rich country where the rich have doubled their wealth in the greatest recession since the 1930's; we were members of the **EU** for over 40 years but shared little of the standards enjoyed by our northern

European cousins. Where has the money gone? Why do our people look
and live so bad? Why do we accept poor standards in everything?

(Comment, 3)

Similarly, in four cases (11 per cent) commenters challenged the idea that
people in the United Kingdom are lazy (put forward in the headline and lead
paragraph of article 11) and instead argued that it is the hard work of people in
the United Kingdom that 'supplement[s] the rest of the world'.

How can we be the laziest people in Europe ? That story has been going the
rounds before we even joined the **EU** nearly 50 years ago. People here work
longer hours than any other **EU** country would. Work here is a treadmill to
keep UK.Ltd going so that it can supplement the rest of the world. What an
insulting article to the hard working people of this country.

(Comment, 11)

Seven mentions of *EU* (20 per cent) occur in comments that can be interpreted
as humorous. The majority of these (7) seem to express anti-EU sentiments,
particularly in relation to the outcome of the then-recent referendum on
EU membership in the United Kingdom, which delivered a verdict that the
country should leave. These comments also criticized the EU's perceived
bureaucratic nature.

Us Brits are such a dreadful lot one would think the **EU** would be glad to
see the back of us :-)

(Comment, 11)

However, seven uses of *EU* (20 per cent) indicated a counter-discourse which
challenged notions that the EU was at fault for UK obesity rates.

Yep, all the fault of the **EU**, health tourism, immigrants, anything but
our fault.

(Comment, 3)

So, uses of *EU* were very different in the comments compared to the articles,
and arguably more ideologically charged. This helps to explain why *Brexit*
(referring to the *Br*itish *exit* from the EU) was key in the comments (eighteen
mentions) but was not mentioned even once in the articles. Of its eighteen uses
in the comments, fifteen accompanied article 11, titled 'UK's obesity shame:
Britain has highest numbers of overweight people in the EU (and we're also
lazy and drink too much)'. In over a third (6) of these, commenters imply that
people who voted to leave the EU are obese (amongst other things) and so are
responsible for the country's high obesity rates.

Thick fat drunk and lazy – typical **brexit** voter

(Comment, 11)

Most responses to these comments (4) took issue with the assertion that people who voted to leave are more likely to have obesity or to be unintelligent.

> I voted **Brexit** and have a BMI of 19.5
>
> (Comment, 11)

But there was also evidence of support for the original comments in three of the responses.

> These are the people who voted **Brexit**.
>
> (Comment, 11)

> Getting into shape for **Brexit**.
>
> (Comment, 11)

So, the EU and Brexit appear to be as controversial in the comments sections of obesity-related articles on *Mail Online* as they are in other online and offline contexts. In most cases, the EU (and the United Kingdom's membership of it) is blamed as one of the reasons for the country's high and rising obesity rates reported in the articles. While *EU* was key in both the articles and the comments, it was only in the latter that we found evidence of such ideologically charged rhetoric, both in favour of and against the EU. Furthermore, the word *Brexit* only occurred in the comments, and its use seemed to have little to do with obesity but, rather, the accusation that someone was obese seemed to constitute a way for users to troll, make assumptions about and generally insult one another on the grounds of their political views. The *Mail* has made its anti-EU position clear in articles it has published in the years running up to and following the 2016 referendum, so the generally anti-EU sentiments articulated in the comments, while going further than the articles in our sample, are not discordant with the newspaper's general stance on this issue. Rather, this could suggest more about the ways that journalists are adapting to new media formats and specifically about how articles are written in ways that are designed to ignite passions, elicit comments and ultimately increase engagement from readers and website users.

The final set of keywords we look at here are all grammatical and reveal both similarities and differences in preferences for the types of modality employed in the articles and the comments. These words are more useful for considering style than theme, including how arguments and claims are presented. The articles' keywords include *likely* and *may* – words which imply a tempered modality by expressing likelihood and possibility rather than certainty. Of the twenty-two instances of *likely* in the articles, half (11) are used to express the likelihood that certain factors, namely, gender, trauma, having parents with obesity and being overweight as a child, make people more susceptible to obesity.

The rate of either condition is higher among men, but women are more **likely** to be obese or extremely obese than are men.

(Article, 4)

In the remaining cases, *likely* is used in the articles to describe men as being less *likely* to believe they are obese than women (2), more *likely* to develop diabetes (2) and less *likely* to seek treatment for diabetes (2). Women are presented as being more *likely* to develop certain types of cancer (2) and as more *likely* to experience trauma and PTSD (2), while people pursuing alternative remedies for cancer are presented as being more *likely* to die of the disease (1).

The other keyword in this category, *may*, requires the caveat that almost half of its uses (8) are nouns referring seven times to the month and once to the former British Prime Minister, Theresa May, so we have to exercise some caution when interpreting differences between the articles and the comments here. When used as a modal verb in the articles (nine cases), *may* is used twice to express the possibility that pregnant women's weight *may* have consequences for their babies' health.

Like avoiding smoking during pregnancy, this review of over 40 articles suggests that maintaining a healthy weight during pregnancy **may** also be important to a child's brain development.

(Comment, 8)

Two further cases are used to express the possibility that obesity *may* cause cancer in people with diabetes, while other instances are used to express the view that obesity *may* have become normalised, that drinking culture and exercise *may* be to blame for obesity rates, that children's hips *may* require replacements due to obesity, and when discussing the health risks that *may* be associated with different types of birth (all one occurrence each). Finally, the remaining case of *may* features as part of a broader rhetorical device in a quote attributed to Tam Fry, whereby a concessive is used to ultimately argue that obesity rates are a cause for concern.

Although today's numbers **may** appear small, they hide a near certainty that they will escalate in the years to come

(Article, 6)

The fact that *likely* and *may* are key in the articles but not the comments could suggest that the articles employ a more hedged style, with claims being presented in a more moderated way. One explanation for this is that some of the articles in our sample are based on published reports and scientific evidence. We have already seen how the articles defer more to research and experts than the comments, and it is possible that the more nuanced modality of this genre of writing then translates, to an extent, into the reporting style. Indeed, many of the uses of *likely* and the modal *may* in the articles occur in direct quotations, while even those that do not involve this could have been introduced through researchers editing and approving segments relating to their work. Whatever the case, it is notable that this more tempered modality does not seem to have translated into the comments, at least to the same extent, since neither of these words were key in that corpus.

While *likely* and *may* were key in the articles, the modal auxiliary verb *should* (123) was key in the comments. *Should* carries a deontic modality, indicating how the world or something in it 'ought to be'. This keyword thus indicates an important function of the comments, specifically that commenters use this space to proffer suggestions and solutions to the perceived 'problems' – in this case, of obesity – that they read about in the corresponding articles. Most of the solutions focussed on personal responsibility and punishment for those who failed at this. Examining uses of *should*, we found the most prevalent pattern (twenty uses) to be comments relating to the *NHS* (a word that is key in both the articles and comments), with some readers suggesting that people with obesity should be refused treatment for obesity-related illnesses (or at least that it be made conditional) and others suggesting that people with obesity should be made to pay for their treatment. In such passages, people with obesity are constructed as irresponsible and burdensome on the NHS and taxpayers.

> Obese people **should** pay more national insurance, I'm sick of subsidising these lazy, greedy people.
>
> (Comments, 3)

> they **should** not be granted bariatric surgery at tax payers expense to sort out their problem when they can do so by closing their mouths to another cream cake
>
> (Comment, 11)

The second most common pattern, evident in fifteen uses of *should*, was the suggestion of solutions focussed on increased parental responsibility and accountability for their children's health. These comments were not exclusive to articles about childhood obesity, and the solutions included parents being made to pay for their children's obesity treatment, being treated as criminals, having their children taken away from them and being prevented from having children in the future.

> The parents **should** be held responsible unless they can convince the healthcare people that there is another cause. It **should** fall under the category of poor child care and maybe considered taking the child into care for its future good.
>
> (Comment, 6)

No Prue, idiot adults with no sense of responsibility **should** be prevented from having children.

(Comment, 9)

Other individualised suggestions manifested in uses of *should* include implorations to people with obesity to practice better self-care (5), limiting unhealthy food (11), stopping using what they perceive to be 'excuses' for not taking responsibility for their health (6), limiting availability of unhealthy food or larger clothing items (4) and shaming people with obesity (4).

Fat shaming **should** be the norm and not ostracised and it might encourage people to do something about it.

(Comment, 11)

In three cases, commenters suggested that people with obesity should have their unemployment benefit reduced or stopped.

why do we run ourselves down? and why are there benefits at all? in a good world where everbody enjoys work and views it as a privilege, there would be no hand outs! i don't think there **should** be even one! get a job for god's sake.

(Comment, 11)

Not all the suggestions encoded through use of *should* were so individualising, though, as some commenters focussed on solutions centred on regulating food advertising (4).

Adverts **should** be banned for unhealthy food, they **should** be still available so people can make the informed choice but not advertised to everywhere you look.

(Comment, 3)

While others focussed on what *should* be done to reduce the number of fast food outlets on high streets, with the (implied) agent of change here presumably being government and/or local authorities (though this is never made explicit).

Maybe something **should** be done with regards to the amount of cheap takeaways that are around. There are about 15 pizza takeaways within a ten minute walk from where I live, and then there is the southern fried chicken places that seem to be everywhere.

(Comment, 9)

In three cases of *should*, commenters expressed criticism of the 'promot[ion]' of larger bodies, in two instances relating this to 'political correctness'.

Political correctness hasn't helped matters. Those promoting curves as real women **should** stop doing so. Curvy women are fat or obese women

(Comment, 3)

In nine cases, commenters bemoaned what they perceived as individuals and authorities telling them how to live their lives. Such comments recall the 'nanny state' discourses described in the previous chapter and were directed, variously, at other commenters, the Government, the *Mail* itself and, in comments below Article 9, Prue Leith.

> They're my kids not the governments. Get out of my life. The day you ban me from giving my kids cakes is the day I give my kids cakes every day (currently they're a treat). Why **should** normal responsible families be punished and controlled !?!
>
> (Comment, 9)

Mostly in response to article 9, other commenters argued that children *should* be allowed treats (3), while a further two argued that children *should* be allowed to continue eating treats provided that they exercised and did so as part of a balanced diet.

Finally, in four uses of *should*, commenters articulated the stance that people with obesity should not have to explain themselves to the Government and should be allowed to live their lives as they see fit, which in one comment included questioning why the media and other readers should be so interested in, and angered by, the lives and choices of others.

> What intrigues me though, is why the subject causes anger. I mean, why **should** it be of interest to anyone else apart from the person. Or perhaps their family. Surely no one else.
>
> (Comment, 7)

Conclusion

Focussing on the *Mail Online*, the analysis in this chapter has revealed numerous similarities and differences between reader comments and the articles to which they relate, as well as demonstrating some interesting features of reader comments in their own right. Overall, the comments provided arguably more stigmatising and responsibilising discourses than the articles, as well as dismissing non-individualising explanations for obesity as *excuses*. As well as focussing much more on food and eating, commenters also framed obesity in the context of *benefit* dependency and irresponsible parenting in a way that the articles in our sample did not. For these *Mail Online* commenters, then, neoliberal notions of personal responsibility seem to constitute a powerful set of discourses with which they understand, make value judgments on and communicate about, obesity and people with it. Such is the seeming commitment to this perspective – that individuals cause their own obesity through failed self-care and should therefore be responsible for remedying it – that most commenters challenged and rejected other explanations for obesity, including those that were put forward both by the articles and by other commenters, such as stress and trauma and the roles of more powerful institutions like the Government and food marketers and manufacturers. Though pervasive, the personal responsibility discourses were not absolute, as some commenters countered such positions, for example through explanations which focussed precisely on those more powerful institutions. However, in all cases these constituted a small minority of the comments overall.

Our analysis has also revealed some interesting features regarding the style of the comments and the types of discursive and rhetorical strategies comment-ers use to legitimise the (mainly) neoliberal perspectives they put forward. Compared to the comments, the articles exhibited a significantly higher use of terminology denoting scientific research and enumeration, which we inter-preted as invoking the authority of expertise and quantification to legitimise their propositions. Similarly, the articles used more moderated forms of modality, which had a hedging effect on the claims being made. By contrast, the commenters tended to under-use such language and instead relied on mythopoetic forms of legitimation, for example drawing on personal observa-tions and experiences, rendering these more widely applicable through impre-cise yet more generalising forms of quantification (e.g. *most*), backed up by markedly stronger epistemic modality.

Another function of the comments was to diagnose the *cause* of obesity and then to recommend remedies, as indicated through the deontic modal verb *should*. The solutions advocated by the *Mail Online* commenters could be interpreted as revealing a great deal about their attitudes towards obesity and included, among other things, introducing forms of 'fat shaming', charging people with obesity fees for healthcare, making people with obesity pay more tax and even withholding healthcare from them. For parents of children with obesity, commenters recommended that they should be made to pay for their children's healthcare, face criminal charges for child neglect and even be prevented from having children in the future.

On the basis of this analysis, we could conclude that the comments sitting beneath obesity articles on the *Mail Online* are even more shaming and even more entrenched within a neoliberal perspective on obesity than the articles themselves. However, our analysis over previous chapters has demonstrated the commitment of certain sections of the press, not least the *Mail* and other right-leaning tabloids, to precisely these types of discourses and the stigmatis-ing representations they entail. So, it is surely too simplistic to claim that the press, and especially the *Mail*, provides a balanced view of obesity that is then rejected wholesale by readers. Instead, it seems that articles are likely to be designed in such a way that they engender precisely the types of responses to obesity that we have encountered in this chapter. The discourses in the *Mail Online* readers' comments are generally consistent with what we have seen from the *Mail* and other right-leaning newspapers, but particularly tabloids, throughout this book. The fact that they appear to be muted in the sample of articles examined in this chapter, at least relative to their accompanying comments, speaks, we would argue, to the subtlety with which the press is now able to operate when inciting weight stigma. As discussed at the beginning of this chapter, comments sections should be viewed as part of the news text. As well as serving a commercial purpose, eliciting comments from readers allows a news story to say much more than the news outlet may itself dare, as less accountable members of the public, who are not placed under the same scrutiny or held to the same standards as news outlets, can build on a news story by adding their own interpretations of it and by recontextualising the issue in question in their comments, in the process applying their own ideological gloss.

As our analysis has demonstrated, readers who leave comments can, wittingly or otherwise, perform much of the ideological work for news outlets, who can instead operate under a veneer of relative passivity and even objectivity. For example, while the news articles rely more on scientific and quantitative evidence, more moderated modality and little explicit evaluation, the comments appear to rely on anecdotal evidence, to be prone to exaggeration and offer more explicit evaluations of the people and things being discussed (in our case, mainly obesity and people with it). However, the less explicitly evaluative style that the *Mail Online* seems to have adopted in these cases allows it to create some distance between itself and the object of the story. In many of the articles we have analysed in this chapter, the stories are based on reports of scientific research. In these contexts, the *Mail Online* does not offer much of an evaluation of the findings but instead simply reports them, often using long, verbatim extracts. It is readers who then provide the more evaluative take in their comments. Crucially here, the studies and stories that are reported are, of course, not chosen at random but, rather, represent precisely the types of stories and embedded propositions that the *Mail* knows will be likely to engender impassioned, even angry responses from readers, drawing on news values such as negativity or unexpectedness. Such stories include those that posit that stress causes obesity, that present the United Kingdom as inferior or as in some way doing worse than other (EU) countries, or that involve some expense to the NHS and taxpayers. Sometimes this backfires and commenters seem to accuse the *Mail* of advocating the proposition or action being reported, for example accusing the newspaper of being unpatriotic for reporting stories about UK obesity rates being the highest in Europe. However, in most cases commenters' ire is directed at the person, group or thing in the article and the messenger – i.e. the *Mail* – is not shot.

Of course, the *Mail Online* commenters in our corpus have not arrived at the weight shaming, anti-obesity views evident in their comments alone, let alone without help from the media. The analysis presented over previous chapters allows us to draw parallels between the types of discourses we have seen in *Mail Online* readers' comments here and many of those that we have seen across the press, but particularly in the right-leaning tabloids, over the decade under study. In this general sense, the media is at least partially responsible for the discourses in the reader comments, most of which are recycled and repurposed by *Mail Online* readers in their responses to specific stories. Yet this does not mean to say that these readers cannot also be persuaded to such views at the very point of reading and commenting on particular stories. As we noted towards the beginning of this chapter, reader comments have been shown to influence other readers' interpretations of news stories, so it could be the case that some comments motivate and shape others that follow them. Further research is required to explore this hypothesis, but it is a worthwhile consideration. As well as that, certain discourses within the articles themselves, when carried over into the comments, could be viewed as providing a more local inspiration or motivation for the comments. A good example of this is the construction of obesity and people with it as burdens on the NHS and as costing the country money. This was one of the few overtly negative representations of obesity and people with it that was shared by both the articles and the comments and could even be interpreted as giving rise to a set of spin-off discourses in the comments which associated obesity with welfare benefits and which advocated a series of money-saving solutions, such as charging people with obesity for treatment and withholding benefit payments and even medical care. It could be the case that certain discourses, perhaps around the NHS and taxpayers' money among others, serve as a bridge between the articles and the comments, with such emotive issues being particularly likely to trigger comments and negative responses. This hypothesis would need to be tested by further research, ideally based on a larger dataset representing comments on a wider range of topics.

To conclude this chapter on a more positive note, our analysis suggests reader comments sections, at least on the *Mail Online* website, do appear to grant opportunities for more democratic forms of journalism in which readers can challenge journalists and each other and engage in important debates on topical social issues. The *Mail Online* comments section was far from an echo chamber, and while most of the comments offered a relatively negative take on obesity, a minority did provide counter discourses. Although such cases were few in number and met with opposition and sometimes even abuse, without the comment facility, these voices (and the perspectives they represent) would have been silenced from this context altogether.

10   Conclusion

Introduction

The analysis presented over the foregoing chapters has explored press representations of obesity from a range of perspectives. As well as comparing language use across different sections of the press (Chapters 2 and 3) and over time (Chapter 4), we have also adopted a more targeted approach to address themes such as shaming (Chapter 5) and the representation of weight loss activities (Chapter 6). In Chapters 7 and 8 we explored how obesity representations intersect with aspects of social identity, respectively gender and social class, while our final analytical chapter involved a different perspective altogether, as we considered how readers responded to obesity representations, and in turn provided their own representations, on the *Mail Online*. This range of thematic and methodological perspectives has yielded a wide range of insights into the discourses that surround obesity in the news. This final chapter concludes the book by critically reflecting on our findings with respect to two significant and overlapping themes that have emerged across our analysis – personal responsibility and shaming – considering the potential motivations and consequences of these pervasive themes and how their potentially harmful effects can be challenged in the future. Before discussing our findings, we first consider the study itself, including its limitations and ideas for possible follow-up research.

Methodological Reflections

The methodological approach adopted in this book can be described as combining techniques from corpus linguistics with concepts from Critical Discourse Studies. We collected a decade's worth of national press articles about obesity and then used specialist computer software to identify frequent or salient language patterns, subjecting such patterns to more detailed qualitative analysis in order to interpret and explain their existence. Such an approach means that we can be reasonably confident that we are able to give a fair account of the data, as opposed to simply picking out the cases that we thought were notable (but which may not have been typical). The approach has also meant that we were able to quantify our findings where appropriate, and as well as cover the whole dataset (Chapter 2) we could make different sorts of comparisons, including type of newspaper (various chapters, but particularly in Chapter 3) and time of publication (Chapter 4).

Across numerous chapters, we have relied on the keywords approach, which identifies words which occur with statistically significant frequency in one corpus (or sub-corpus/section of a corpus) compared against another. This is a robust and well-tested approach in corpus linguistics methodology which is especially useful for identifying salient language use in large datasets. However, it is not without problems. One is that the analyst has to impose their own cut-off points for significance and then make decisions about which keywords to focus on, and in how much detail. A keyword analysis is thus always going to be driven to an extent by researcher decisions, even though the process itself is computational. We have tried, at least, to be as explicit as possible regarding this process, although we acknowledge that in some of the tables of keywords we have presented, there was not enough space to discuss all of them. Instead, we have attempted to cover as broad and representative a range of keywords as possible, as opposed to making the same analytical point multiple times.

One aspect that we did *not* cover in our research was the fact that newspaper articles are characteristically multimodal and typically contain a mixture of text and visuals, as well as online editions often making use of hyper-links and videos. Our analysis only considered what was communicated through the written parts of the news texts in our corpus, and we must acknowledge that, in the news, meaning can be co-created through associations between writing and image. For example, a seemingly 'well-meaning' article about obesity may be interpreted in a meaner light if the image associated with it provides a negative representation of a person with obesity. Studies that have examined visuals in news about obesity have indicated that such images are less likely to show people with obesity as wearing professional clothing, fully clothed or exercising compared to pictures of people who do not have obesity (Heuer et al. 2011). Unfortunately, the corpus linguistic approach to Critical Discourse Studies we have taken, like most other corpus-informed approaches to discourse more broadly, is one which works primarily on written text, and although there is a small amount of work which has considered how visual images can be incorporated into corpus analysis (e.g. Caple et al. 2019), the database we used to collect our corpus did not include any images. This is an area for future research which we believe is worth undertaking.

Another aspect to consider is reader comments. While Chapter 9 examined a small corpus of such comments, these were drawn from the website of one newspaper only (*Mail*) and covered comments relating to just thirteen articles from a single month. The findings emerging from that analysis are certainly revealing about the ways in which readers react to news articles about obesity but, due to the small size and thus restricted representativeness of this corpus, we are not able to make the same kinds of generalising claims about this analysis that we made in the other analysis chapters. As with the visuals, the issue here related to accessibility and availability of retrieving comments from the online versions of news websites, and after experimenting with different options, we decided to take a smaller sample from the newspaper that made up the largest part of our corpus, as opposed to trying to examine a range of comments from lots of different newspapers - something which has the potential to be a book-length analysis in itself.

There are other potential extensions to the study reported in this book, such as comparing our findings against a corpus of similar articles collected from the press of a different country, or extending the time period forward or backwards to further chart the changing representations of obesity over a longer period of time. We hope that this book will inspire other researchers not only to adopt similar methods but to carry out related studies that can complement this one.

Blaming and Shaming

The discourse of personal responsibility is central to the press's representation of obesity. In Chapter 2, we saw how it is pervasive across the entirety of the British press, though in Chapter 3 we saw that it was particularly characteristic of articles from the right-leaning tabloids, especially in the context of narratives about people who have lost weight through diet and exercise. In Chapter 4, we demonstrated that it has grown in dominance, over time taking up more space in obesity articles across all sections of the press, with alternative explanations for obesity decreasing, even in the left-leaning broadsheets (where these are most likely to be found). Some of the most explicit manifestations of the personal responsibility discourse were found in Chapter 6, where we explored the ways in which the press reported on a wide range of weight loss methods, including diet and exercise, with such articles targeting readers directly and advising a multitude of ways to lose weight and maintain a 'healthy' body.

Yet, such was the power and pervasiveness of the personal responsibility discourse that it also influenced the representation of obesity in more complex and subtle ways, and in relation to other themes in the obesity coverage. For example, in Chapter 2 we saw how, although obesity was described using medical terminology and in terms of medical concepts, the press rarely went as far as describing obesity as a 'disease', despite the fact that it is defined as such by the World Health Organisation. This, we argued, is because in medicalising a phenomenon such as obesity, and labelling it as a 'disease', there is the potential to alleviate some of the blame and accountability that is otherwise attributed to people with it (Conrad 2007). Therefore, by construing obesity as a medical problem but *not quite* a disease, journalists are able to draw on dominant medical terminology and concepts, such as the BMI, with which they and their readers will be familiar, but without compromising the personal responsibility discourse they draw on in their treatment of this topic. Similarly, by presenting obesity in medical terms, the press (and particularly the right-leaning tabloids) can foreground its connection to other health problems, such as diabetes and heart disease, thereby constructing it as a threat to health and even life, in the process producing more dramatic and sensationalistic headlines.

In Chapter 3, we saw how surgical forms of weight loss tend to be depicted negatively in the press, presented as being both expensive to taxpayers and dangerous to those who undergo them. People who have weight loss surgery are represented as something of an antithesis to those who achieve weight loss in ways that demonstrate the neoliberal 'gold standard' of the rational individual who makes good choices and practices self-control and restraint, such as through diet and exercise. Those who meet this standard are able to ensure that they do *not* rely on the state, or that they at least rely on it less, compared to those who depend on state-funded surgical procedures (and other healthcare interventions) to reduce and control their weight. We have also seen how the discourse of personal responsibility intersects with representations of particular social identities. For example, our analysis in Chapter 7 showed how women, and particularly mothers, were responsibilised for the health of their families, including their (unborn) children, but also the health of male relatives such as their husbands, and indeed other women beyond their family. Meanwhile, in Chapter 8 we saw how the right-leaning press largely backgrounded the influence of social class in explanations of the causes of obesity, again perhaps because to have depicted obesity risk as contingent on something that is largely beyond individual control, such as social class, would risk undermining representations of obesity as being determined by personal responsibility and individual control.

The personal responsibility discourse can also be linked to another pervasive feature of the press's coverage under study; namely, representations which *shame* people with obesity. The specific representations and linguistic choices to this effect described throughout the foregoing chapters are too many to list here. However, the perhaps most obvious examples can be found in Chapter 5, which focussed specifically on shaming language, and identified the use of labels such as *gut-bucket*, *lard-arse*, *porker* and *fatso*, which dehumanise people with obesity and reduce them to repositories of fat. In this chapter, we also noted how certain eating behaviours were presented as wrong, even sinful, through verbs such as *gorge, bolt* and *wolf*, which depict their referents as animalistic and greedy. We also noted how obesity tended to be indexed with reference to unhealthy foods, such as *pies*, featuring, for example, in puns and word-play in article headlines to present people with obesity as (sometimes criminally) addicted to sugary, fatty, processed food. Yet shaming can occur in more subtle ways, too, such as through use of reductive terms such as *the obese*, knowing use of euphemisms such as *big-boned* or *voluptuous* or employment of stereotypes such as the funny or jolly fat person. If the same kind of language, which expresses disgust towards people with obesity, was employed to describe other groups in society, for example based on their race, sexuality or gender, we suspect that there would likely (and rightly) be public outcry. Yet the tabloids have used such terms in relation to obesity with seemingly little consequence.

To try to explain why the press is able to shame people with obesity so explicitly and seemingly without challenge, it is useful to consider the ways in which shaming is related to responsibility. As noted previously, the discourse of personal responsibility is linked to shaming representations and we would argue that these enjoy a mutually enforcing relationship in the context of press coverage of obesity. Specifically, the construction of obesity as something that individuals inflict on themselves conceives of it as a kind of moral failing which, in turn, gives license to the press but also others in society more broadly to berate and shame people with obesity. Individual accountability is key here, as the understanding of obesity as something that is preventable and, so, self-inflicted, renders people with obesity as 'fair game', as they are perceived to have 'brought it on themselves'. Indeed, it is hard, if not impossible, to imagine the journalists who wrote the articles contained in our corpus representing people with cancer or dementia in the same ways that they talk about people with conditions that are perceived to be preventable, such as obesity and diabetes. Of course, one's risk of most illnesses – cancers and dementias included – can be inflated or reduced through certain lifestyle choices. It is thus *perceptions* of preventability, themselves brought about through societal discourses, that underpin such representations. And as we have seen in our analysis, the perception of obesity as preventable, both in the press and in society more widely, can be used to legitimate the shaming of people with obesity, with the defence that it is intended to encourage positive lifestyle changes and is 'for their own good'.

Though dominant, it is important to note that the discourse of personal responsibility was not unchallenged in our corpus, as we also found some evidence of counter-discourses, for example which located the responsibility for the causes and responses to obesity with wider social forces and more powerful institutions, such as the Government and food marketers and manufacturers. Such representations were in the minority, though, and tended to be found in the left-leaning newspapers, and the broadsheets in particular. In general, such discourses were much more likely to be challenged or undermined than propagated.

Though such minority discourses can be considered to counter the dominant personal responsibility position, both these positions nevertheless share a view of obesity as a problem for which 'blame' has to be attributed and a solution found. Counter discourses in the sense of those which promoted fat acceptance or body positivity, and/or which questioned or argued against the existence of obesity as a medically diagnosable phenomenon in the first place, were so infrequent in the press that we hardly encountered them in our analysis at all. Body positivity is aimed at countering shaming messages so that people with larger bodies feel able to reclaim that identity as a positive one. It is a form of resistance which rejects mainstream thinking and has been effective in reducing guilt and self-hatred in other stigmatised groups such as LGBT+ people. However, our analysis found that this perspective received relatively little attention in the press, and when it did, it tended to be framed as controversial. So, discourses advocating views other than that of obesity as a matter of personal responsibility are at-best problematised in the press and, at-worst, elided altogether.

So, if obesity is, as most of the UK press would seem to agree, a problem that needs to be solved, then we can ask how conducive these representations are likely to be to finding a solution. Critiques of neoliberal models of public health are comprehensive and long-standing (e.g. Lupton 1995). One of the main problems of such approaches is that, even if we accept that obesity is brought on by individual lifestyle choices, neoliberal frameworks tend to ignore the fact that personal life circumstances can lead to ill-health. In the context of obesity, such factors include people having insufficient financial resources to afford increasingly expensive fresh fruit and vegetables, forcing them to buy and eat the nutritionally poorer alternatives that they *can* afford, and people living in built environments that do not permit much walking or cycling, which forces them to drive or take public transport to work or school. In fact, in Chapter 8 we saw how such issues, which are closely tied to issues of social class, are largely obscured from press coverage, with obesity risk instead tending to be presented as something that transcends class divisions and rests almost entirely on individual choices. Implorations to individuals to 'take responsibility' for their lives and to make 'better choices' thus risk overlooking the fact that the amount of exercise that people engage in and the types of food they eat are likely to be strongly influenced by factors which lie beyond individual control. It is likely for this reason that public health campaigns and initiatives which assume that individuals are self-determining in their life circumstances often fail to instigate the desired (positive) behavioural changes in the populations they target (Whitehead and Crawshaw 2012).

Even if one successfully follows the neoliberal doxa of personal responsibility, on the basis of the weight loss advice given in the press, this will not necessarily equate with 'health'. The relationship between obesity and health is, as we discussed at the beginning of this book, uncertain and contested. It is beyond the scope of this book to contribute to such debates. However, even if we set this contentious issue to one side and assume that reduction in calories and increased physical activity do reduce one's chances of developing obesity, these methods are not equally effective for all. In fact, on a practical note, the analysis in Chapter 6 showed that the weight loss advice given to readers varies substantially across the press and over time. That advice is also often framed by the press in ways that encourage a view of the body as something that is separate from the self, mechanical even, and which can be subjected to painful and gruelling diets and exercise regimes to ensure good health. Even if such methods do reduce one's weight, we can question whether or not the view of the body and the self that they advocate, and the ways of treating the body that they normalise, are likely to produce contented and 'healthy' attitudes towards the body and the self in the long term.

Another issue with neoliberal frameworks is that if we understand health to be a result of an individual's ability to look after themselves, then ill-health can consequently be viewed as resulting from individuals' (moral) failure to take responsibility for themselves and their lives (or, indeed, those of their family). As we have argued in this chapter, such conceptions of health issues – obesity included – are likely to give rise to negative responses, including those which shame and stigmatise, sometimes with the aim of 'motivating' those at-risk to make 'better' life choices. Shaming is unkind and, we feel, unlikely to produce populations of people who are in better health and have more contented attitudes towards themselves and their bodies. The use of shaming as a motivational tool may work for some. However, when applied broad-brush, as in the national press, it assumes that everyone enjoys the same capacity for self-determination. In contexts where people do not respond positively to such discourse, either because it does not appeal to them or precisely because they cannot alter their life circumstances even if they so-wished, it seems more likely that shaming will be internalised and then potentially have an adverse effect on individuals' mental and physical health (see also: Brookes and Harvey 2015). Indeed, a 2020 survey on obesity attitudes in the United Kingdom by Novo Nordisk (cited in Obesity UK 2020) reported that 58 per cent of people with obesity find coverage of it in the media to be negative, while 60 per cent would like to see this coverage improved.

Yet the shaming of people with obesity is not just carried out by the press but society at-large, with the media reflecting but also potentially fuelling such discriminatory practices. The aforementioned survey carried out by Novo Nordisk showed that two-thirds of the general public view obesity as a lifestyle choice, while a quarter believe that people with obesity are selfish and lack self-control. The same survey showed that such perceptions can also tangibly harm the life chances of people with obesity, as around a third of people were reported as believing that people with obesity are less effective at work compared to people perceived to be a 'healthy weight' (*ibid.*). A similar picture emerges from our analysis of readers' comments in Chapter 9, which also provides evidence for the pervasiveness of the personal responsibility discourse around obesity beyond the pages of the newspapers. In fact, the readers in our sample not only adopted personal responsibility and shaming discourses in their comments but arguably went further than the articles in the extent to which they adopted such discourses, doing so more explicitly, including advocating 'fat shaming' along with more severe forms of punishment against people with obesity. For people with obesity, shaming discourses not only shape the ways that they are represented in the press but also have the potential to influence their relationships with others and the ways that they are perceived within society.

Changing the Discourse

Given that the media has the power to shape social attitudes and can influence government policy, it is important to look closely at the way the media talks about an issue such as obesity and to consider any changes to the discourse that could reduce the shaming and stigmatisation of the group(s) concerned. However, it is also important that we do not give too much credence to shaming language as being the only problem. Campaigns that are simply based on not using words such as *fatty*, without addressing the underlying harmful attitudes around obesity, will just result in new words being invented (or existing ones reappropriated) that have similar functions to the old banned ones, as well as potentially creating a backlash about language policing which is likely to be counter-productive, as has been observed in relation to sexist language and debates around 'political correctness' (Mills 2008).

Another area where we need to tread with caution relates to the extent to which we attribute negative attitudes towards obesity to the media alone. Newspapers are not single-handedly responsible for creating shaming representations of people with obesity; they often draw on widespread tropes that date back to at least the end of the Victorian era (Matthews 2016). For example, a book by Cesare Lombroso (1897), titled *The Female Offender*, makes a link between obesity, prostitution and insanity, claiming that prostitutes and insane women were more likely to be obese. Another book, *The Woman Beautiful*, by Adelia Fletcher (1899) claims that the woman who makes a god of her stomach is incorrigible, and that excessive weight is a result of the indolence of the mind. The English language contains numerous negative idioms involving the word *fat*: *cut the fat, trim the fat, fat lot of good/ use, fat head, work off the fat, run to fat, fat-cat.* It is not surprising that even by the age of three, we discriminate against people with obesity (Cramer and Steinwert 1998). Perhaps the uncomfortable reason why some newspapers engage in shaming and negative representations of obesity is because such representations are familiar and unchallenging to reasonably large numbers of people. Indeed, as noted, the analysis of readers' comments in Chapter 9 found that audience responses tended to go even further than the articles themselves, with more use of terms such as *fat*, calling people with obesity lazy and advocating shaming as well as assigning more blame and responsibility to individuals. It could therefore be argued that when newspapers engage in these kinds of negative representations themselves, they are reinforcing a commonly held worldview, and that it may be economically advantageous for them to do so. So it is important to note that it is not newspapers alone who ought to be held to account but the views of wider society, of which we are all part.

We should also bear in mind that the entire picture across the UK press was not equally negative or without more positive representations. The *Guardian*, *Independent*, *i* and *Morning Star* tended to engage less in such shaming and responsibilising representations relative to the other newspapers in our corpus and reported less on inspirational diet narratives or discussion of faddy weight loss activities, instead being more likely to take social, economic and political factors into account. Such representations are at least more varied than those offered by their right-leaning counterparts and were better at conveying the complexity of obesity, even if such representations do, unfortunately, appear to be decreasing over time. Imagined audiences are important, then, as these newspapers cater to a more liberal or left-of-centre audience which would be more likely to be receptive to such messages. It is thus somewhat ironic that the tabloids, which tend to be chosen over broadsheets by working class readers (Baker et al. 2013: 69), who are likely to have less control over their lives generally, are the ones that push personal responsibility the most, and even more ironic that the people reading tabloids may hold even stronger views to that end.

With these caveats in mind, what can be done to change press discourse around obesity, and how? Some attempts have been made to improve the situation and to 'change the discourse', so to speak, of obesity in the media. A recent example of this is the set of guidelines produced by the charity *Obesity UK*, titled, 'The Responsible Reporting of Obesity: Media Guidelines' (2020). Some of these recommendations relate to language use directly, such as avoiding use of language which stigmatises and has negative connotations; adopting person-first language (i.e. *people with obesity* rather than *obese people*); avoiding phrases that imply a one-size-fits-all approach to weight loss such as 'eat less, move more'; and avoiding connotative language such as describing people with obesity as 'bubbly', 'jolly' or as having a 'big personality'. Other recommendations orient more to general principles when reporting on obesity, such as avoiding simplistic explanations; thinking about how people living with obesity would feel about your language use; and avoiding the 'blame game'. The guidelines also encourage journalists to increase the visibility of people with obesity and to give them a voice on issues *other than* obesity, for example by publishing interviews with and comments from them on other topics. These recommendations address many of the most problematic forms of language use we have observed in our corpus of press articles, particularly those which advise against euphemistic and connotative language and to avoid the 'blame game' and providing overly simplistic explanations of what is, in obesity, a complex health and social issue. Meanwhile, more engagement with empathetic journalistic practices and dedicating more page space to the voices of people with obesity themselves seem like worthwhile principles that could help to reduce shaming language.

This is not the first attempt to change the language around obesity in the media, as others have tried but with limited (if any) apparent success. Any initiative will require time to become effective. The take-up of the guidelines described in this section can only be properly evaluated in the coming years, though we think that adherence to these principles by journalists could lead to a kinder and more person-centred style of reporting. We would add to these guidelines our view that the press would benefit from a diversification in the discourses on which it draws when communicating about obesity. It is, as noted, beyond the scope of this book to engage in debates around what the best approach to obesity is or even about how it should be defined and viewed by society. However, more balanced reporting which does not present obesity just as a matter of personal responsibility but which engages in debate about social and political factors, as well as giving voice to marginalised perspectives such as fat acceptance, would at least reflect more faithfully obesity's complexity while helping to acknowledge that there are a range of ways of conceptualising and approaching it. Such reporting would also help to denaturalise the personal responsibility discourse, enabling readers to view it as just one way of perceiving obesity while at the same time availing them of a wider range of discourses from which they can make an informed choice about which ones make the most sense to them and which ones help them to better understand obesity and their own relationships with their bodies and their weight. It is naïve to expect that getting newspapers to change their reporting on obesity will result in its levels going down from 30 per cent to the 10–15 per cent that they were before the rise that occurred in the 1990s. However, if it is the aim of newspapers to report on obesity in ways that better equip the public and the Government to arrest the so-called 'obesity epidemic', then reportage that advocates multiple approaches, including those that involve greater accountability on the part of powerful institutions such as the Government and food manufacturers and marketers, should be welcomed.

The Trouble with News Values

Studies of problematic news representations, and particularly those which advocate or seek to instigate changes to journalistic practices, need to acknowledge the pressures and restraints that are placed on journalists and the industry, particularly during a period where traditional print newspapers are facing increasing competition from a wide range of online sources which are sometimes free to view. Journalists must carefully cater to audiences who will only continue to buy a newspaper if they feel that it reflects back to them a worldview that is reasonably congruent with their own. The relationship between news producer and news receiver has become ever more symbiotic in recent years. For example, with online versions of newspapers it is possible for editors to identify with painstaking accuracy the kinds of headlines that get 'clicked' on most frequently and how long people spend reading an article. This information can be used to further tailor the news, creating the kind of content that is most likely to engage readers. The trends across a decade that we saw in Chapter 4 are likely to have been affected to an extent by this kind of 'responsive' journalism, which aims to do whatever it can to attract and retain readers.

And news values, which are engendered towards getting people to engage with a news article, help to contribute towards some of the more problematic aspects of the reporting that we have highlighted in our analysis. For example, articles which draw on or construct the news value of unexpectedness can result in stories about obesity or weight loss which go against received wisdom, resulting in confusion and readers being encouraged to keep changing their diets as a result of all the different kinds of advice that they are presented with. As we saw in Chapter 6, the British press can be characterised as presenting to readers a great deal of conflicting information around what counts as healthy, what are good and bad diets, and what type of exercise should be done to lose weight. Once people with obesity have been shamed by the press, they are then given confusing messages about what they should do about it.

Other news values can also mean that certain perspectives on obesity receive more attention than others. For example, celebrities can be hugely influential in terms of the types of diet that people adopt, and stories about celebrities sell newspapers, even if the celebrity is associated with an unproven or even potentially dangerous weight loss product or program. As Chapter 4 also showed, the news value of timeliness/recency means that journalists represent stories around obesity and weight loss in different ways at different times of the year. A flurry of dietary advice occurs in January, after people traditionally consume more and move less during December. This eases off gradually over the coming months, until people are reminded that their summer holidays are coming and that if they want to have beach bodies, they had better do something about it, with May being the month when the press collectively write about obesity the most. As a result, the frequency and types of advice given by the press, and the exhortations to readers to think about their bodies and their weight, are in perpetual fluctuation, with the result being a cycle of inconsistency.

Being positioned by the press as the main caregivers within families (see Chapter 7), women's anxieties are particularly prey to the annual news cycle – how many Easter Eggs to give to your children in March–April; the pressure to look good in a bikini during the summer holiday; the humiliation of realising that your children will have to wear extra-large school uniforms in September for the new school year; balancing the desire to provide Christmas fayre (mince pies, Christmas pudding, turkey, plenty of alcohol) for the family with ensuring nobody puts on too much weight. The domestic routines of family life put women in a perpetual state of worry as a result of the conflicting pressures from month to month. The press is certainly not to blame for phenomena such as annual weather fluctuations or the occurrence of seasonal holidays and it is unlikely that news stories will ever stop trying to be relevant to such events. Therefore, it is important to equip readers with a critical awareness of how different kinds of news values can impact on the way that a topic such as obesity is written about at different times of the year, and to be fair to some sections of the press, we did identify a fair amount of self-reflection, with journalists indicating awareness that people start diets in January but that these often don't last.

So, while academics may be tempted to make lofty recommendations about how newspapers should approach writing about certain social groups or topics, they should also bear in mind that such advice may have little effect, as newspapers acting on it may risk losing readers. With that said, readers have more affordances than ever before to respond to articles that they like or dislike, either through comments sections of newspapers (see Chapter 9) or by sharing articles on social media platforms such as Twitter, in the process applying their own interpretive gloss. An organisation called Stop Funding Hate encourages readers to engage with advertisers to highlight problematic articles, the reasoning being that if advertisers withdraw their business, then newspapers will be fearful of losing advertising revenue and will thus be compelled to change their tone. It is an argument that makes use of neoliberal values (i.e. change or risk losing money) as opposed to moral ones (i.e. change because it's the right thing to do). This represents another irony, considering that we found the most popular discourse around obesity to be that of personal responsibility, which also keys into a neoliberal mindset. So while we acknowledge that the kinds of recommendations made in this chapter and elsewhere in the book are unlikely to cause newspaper editors to instigate a revelatory change of policy, we believe that change can be encouraged in a more gradual and incremental way. This can be achieved by helping to raise awareness for individuals and organisations about the types and extent of problematic press reporting on obesity, both in terms of the clearly stigmatising techniques but also the more subtle tactics that may otherwise go overlooked.

Concluding Remarks

To conclude this chapter and, with it, this book, if we had to point to just three problematic areas of news reporting on obesity that we found across our analysis they would be (i) the use of explicit and subtle shaming representations of people with obesity while ignoring the voices of such people; (ii) the large amount of confusing and conflicting information regarding weight loss or what counts as a 'healthy' weight; and (iii) the over-simplification of obesity in terms of it being presented mostly as a mere matter of personal responsibility, to the detriment of consideration of wider social, political and economic factors. Our analysis has indicated that not all newspapers engage in these three problematic practices to the same extent – they are more commonly found in the tabloids and/or right-leaning newspapers. However, we also found them in broadsheets and liberal newspapers, to a lesser extent, and our analysis in Chapter 4 indicated that even the left-leaning broadsheets were engaging less with social factors over time, indicating the direction of travel for the national conversation around obesity. As we mentioned in that chapter, although levels of obesity in the United Kingdom hardly increased between 2008 and 2017, the framing of obesity as an epidemic and a problem increased during this period.

At the time of writing, the current Prime Minster of the United Kingdom, Boris Johnson, has recently unveiled a £10 million advertising campaign called 'Better Health' to reduce obesity levels in the United Kingdom. The 'upbeat, energising' campaign is described as having a particular focus on people from black, Asian and minority backgrounds, who suffered disproportionately high death rates as a result of the COVID-19 pandemic. Johnson himself, who was hospitalised with the virus, is believed to have become convinced that his weight was part of the reason why he became so unwell. £10 million is not a huge amount (as a comparison, there are currently 135 houses in central London for sale at that price or above) but it is a start and could represent a shift in Johnson's own attitude. The media reported him as saying, 'I'm not normally a believer in nannying, or bossing type of politics. But the reality is that obesity is one of the real co-morbidity factors. Losing weight is, frankly, one of the ways that you can reduce your own risks from Covid.' (*Guardian*, 25 July 2020). It will be interesting to see if journalists, particularly those who berated the likes of Jamie Oliver and Emily Thornberry for being bossy, also signal a change in tone in the future. We would certainly characterise the decade we studied as, at best, a wasted opportunity and, at worst, a step in the wrong direction in terms of how the majority of the British national press has contributed to discussions of obesity. We can only hope that the following decade is better.

References

Allison, D., Fontaine, K., Manson, J., Stevens, J. and Van Itallie, T. (1999). Annual deaths attributable to obesity in the United States. *JAMA*, 282(16), 1530–1538.

Anthony, A., Gatrell, C., Popay J. and Thomas, C. (2004). Mapping the determinants of health inequalities in social space: Can Bourdieu help us? *Health and Place*, 10(3), 203–291.

Aston, G. and Burnard, L. (1998). *The BNC Handbook: Exploring the British National Corpus*. Edinburgh: Edinburgh University Press.

Atanasova, D., Gunter, B. and Koteyko, N. (2013). Ways of seeing obesity: A visual content analysis of British and German online newspapers, 2009–2011. *The International Journal of Communication and Health*, 1, 1–8.

Atanasova, D. and Koteyko, N. (2017). Obesity frames and counter-frames in British and German online newspapers. *Health*, 21(6), 650–669.

Atanasova, D., Koteyko, N. and Gunter, B. (2012). Obesity in the news: Directions for future research. *Obesity Reviews*, 13(6), 554–559.

Baek, H., Ahn, J. and Choi, Y.-S. (2012). Helpfulness of online consumer reviews: Readers' objectives and review cues. *International Journal of Electronic Commerce*, 17(2), 99–126.

Baker, C. (2019). Obesity Statistics. House of Commons Briefing Paper 3336.

Baker, P. (2006). *Using Corpora in Discourse Analysis*. London: Continuum.

    (2010a). Representations of Islam in British broadsheet and tabloid newspapers 1999–2005. *Journal of Language and Politics*, 9(2), 310–338.

    (2010b). *Sociolinguistics and Corpus Linguistics*. Edinburgh: Edinburgh University Press.

Baker, P., Brookes, G. and Evans, C. (2019). *The Language of Patient Feedback: A Corpus Linguistic Study of Online Health Communication*. London: Routledge.

Baker, P., Gabrielatos, C., KhosraviNik, M, Krzyżanowski, M., McEnery, T. and Wodak, R. (2008). A useful methodological synergy? Combining critical discourse analysis and corpus linguistics to examine discourses of refugees and asylum seekers in the UK press. *Discourse & Society*, 19(3), 273–306.

Baker, P., Gabrielatos, C. and McEnery, T. (2013). *Discourse Analysis and Media Attitudes: The Representation of Islam in the British Press*. Cambridge: Cambridge University Press.

Baker, P. and Levon, E. (2016). 'That's what I call a man': Representations of racialised and classed masculinities in the UK print media. *Gender & Language*, 10(1), 106–139.

Baker, P. and McEnery, T. (2014). 'Find the doctors of death: Press representation of foreign doctors working in the NHS, a corpus-based approach'. In: A. Jaworski and N. Coupland (Eds.), *The Discourse Reader* (3rd edition). London: Routledge, pp. 465–480.

(2015). 'Who benefits when discourse gets democratised? Analysing a Twitter corpus around the British Benefits Street debate'. In: P. Baker and T. McEnery (Eds.), *Corpora and Discourse Studies: Integrating Discourse and Corpora*. Basingstoke: Palgrave, pp. 244–265.

Baker, P. and McGlashan, M. (2020). 'Critical discourse analysis'. In: S. Adolphs and D. Knight (Eds.), *The Routledge Handbook of English Language and Digital Humanities*. London: Routledge, pp. 220–241.

Baron, A. (2011). Dealing with spelling variation in early modern English texts. Unpublished PhD thesis, Lancaster University.

Baum F. and Fisher, M. (2014). Why behavioural health promotion endures despite its failure to reduce health inequities. *Sociology of Health and Illness*, 36(2), 213–225.

Beck, U. (1992). *Risk Society: Towards a New Modernity*. London: Sage.

Becker, H. (1963). *Outsiders: Studies in the Sociology of Deviance*. New York: Macmillan.

Bednarek, M. and Caple, H. (2017). *The Discourse of News Values*. Oxford: Oxford University Press.

Bell, A. (1991). *Language of News Media*. Oxford: Blackwell.

Bennett, E. and Gough, B. (2013). In pursuit of leanness: The management of appearance, affect and masculinities within a men's weight loss forum. *Health*, 17 (3), 284–299.

Bennett, J. (2013). Moralising class: A discourse analysis of the mainstream political response to Occupy and the August 2011 British riots. *Discourse & Society*, 24(1), 27–45.

Biber, D. and Conrad, S. (2009). *Register, Genre, and Style*. Cambridge: Cambridge University Press.

Bissell, P., Peacock, M., Blackburn, J. and Smith, C. (2016). The discordant pleasures of everyday eating: Reflections on the social gradient in obesity under neo-liberalism. *Social Science & Medicine*, 159, 14–21.

Block, D. (2013). *Social Class in Applied Linguistics*. London: Routledge.

Blüher, M. (2012). Are there still healthy obese patients? *Current Opinion in Endocrinology, Diabetes and Obesity*, 19(5), 341–346.

Boero, N. (2007). All the news that's fat to print: The American 'obesity epidemic' and the media. *Qualitative Sociology*, 30(1), 41–60.

(2012). *Killer Fat: Media, Medicine, and Morals in the American 'Obesity Epidemic'*. New Brunswick: Rutgers University Press.

(2013). Obesity in the media: Social science weighs in. *Critical Public Health*, 23(3), 371–380.

Bonfiglioli, C., King, L., Smith, B., Chapman, S. and Holding, S. (2007). Obesity in the media: Political hot potato or human interest story? *Australian Journalism Review*, 29(1), 53–61.

Bordo, S. (1993). *Unbearable Weight: Feminism, Western Culture, and the Body*. Berkeley and Los Angeles: University of California Press.

Brewis, A. (2014). Stigma and the perpetuation of obesity. *Social Science & Medicine*, 118, 152–158.

(2017). 'Introduction – Making Sense of the New Global Body Norms'. In: E. Anderson-Fye and A. Brewis (Eds.), *Fat Planet: Obesity, Culture, and Symbolic Body Capital*. Albuquerque: University of New Mexico Press, pp. 1–4.

Brewis, A., Wutich, A., Falletta-Cowden, A. and Rodríguez-Soto, I. (2011). Body norms and fat stigma in global perspective. *Current Anthropology*, 52(2), 269–276.

Brezina, V., McEnery, T. and Wattam, S. (2015). Collocations in context: A new perspective on collocation networks. *International Journal of Corpus Linguistics*, 20(2), 139–173.

Brookes, G. (2018). Insulin restriction, medicalisation and the Internet: A corpus-assisted study of diabulimia discourse in online support groups. *Communication & Medicine*, 15(1), 14–27.

(2020). 'Corpus linguistics in illness and healthcare contexts: A case study of diabulimia support groups'. In: Z. Demjén (Ed.), *Applying Linguistics in Illness and Healthcare Contexts*. London: Bloomsbury, pp. 44–72.

Brookes, G., Atkins, S. and Harvey, K. (forthcoming). 'Corpus linguistics and health communication: Using corpora to examine the representation of health and illness'. In: A. O'Keeffe and M. McCarthy (Eds.), *The Routledge Handbook of Corpus Linguistics* (2nd edition). London: Routledge, In Press.

Brookes, G. and Baker, P. (2021). Fear and responsibility: Discourses of obesity and risk in the UK press. *Journal of Risk Research*. Online First. DOI: 10.1080/13669877.2020.1863849.

Brookes, G. and Harvey, K. (2015). Peddling a semiotics of fear: A critical examination of scare tactics and commercial strategies in public health promotion. *Social Semiotics*, 25(1), 57–80.

Brookes, G., Harvey, K. and Mullany, L. (2016). 'Off to the best start'? A multimodal critique of breast and formula feeding health promotional discourse. *Gender & Language*, 10(3), 340–363.

Brookes, G. and McEnery, T. (2020). Correlation, collocation and cohesion: A corpus-based critical analysis of violent jihadist discourse. *Discourse & Society*, 31(4), 351–373.

Brookes, G. and Wright, D. (2020). 'From burden to threat: A diachronic study of language ideology and migrant representation in the British press'. In: P. Rautionaho, A. Nurmi and J. Klemola (Eds.), *Corpora and the Changing Society: Studies in the Evolution of English*. Amsterdam: John Benjamins, pp. 113–140.

Brown, B. and Baker, S. (2012). *Responsible Citizens: Individuals, Health and Policy under Neoliberalism*. London: Anthem Press.

Buchbinder, D. (2010). *Studying Men and Masculinities*. London: Routledge.

Burchell, G. (1993). Liberal government and techniques of the self. *Economy and Society*, 22(3), 267–282.

Burns, M. and Gavey, N. (2008). 'Dis/orders of weight control: Bulimic and/or "healthy weight" practices'. In: S. Riley, M. Burns, H. Frith, S. Wiggins and P. Markula (Eds.), *Critical Bodies: Representations, Identities and Practices of Weight and Body Management*. Basingstoke: Palgrave Macmillan, pp. 139–154.

Campos, P., Saguy, A., Ernsberger, P., Oliver, E. and Gaesser, G. (2006). The epidemiology of overweight and obesity: Public health crisis or moral panic? *International Journal of Epidemiology*, 35(1), 55–60.

Candlin, C. N., Maley, Y. and Sutch, H. (1999). 'Industrial instability and the discourse of enterprise bargaining'. In: S. Sarangi and C. Roberts (Eds.), *Talk, Work and Institutional Order: Discourse in Medical, Mediation and Management Settings*. Berlin: Mouton De Gruyter, pp. 323–349.

Caple, H., Anthony, L. and Bednarek, M. (2019). Kaleidographic: A data visualization tool. *International Journal of Corpus Linguistics*, 24(2), 245–261.

Carnethon, M., De Chavez, P., Biggs, M., Lewis, C., Pankow, J., Bertoni, A., Golden, S., Liu, K., Mukamal, K., Campbell-Jenkins, B. and Dyer, A. (2012). Association of weight status with mortality in adults with incident diabetes. *JAMA*, 308(6), 581–590.

Caulfield, T., Alfonso, V. and Shelley, J. (2009). Deterministic?: Newspaper Representations of Obesity and Genetics. *The Open Obesity Journal*, 1(1), 38–40.

Charteris-Black, J. and Seale, C. (2010). *Gender and the Language of Illness*. Basingstoke: Palgrave Macmillan.

Chrysochu, P. (2010). Food health branding: The role of marketing mix elements and public discourse in conveying a healthy brand image. *Journal of Marketing Communications*, 16(1–2), 69–85.

Collins, L. (2019). *Corpus Linguistics for Online Communication*. London: Routledge.

Collins, L. and Nerlich, B. (2015). Examining user comments for deliberative democracy: A corpus-driven analysis of the climate change debate online. *Environmental Communication*, 9(2), 189–207.

Conboy, M. (2005). *Tabloid Britain: Constructing a Community through Language*. London: Routledge.

Connell, R. (1995). *Masculinities*. Sydney: Allen & Unwin.
  (2000). *The Men and the Boys*. Sydney: Allen & Unwin.

Connell, R. and Messerschmidt, J. W. (2005). Hegemonic masculinity: Rethinking the concept. *Gender and Society*, 19(6), 829–859.

Conrad, P. (2007). *The Medicalization of Society: On the Transformation of Health Conditions into Treatable Disorders*. Baltimore: The Johns Hopkins University Press.

Conrad, P. and Schneider, J. (1980). *Deviance and Its Medicalization: From Badness to Sickness*. St. Louis: Mosby.

Corrigan, D. and Scarlett, M. (2020). *Health Survey (NI): First Results 2018/19*. Northern Ireland: Department of Health. www.health-ni.gov.uk/sites/default/files/publications/health/hsni-first-results-18-19_1.pdf

Cotter, C. (2010). *News Talk: Investigating the Language of Journalism*. Cambridge: Cambridge University Press.

Couch, D., Thomas, S. L., Lewis, S., Blood, R. W. and Komesaroff, P. (2015). Obese adult's perception of news reporting on obesity. The panopticon and synopticon at work. *Sage Open*, 5(4), 2158244015612522.

Courtenay, W. H. (2000). Constructions of masculinity and their influence on men's well-being: A theory of gender and health. *Social Science & Medicine*, 50(10), 1385–1401.

Cramer, P. and Steinwert, T. (1998). Thin is good, fat is bad: How early does it begin? *Journal of Applied Developmental Psychology*, 19(3), 429–451.

Crawford, R. (1980). Healthism and the medicalization of everyday life. *International Journal of Health Services*, 10(3), 365–388.

Crawford, P., Brown, B. and Harvey, K. (2014). 'Corpus linguistics and evidence-based health communication'. In: H. E. Hamilton and W. S. Chou (Eds.), *The Routledge Handbook of Language and Health Communication*. London: Routledge, pp. 75–90.

De Rossi, P. (2010). *Unbearable Lightness: A Story of Loss and Gain*. New York: Simon and Schuster.

Dunning, T. (1993). Accurate methods for the statistics of surprise and coincidence. *Computational Linguistics*, 19(1), 61–74.

Durkheim, E. (1895). *Rules of the Sociological Method*. New York: The Free Press.

Durrant, P. and Doherty, A. (2010). Are high frequency collocations psychologically real? Investigating the thesis of collocational priming. *Corpus Linguistics and Linguistic Theory*, 6(2), 125–155.

Eckert, P. and McConnell-Ginet, S. (2003). *Language and Gender*. Cambridge: Cambridge University Press.

Epstein, S. (1998). 'Gay politics, ethnic identity: The limits of social constructionism'. In: P. Nardi and B. Schneider (Eds.), *Social Perspectives in Lesbian and Gay Studies*. London: Routledge, pp. 134–159. Reprinted from *Socialist Review 93/94* (May–August 1987), pp. 9–54.

Evans, B. (2006). 'Gluttony or sloth': Critical geographies of bodies and morality in (anti)obesity policy. *Area*, 38(3), 259–267.

Evert, S. (2008). 'Corpora and collocations'. In: A. Lüdeling and M. Kytö (Eds.), *Corpus Linguistics: An International Handbook*. Berlin: Mouton de Gruyter, pp. 1212–1248.

Fairclough, N. (1992). 'Introduction'. In: N. Fairclough (Ed.), *Critical Language Awareness*. London: Pearson, pp. 1–30.

   (1995). *Critical Discourse Analysis*. Boston: Addison Wesley.

   (2003). *Analysing Discourse*. London: Routledge.

   (2015). *Language and Power* (3rd edition). London: Routledge.

Falk, G. (2001). *Stigma: How We Treat Outsiders*. Prometheus Books.

Farrell, A. (2011). *Considering Fat Shame*. New York: NYU Press.

Faulconbridge, L. and Bechtel, C. (2014). Depression and disordered eating in the obese person. *Current Obesity Reports*, 3(1), 127–136.

Filc, D. (2004). The medical text: Between biomedicine and hegemony. *Social Science & Medicine*, 59(6), 1275–1285.

Flint, S., Hudson, J. and Lavallee, D. (2016). The portrayal of obesity in U.K. national newspapers. *Stigma and Health*, 1(1), 16–28.

Flynn, R. (2006). 'Health and risk'. In: G. Mythen and S. Walklate (Eds.), *Beyond the Risk Society: Critical Reflections on Risk and Human Security*. Maidenhead: Open University Press, pp. 77–95.

Fothergill, E., Guo, J., Howard, L., Kerns, J. C., Knuth, N. D., Brychta, R., Hall, K. D. (2016). Persistent metabolic adaptation 6 years after 'The Biggest Loser' competition. *Obesity*, 24(8), 1612–1619.

Foucault, M. (1972). *The Archaeology of Knowledge*. New York: Pantheon.

   (1976). *The History of Sexuality: An Introduction*. Harmondsworth: Penguin.

   (1979). *Discipline and Punish*. Harmondsworth: Penguin.

Fowler, R. (1991). *Language in the News: Discourse and Ideology in the Press*. London: Routledge.

Fox, N. (1993). *Postmodernism, Sociology and Health*. Maidenhead: Open University Press.

Freebody, P. and Baker, C. (1987). 'The construction and operation of gender in children's first school books'. In: A. Pauwels (Ed.), *Women, Language and Society in Australia and New Zealand*. Sydney: Australian Professional Publications, pp. 80–107.

Gablasova, D., Brezina, V. and McEnery, T. (2017). Collocations in corpus-based language learning research: Identifying, comparing and interpreting the evidence. *Language Learning*, 67(1), 155–179.

Galasiński, D. (2004). *Men and the Language of Emotions*. Basingstoke: Palgrave Macmillan.

Galtung, J. and Ruge, M. (1965). The structure of foreign news: The presentation of the Congo, Cuba and Cyprus crises in four Norwegian newspapers. *Journal of Peace Research*, 2(1), 64–90.

Gard, M. (2011). *The End of the Obesity Epidemic*. London: Routledge.

Gard, M. and Wright, J. (2005). *The Obesity Epidemic: Science, Morality and Ideology*. London: Routledge.

Giddens, A. and Pierson, C. (1998). *Making Sense of Modernity: Conversations with Anthony Giddens*. Stanford, CA: Stanford University Press.

Gill, R. (2008). 'Body Talk: Negotiating Body Image and Masculinity'. In: S. Riley, M. Burns, H. Frith, S. Wiggins and P. Markula (Eds.), *Critical Bodies: Representations, Identities and Practices of Weight and Body Management*. Basingstoke: Palgrave Macmillan, pp. 101–116.

Gill, R., Henwood, K. and McLean, C. (2000). 'The tyranny of the "six-pack"? Culture in Psychology'. In: C. Squire (Ed.), *Culture in Psychology*. London: Routledge, pp. 100–117.

Glasgow, S. (2012). The Politics of Self-Craft: Expert Patients and the Public Health Management of Chronic Disease. *Sage Open*, 2(3), 1–11.

Glass, T. (2000). 'Psychosocial interventions'. In: L. Berkman and I. Kawachi (Eds.), *Social Epidemiology*. Oxford: Oxford University Press, pp. 267–305.

Glenn, N. M., Champion, C. C. and Spence, J. C. (2012). Qualitative content analysis of online news media coverage of weight loss surgery and related reader comments. *Clinical Obesity*, 2(5–6), 125–131.

Goffman, E. (1963). *Stigma*. Englewood Cliffs, NJ: Prentice-Hall.

(1974). *Frame Analysis: An Essay on the Organization of Experience*. New York: Harper & Row.

Gollust, S., Lantz, P. and Ubel, P. (2009). The polarizing effect of news media messages about the social determinants of health. *American Journal of Public Health*, 99(12), 2160–2167.

Goodman, L. A. (1961). 'Snowball sampling'. *Annals of Mathematical Statistics*, 32(1), 148–170.

Gough, B. (2006). Try to be healthy, but don't forgo your masculinity: Deconstructing men's health discourse in the media. *Social Science & Medicine*, 63(9), 2476–2488.

(2007). 'Real men don't diet': An analysis of contemporary newspaper representations of men, food and health. *Social Science & Medicine*, 64(2), 326–337.

(2010). 'Promoting 'masculinity' over health: A critical analysis of men's health promotion with particular reference to an obesity reduction manual'. In: B. Gough and S. Robertson (Eds.), *Men, Masculinities and Health: Critical Perspectives*. Basingstoke: Palgrave Macmillan, pp. 125–142.

Guy, G. (2011). 'Language, social class, and status'. In: R. Mesthrie (Ed.), *The Cambridge Handbook of Sociolinguistics*. Cambridge: Cambridge University Press, pp. 159–185.

Gwyn, R. (2002). *Communicating Health and Illness*. London: Sage.

Hall, S. (1997). *Representation: Cultural Representations and Signifying Practices*. London: Sage.

Halliday, M. A. K. (1978). *Language as a Social Semiotic: The Social Interpretation of Language and Meaning*. London: Edward Arnold.

Hamilton, K. (2012). Low-income families and coping through brands: Inclusion or stigma? *Sociology*, 46(1), 74–90.

Hamilton, C., Adolphs, S. and Nerlich, B. (2007). The meanings of 'risk': A view from corpus linguistics. *Discourse & Society*, 18(2), 163–181.

Harcup, T. and O'Neill, D. (2001). What is news? Galtung and Ruge revisited. *Journalism Studies*, 2(2), 261–280.

(2017). What is news? News values revisited (again). *Journalism Studies*, 18(12), 1470–1488.

Hardie, A. (2012). CQPweb – combining power, flexibility and usability in a corpus analysis tool. *International Journal of Corpus Linguistics*, 17(3), 380–409.

Harvey, D. (2005). *A Brief History of Neoliberalism*. Oxford: Oxford University Press.

Harvey, K. and Brookes, G. (2019). Looking through Dementia: What do commercial stock images tell us about aging and cognitive decline? *Qualitative Health Research*, 29(7), 987–1003.

Heuer, C., McClure, K. and Puhl, R. (2011). Obesity stigma in online news: A visual content analysis. *Journal of Health Communication*, 16(9), 976–987.

House of Commons. (2004). *Health Select Committee Report: Obesity*. London: The Stationary Office.

Hunston, S. (2002). *Corpora in Applied Linguistics*. Cambridge: Cambridge University Press.

Hunt, D. and Brookes, G. (2020). *Corpus, Discourse and Mental Health*. London: Bloomsbury.

Iggers, J. (1999). *Good News, Bad News: Journalism Ethics and the Public Interest*. Boulder, CO: Westview Press.

Irvine, L. (1999). *Codependent Forevermore: The Invention of Self in a Twelve Step Group*. Chicago: University of Chicago Press.

Jewell, J. (2014). Love them or hate them, BTL comments have changed journalism forever. *The Conversation*. Online. https://theconversation.com/love-them-or-hate-them-btl-comments-have-changed-journalism-forever-33816.

Johnson, J. and Partington, A. (2017). 'A corpus-assisted discourse study (CADS) of representations of the 'underclass' in the English-language press: Who are they, how do they behave, and who is to blame for them?'. In: E. Friginal (Ed.), *Studies in Corpus-Based Sociolinguistics*. London: Routledge, pp. 293–318.

Jones, A. (2018). I was on a diet for 18 years. Here's what a learnt. Online article at www.bbc.co.uk/bbcthree/article/6b0548de-903f-4b15-8dd8-5c11bed79efc

Jones, O. (2012). *Chavs: The Demonization of the Working Class*. London: Verso.

Jutel, A. (2009). Sociology of diagnosis: A preliminary review. *Sociology of Health & Illness*, 31(2), 278–299.

Kim, S. and Popkin, B. (2006). Commentary: Understanding the epidemiology of overweight and obesity – A real global public health concern. *International Journal of Epidemiology*, 35(1), 60–82.

Kimmel, M. S. (2000). *The Gendered Society*. Oxford: Oxford University Press.

Kovach, B. and Rosenstiel, T. (2007). *The Elements of Journalism: What Newspeople Should Know and the Public Should Expect*. California: Three Rivers Press.

Kwan, S. and Graves, J. (2013). *Framing Fat: Competing Constructions in Contemporary Culture*. New Brunswick, NJ: Rutgers University Press.

Kyle, T. K. and Puhl, R. M. (2014). Putting people first in obesity. *Obesity*, 22(5), 1211–1211.

Labov, W. (2006). *The Social Stratification of English in New York City* (2nd edition). Cambridge: Cambridge University Press.

(2013). *The Language of Life and Death: The Transformation of Experience in Oral Narrative*. Cambridge: Cambridge University Press.

Lakoff, G. and Johnson, M. (1980). *Metaphors We Live By*. Chicago: University of Chicago Press.

Le Grand, J. and New, B. (2015). *Government Paternalism: Nanny State or Helpful Friend?* Princeton, NJ: Princeton University Press.

Ledin, P. and Machin, D. (2015). How lists, bullet points and tables recontextualize social practice: A multimodal study of management language in Swedish universities. *Critical Discourse Studies*, 12(4), 463–481.

Lee, E-J (2012). That's not the way it is: How user-generated comments on the news affect perceived media bias. *Journal of Computer-Mediated Communication*, 18 (1), 32–45.

Levay, C. (2014). Obesity in organizational context. *Human Relations*, 67(5), 565–585.

Love, R., Dembry, C., Hardie, A., Brezina, V. and McEnery, T. (2017). The Spoken BNC2014: Designing and building a spoken corpus of everyday conversations. *International Journal of Corpus Linguistics*, 22(3), 319–344.

Lupton, D. (1995). *The Imperative of Health: Public Health and the Regulated Body*. London: Sage.

(2013). *Risk* (2nd edition). London: Routledge.

(2017). *Digital Health: Critical and Cross-Disciplinary Perspectives*. London: Routledge.

(2018). *Fat* (2nd edition). London: Routledge.

Lynott, D., Walsh, M., McEnery, T., Connell, L., Cross, L. and O'Brien, K. S. (2019). Are you what you read? Predicting implicit attitudes to immigration based on linguistic distributional cues from newspaper readership: A pre-registered study. *Frontiers in Psychology*, 10, 842.

Madden, H. and Chamberlain, K. (2004). Nutritional health messages in women's magazines: A conflicted space for women readers. *Journal of Health Psychology*, 9(4), 583–597.

Mair, C. (2002). 'Three changing patterns of verb complementation in Late Modern English: A real-time study based on matching text corpora'. *English Language and Linguistics*, 6(1), 105–131.

Mann, T., Tomiyama, A. J., Westling, E., Lew, A.M., Samuels, B. and Chatman, J. (2007). Medicare's search for effective obesity treatments: Diets are not the answer. *American Psychologist*, 62(3), 220–233.

Markula, P., Burns, M. and Riley, S. C. E. (2008). 'Introducing critical Bodies: Representations, identities and practices of weight and body management'. In: S. C. E. Riley, M. Burns, H. Frith and P. Markula (Eds.), *Critical bodies: Representations, Practices and Identities of Weight and Body Management*. Basingstoke: Palgrave Macmillan, pp. 1–23.

Marsh, P. (2004). Poverty and Obesity. *Social Issues Research Centre*. Online. www .sirc.org/articles/poverty_and_obesity.shtml.

Matthews, M. (2016) Victorian Fat Shaming: Harsh Words on Weight from the 20th Century. Online. www.mimimatthews.com/2016/04/25/victorian-fat-shaming-harsh-words-on-weight-from-the-19th-century/.

McAdams, D. (2006). *The Redemptive Self: Stories Americans Live By*. Oxford: Oxford University Press.

McEnery, T. (2006). *Swearing in English: Bad Language, Purity and Power from 1586 to the Present*. London: Routledge.

McEnery, T. and Hardie, A. (2012). *Corpus Linguistics: Method, Theory and Practice*. Cambridge: Cambridge University Press.

McEnery, T. and Wilson, A. (2001). *Corpus Linguistics: An Introduction* (2nd edition). Edinburgh: Edinburgh University Press.

Meadows, A. and Daníelsdóttir, S. (2016). What's in a word? On weight and terminology. *Frontiers in Psychology*, 7, 1527.

Meyerhoff, M. (2006). *Introducing Sociolinguistics*. London: Routledge.

Mills, S. (2008). *Language and Sexism*. Cambridge: Cambridge University Press.

(2017). *English Politeness and Social Class*. Cambridge: Cambridge University Press.

Monaghan, L. (2005). Discussion Piece: A Critical Take on the Obesity Debate. *Social Theory & Health*, 3(4), 302–314.

(2008). *Men and the War on Obesity: A Sociological Study*. London: Routledge.

Mulderrig, J. (2011). The grammar of governance. *Critical Discourse Studies*, 8(1), 45–68.

(2018). Multimodal strategies of emotional governance: A critical analysis of 'nudge' tactics in health policy. *Critical Discourse Studies*, 15(1), 39–67.

Mythen, G. and Walklate, S. (2006). 'Introduction: Thinking beyond the risk society'. In: G. Mythen and S. Walklate (Eds.), *Beyond the Risk Society: Critical Reflections on Risk and Human Security*. Maidenhead: Open University Press, pp. 1–10.

Nash, W. (1985). *The Language of Humour*. Harlow: Longman.

Nath, R. (2019). The injustice of fat stigma. *Bioethics*, 33(5), 577–590.

National Health Service. (2019). Obesity: Causes. Online. www.nhs.uk/conditions/obesity/causes/.

National Obesity Observatory. (2012). Overweight and obesity: Where are we and where are we heading? Online. www.england.nhs.uk/wp-content/uploads/2012/05/Obesity-Review-Group-19-April-2012-Background-Slide-Set-1-Prevalence-and-Trends.pdf.

National Statistics. (2018). *Statistics on Obesity, Physical Activity and Diet*. United Kingdom: NHS Digital. https://files.digital.nhs.uk/publication/0/0/obes-phys-acti-diet-eng-2018-rep.pdf.

Neurauter-Kessels, M. (2011). Im/polite reader responses on British online news sites. *Journal of Politeness Research*, 7(2), 187–214.

NHS Digital (2020). Statistics on Obesity, Physical Activity and Diet, England. Online. https://digital.nhs.uk/data-and-information/publications/statistical/statistics-on-obesity-physical-activity-and-diet/england-2020.

O'Brien, R., Hunt, K. and Hart, G. (2005). Men's accounts of masculinity and help-seeking: 'It's caveman stuff, but that is to a certain extent how guys still operate'. *Social Science & Medicine*, 61(3), 503–516.

O'Rahilly, S. and Farooqi, I. S. (2008). Human obesity: A heritable neurobehavioral disorder that is highly sensitive to environmental conditions. *Diabetes*, 57(11), 2905–2910.

Obesity UK. (2020). The Responsible Reporting of Obesity: Media Guidelines. Online https://static1.squarespace.com/static/5bc74880ab1a6217704d23ca/t/5eac46dc2343c149b76d78a2/1588348718811/MAC01741_NN_UK_Media+Obesity_reporting_A5_RGB_Lo1a.pdf.

Ogden, J. (2003). *The Psychology of Eating: From Healthy to Disordered Behavior.* London: Blackwell.

Orbach, S. (1978). *Fat Is a Feminist Issue: The Anti-Diet Guide to Permanent Weight Loss.* New York: Paddington Press.

Ortega, F., Ruiz, J., Labayen, I., Lavie, C. and Blair, S. (2018). The Fat but Fit paradox: What we know and don't know about it. *British Journal of Sports Medicine*, 52(3), 151–153.

Partington, A. (2009). 'Evaluating evaluation and some concluding thoughts on CADS'. In: J. Morley and P. Bayley (Eds.), *Corpus-Assisted Discourse Studies on the Iraq Conflict: Wording the War.* London: Routledge, pp. 261–304.

Paterson, L. L. (2020). Electronic supplement analysis of multiple texts: Exploring discourses of UK poverty in Below the Line comments. *International Journal of Corpus Linguistics*, 25(1), 62–88.

Pearce, M. (2001). 'Getting behind the image': Personality politics in a Labour Party election broadcast. *Language and Literature*, 10(3), 211–228.

Petruck, M. (1997). 'Frame semantics'. In: J. Verschueren, J-O. Östman, J. Blommaert and C. Bulcaen (Eds.), *Handbook of Pragmatics.* Amsterdam: John Benjamins, pp. 1–13.

Pope, H., Phillips, K. and Olivardia, R. (2000). *The Adonis Complex: The Secret Crisis of Male Body Obsession.* New York: The Free Press.

Public Health England (2020). Childhood Obesity: Applying All Our Health. Online. www.gov.uk/government/publications/childhood-obesity-applying-all-our-health/childhood-obesity-applying-all-our-health.

Puhl, R., Peterson, J. and Luedicke, J. (2013). Fighting obesity or obese persons? Public perceptions of obesity-related health messages. *International Journal of Obesity (London)*, 37(6), 774–782.

Raisborough, J. (2016). *Fat Bodies, Health and the Media.* Basingstoke: Palgrave Macmillan.

Rampton, B. (2006). *Language in Late Modernity: Interaction in an Urban School.* Cambridge: Cambridge University Press.

(2010). Social class and sociolinguistics. *Applied Linguistics Review*, 1, 1–21.

Rayson, P. (2008). From key words to key semantic domains. *International Journal of Corpus Linguistics*, 13(4), 519–549.

Reagle, J. M. (2015). *Reading the Comments: Likers, Haters, and Manipulators at the Bottom of the Web*. Cambridge, MA: MIT Press.

Reisigl, M. and Wodak, R. (2001). *Discourse and Discrimination: Rhetorics of Racism and Antisemitism*. London: Routledge.

Rich, E. and Evans, J. (2005). 'Fat Ethics' – the obesity discourse and body politics. *Social Theory & Health*, 3(4), 341–358.

Richardson, J. E. (2007). *Analysing Newspapers: An Approach from Critical Discourse Analysis*. Basingstoke: Palgrave.

Ries, M., Rachul, C. and Caulfield, T. (2011). Newspaper reporting on legislative and policy interventions to address obesity: United States, Canada, and the United Kingdom. *Journal of Public Health Policy*, 32(1), 73–90.

Ritenbaugh, C. (1982). Obesity as a culture-bound syndrome. *Culture, Medicine, and Psychiatry*, 6(4), 347–364.

Rohloff, A. and Wright, S. (2010). Moral panic and social theory: Beyond the heuristic. *Current Sociology*, 58(3), 403–419.

Saguy, A. and Almeling, R. (2008). Fat in the fire? Science, the news media, and the 'obesity epidemic'. *Sociological Forum*, 23(1), 53–83.

Saguy, A. and Gruys, K. (2010). Morality and health: News media constructions of overweight and eating disorders. *Social Problems*, 57(2), 231–250.

Saguy, A., Gruys, K. and Gong, S. (2010). Social problem construction and national context: News reporting on 'overweight' and 'obesity' in the United States and France. *Social Problems*, 57(4), 586–610.

Savage, M. (2000). *Class Analysis and Social Transformation*. Oxford: Oxford University Press.

Scottish Government. (2017). *Obesity Indicators. Scotland: Official Statistics*. www.gov.scot/publications/obesity-indicators-monitoring-progress-prevention-obesity-route-map/.

Semino, E., Demjén, Z., Demmen, J., Koller, V., Payne, S., Hardie, A. and Rayson, P. (2017). The online use of Violence and Journey metaphors by patients with cancer, as compared with health professionals: A mixed methods study. *BMJ Supportive & Palliative Care*, 7, 60–66.

Shilliam, R. (2018). *Race and the Undeserving Poor: From Abolition to Brexit*. Newcastle Upon Tyne: Agenda Publishing.

Shugart, H. A. (2013). Weight of tradition: Culture as a rationale for obesity in contemporary U.S. news coverage. *Obesity Reviews*, 14, 736–744.

Smith, C. A., Schmoll, K., Konik, J. and Oberlander, S. (2007). Carrying weight for the world: Influence of weight descriptors on judgments of large-sized women. *Journal of Applied Social Psychology*, 37, 989–1006.

Smith, M. D., Patterson, E., Wahed, A. S., Belle, S. H., Berk, P. D., Courcoulas, A. P., Dakin, G. F., Flum, D. R., Machado, L., Mitchell, J. E., Pender, J., Pomp, A., Pories, W., Ramanathan, R., Schrope, B., Staten, M., Ude, A. and Wolfe, B. M. (2011). 30-day mortality after bariatric surgery: Independently adjudicated causes of death in the longitudinal assessment of bariatric surgery. *Obesity Surgery*, 21(11), 1687–1692.

Smith-Stvan, L. (2013). Stress management: Corpus-based insights into vernacular interpretations of stress. *Communication & Medicine*, 10(1), 81–93.

Sproston, K. and Mindell, J. (2006). *Health Survey for England 2004: The Health of Minority Ethnic Groups*. London: The Information Centre.

Statista. (2019). Obesity prevalence among individuals in England from 2000 to 2018, by gender. Online. www.statista.com/statistics/334126/obesity-prevalence-by-gender-in-england-uk/.

Stice, E., Schupak-Neuberg, E., Shaw, H. E. and Stein, R. L. (1994). Relation of media exposure to eating disorder symptomatology: An examination of mediating mechanisms. *Journal of Abnormal Psychology*, 103, 836–840.

Stubbs, M. (2001). *Words and Phrases: Corpus Studies of Lexical Semantics*. Oxford: Blackwell.

Suler, J. (2004). The online disinhibition effect. *Cyberpsychology & Behavior*, 7(3), 321–326.

Sunderland, J. (2004). *Gendered Discourses*. Basingstoke: Palgrave Macmillan.

Synnott, A. (1992). Tomb, temple, machine and self: The social construction of the body. *The British Journal of Sociology*, 43(1), 79–110.

Taylor, C. (2013). Searching for similarity using corpus-assisted discourse studies. *Corpora*, 8(1), 81–113.

Taylor, R. (2013). *God Bless the NHS: The Truth Behind the Current Crisis*. London: Faber and Faber.

Thomas-Meyer, M., Mytton, O. and Adams, J. (2017). Public responses to proposals for a tax on sugar-sweetened beverages: A thematic analysis of online reader comments posted on major UK news websites. *PLoS ONE*, 12(11), e0186750.

Tomiyama, A. J., Ahlstrom, B. and Mann, T. (2013). Long-term effects of dieting: Is weight loss related to health? *Social and Personality Psychology Compass*, 7(12), 861–877.

Trudgill, P. (1974). *The Social Differentiation of English in Norwich*. Cambridge: Cambridge University Press.

Turner, P. (2019). *The No Need to Diet Book*. London: Head of Zeus.

Udry, J. R. (1994). The nature of gender. *Demography*, 31, 561–573.

Ulijaszek, S. (2014). Do adult obesity rates in England vary by insecurity as well as by inequality? An ecological cross-sectional study. *BMJ Open*, 4(5), e004430.

van Dijk, T. (1991). *Racism and the Press*. London: Routledge.

van Leeuwen, T. (1996). 'The representation of social actors.' In: C. Caldas- Coulthard and M. Coulthard (Eds.), *Texts and Practices: Readings in Critical Discourse Analysis*. London: Routledge, pp. 32–70.

(2007). Legitimation in discourse and communication. *Discourse & Communication*, 1(1), 91–112.

(2008). *Discourse and Practice: New Tools for Critical Discourse Analysis*. Oxford: Oxford University Press.

van Leeuwen, T. J. and Wodak, R. (1999). Legitimizing immigration control: A discourse-historical analysis. *Discourse Studies*, 1(1), 83–118.

Vartanian, L. R. and Porter, A. M. (2016). Weight stigma and eating behaviour. *Appetite*, 102, 3–14.

Vigarello, G. (2013). *The Metamorphoses of Fat: A History of Obesity*. New York: Columbia University Press.

Voigt, K., Nicholls, S. and Williams, G. (2014). *Childhood Obesity: Ethical and Policy Issues*. Oxford: Oxford University Press.

Wann, M. (2009). 'Foreword: Fat studies: An invitation to revolution'. In: E. Rothblum and S. Solovay (Eds.), *The Fat Studies Reader*. New York: New York University Press, pp. xi–xxvi.

Weber, P. (2014). Discussions in the comments section: Factors influencing participation and interactivity in online newspapers' reader comments. *New Media & Society*, 16(6), 941–957.

White, A. and Johnson, M. (2000). Men making sense of their chest pain: Niggles, doubts and denials. *Journal of Clinical Nursing*, 9(4), 534–541.

Whitehead, P. and Crawshaw, P. (2012). *Organising Neoliberalism: Markets, Privatisation and Justice*. London: Anthem Press.

Widdowson, H. (2000). On the limitations of linguistics applied. *Applied Linguistics*, 21(1), 3–25.

(2004). *Text, Context, Pretext: Critical Issues in Discourse Analysis*. Oxford: Blackwell.

Williams, R. (1976). *Keywords: A Vocabulary of Culture and Society*. London: Fontana.

World Health Organization. (2018). Global Strategy on Diet, Physical Activity and Health. Online. www.who.int/dietphysicalactivity/childhood_why/en/.

(2019). Obesity. Online. www.who.int/topics/obesity/en/.

Wright, D. and Brookes, G. (2019). 'This is England, speak English!': A corpus-assisted critical study of language ideologies in the right-leaning British press. *Critical Discourse Studies*, 16(1), 56–83.

Zhou, S. (2012). 'Advertorials': A genre-based analysis of an emerging hybridized genre. *Discourse and Communication*, 6(3), 323–346.

Zola, I. K. (1972). Medicine as an institution of social control. *The Sociological Review*, 20(4), 487–504.

Index